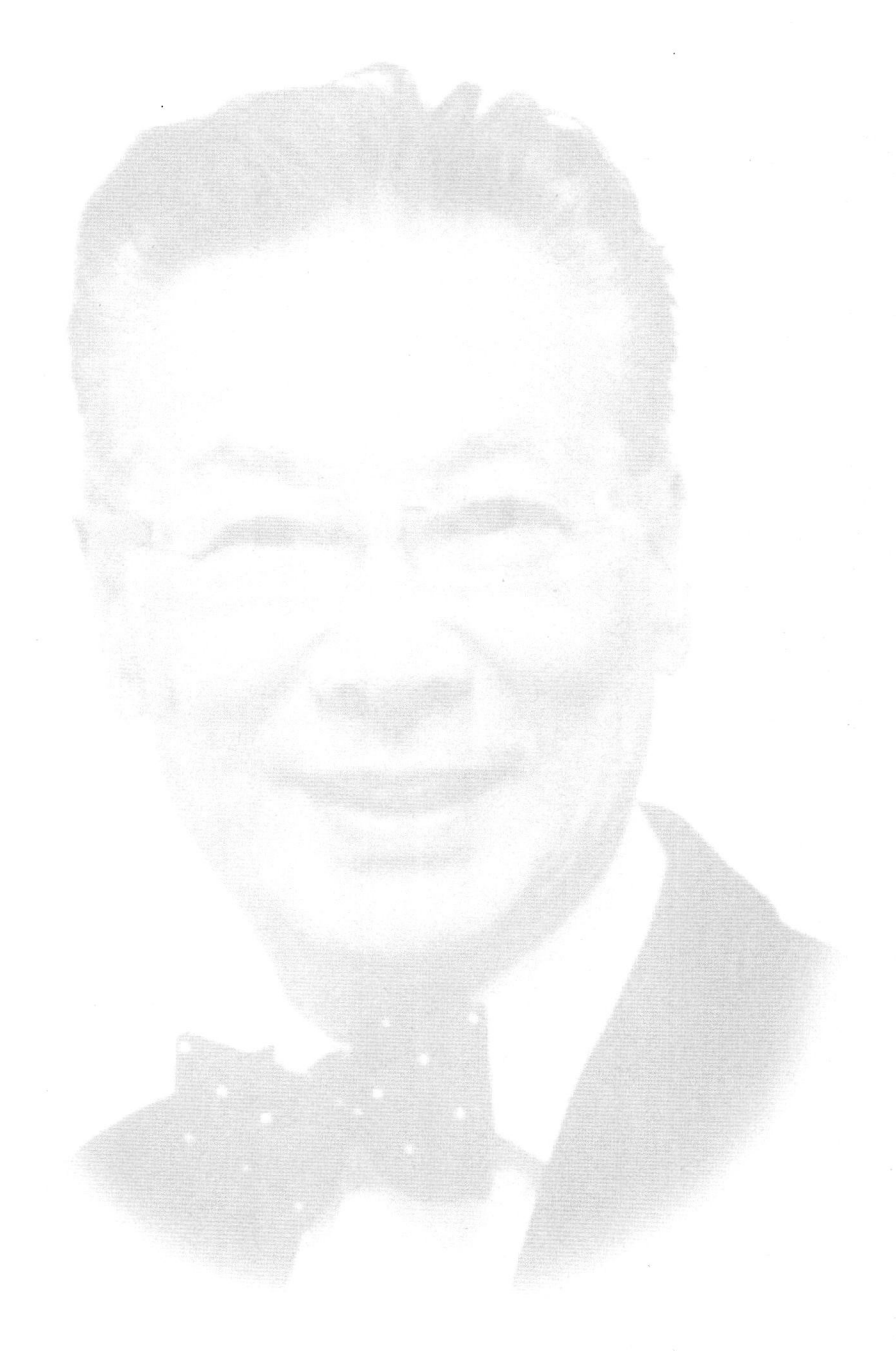

Encyclopedia of Natural Products

Prof. Dr. Paul Ling Tai

D.P.M., FACFS, ABPS, ABAARM

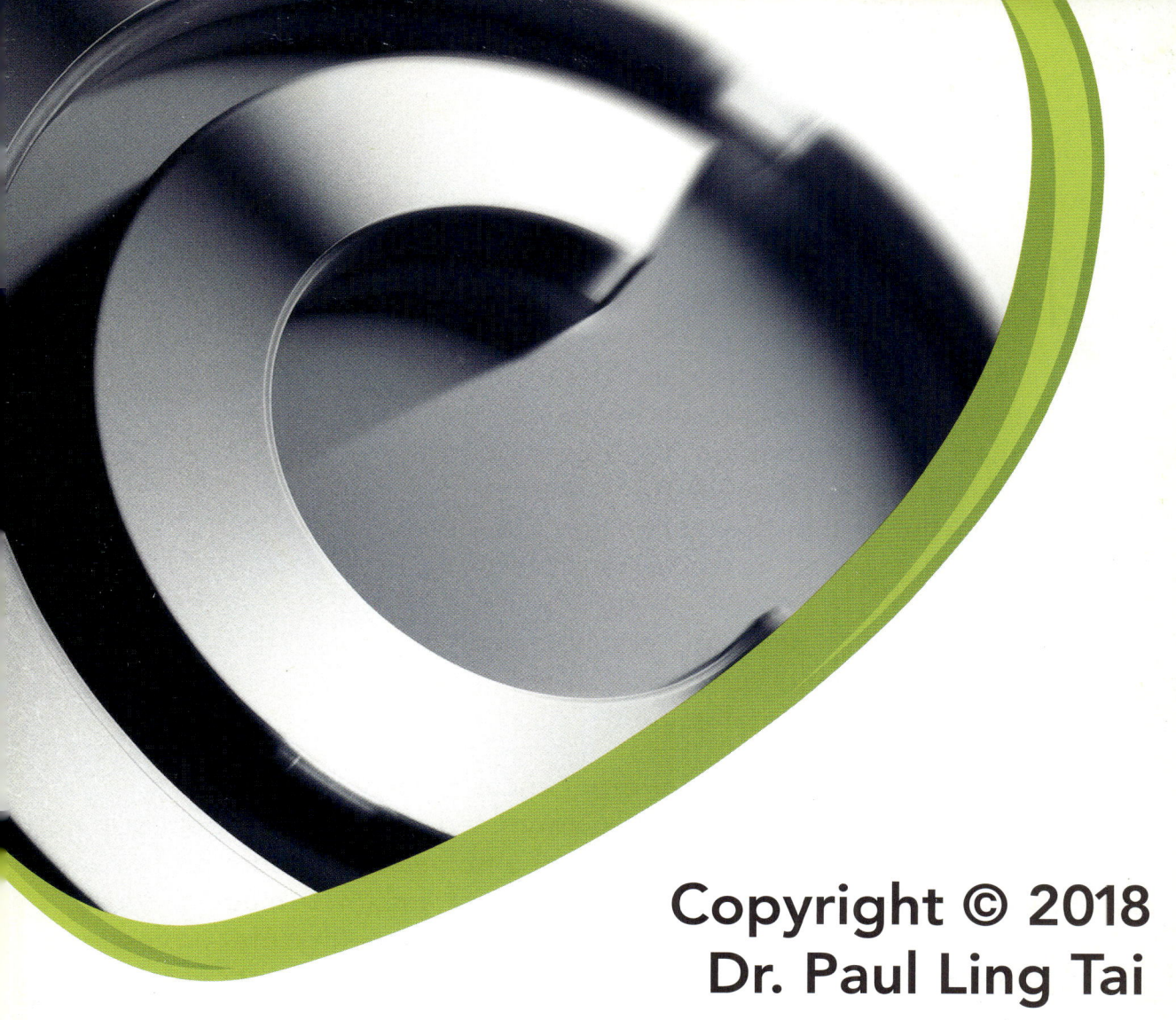

Copyright © 2018
Dr. Paul Ling Tai

Publisher:

BARM PMA Publication

All rights reserved. No part of this book may be reproduced or transmitted in any form or by any means without the written permission of the publisher and/or author.

ISBN: 978-0-9863188-2-5

Disclaimer

This publication is designed to provide scientific, authoritative and personal anecdotal information in regard to the subject matter covered. The reader understands that the author and publisher are not engaged in rendering professional services.

If you require medical, psychological or any other expert assistance, please seek the services of a professional.

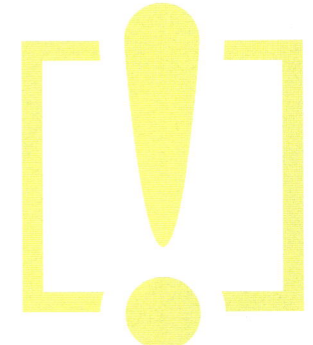

The information, personal experiences, anecdotal stories, procedures and suggestions contained within this book are not intended to replace the services of a trained health care professional or to serve as a replacement for a professional medical doctor's advice and care. You should consult a health care professional regarding any of the information, ideas, personal experiences, anecdotal stories, procedures, supplements, drug therapies or any other information from this book.

The author and publisher hereby specifically disclaim any and all liability arising directly or indirectly from the use or application of any of the products, ideas, procedures, drug therapies, or suggestions contained in this book and any errors, omissions, and inaccuracies in the information contained herein.

The treatment and supplements included in this book are for identification purposes only and are not intended to recommend or endorse the product.

Prof. Dr. Paul Ling Tai
D.P.M., FACFS, ABPS, ABAARM, DACBN

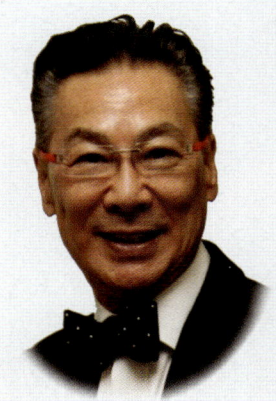

Prof. Dr. Paul Ling Tai is the Chairman & President of the Brasil American Academy of Aging & Regenerative Medicine (BARM), President of Institute of Bones, Joints & Muscle Pain, International Society of Obesity & Metabolic Dysfunction. President of American Academy of Clinical Nutrition & International Society of Stem Cell & Genetics; A past faculty member and lecturer of the American Academy of Anti-Aging Medicine (A4M); Faculty member and former Dean of Post Graduate Medical Education and Chairman of the Department of Medical Research at University of Health Science Antigua (UHSA), School of Medicine & School of Nursing. A Professor of Aging & Regenerative Medicine at University of Paulista (UNIP) in Sao Paulo, Brazil; A frequent lecturer at International Anti-Aging & Health Conferences worldwide. Prof. Dr. Tai was one of the academic contributing authors to the Anti-Aging Medical Therapeutic publications published by the A4M. He is a Board certified Anti-Aging Physician and Diplomate by the American Board of Anti-Aging and Regenerative Medicine; a Diplomate & Certified Clinical Nutritionist of the American Clinical Board of Nutrition. The Head of Research & Coordinator of a Multi-Center Clinical correlation Study on Endocrinology & Saliva Test – A Co-Project with University of UniAmericas, Brazil. Prof. Dr. Tai has been featured in many renowned medical newsletters, television appearances, and radio health talk shows nationwide.

Prof. Dr. Tai is a member of the surgical staff at Annapolis-Oakwood Hospital in Detroit, Michigan, a trained Podiatric Medical Physician and double Board certified surgeon specializing in reconstructive plastic surgery of ankle and foot. He has served under two Michigan State Governors and was recognized with a Vice Chairman's position on the Michigan Board of Podiatric Medical Licensing and as Chief Examiner for new Podiatric physicians. He also served as head of Surgical Residencies. In additional to his various capacities, Prof. Dr. Tai has served as Chairman of the Podiatric Physicians Continuing Education, as well as Chief Compliance Officer for the state of Michigan, supervising doctors. He is the past Coordinator for the Master Degree in Science in Aging and Regenerative Medicine at UHSA. Past Chairman & President of the American Academy of Anti-Aging Medicine (A4M) of Brazil; Past Official Latin American Delegate for the World Anti-Aging Academy of Medicine (WAAAM). A professor in the New York College of Podiatric Medicine's Department of Integrative Medicine; Prof. Dr. Tai is an expert in herbal and cosmetic compound engineering, clinical research and development with Fourteen (14) U.S. Patents credited to his name.

Prof. Dr. Tai is a Knighted Physician, a member of the Royal College of Papal Knights in Americas, granted by the Vatican, His Holiness Pope BENEDICT XVI, and Grand Physician General of the Sovereign Medical Order of Knights Hospitaller. He is also the medical consultant to thousands of doctors on difficult cases all over the world, earning him the title of the "Doctor's doctor" and "Doctor of last resort".

Prof. Dr. Paul Ling Tai is a best seller author of books "Cordyceps Miracles", "8 Powerful Secrets to Anti-Aging" and "Thin Factors" with published Clinical studies completed with Dr. Steven Morganstern, MD on patented technologies and scientific solutions to Weight Loss and Obesity. He also authored: "Fabulously Beautiful You", "Noninvasive Plastic Surgery and Anti-Aging", a textbook revealing the breakthrough technologies in healthy aging skincare, noninvasive plastic surgery, skin restoration and skin fitness, and latest breakthrough US Patent Weight Loss Technologies. His Latest blockbuster book is the "Gold Book of Anti-Aging & Regenerative Medicine" Volume I & II.

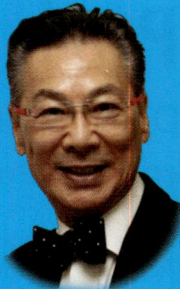

Prof. Dr. Paul Ling Tai
D.P.M., FACFS, ABPS, ABAARM, DACBN

SUMMARY

- Ankle & Foot Surgeon, Orthopedic/Podiatric Surgical Reconstructive Team, Surgery Department Annapolis-Oak wood Hospital, Detroit, Michigan
- Professor and Coordinator of the Anti-Aging Post-Graduate Master Degree, University of Paulista (UNIP), Sao Paulo, Brazil
- Past Chairman of the Department of Post Graduate Medical Education, University of Health Sciences Antigua Medical & Nursing School (UHSA)
- Past Chairman of the Department of Medical Research, University of Health Sciences Antigua Medical & Nursing School (UHSA)
- Past Professor of Master Degree in Science of Aging & Regenerative Medicine & Clinical Nutrition
- Past Professor of Integrative Medicine. NYCPM, New York, New York
- Past Coordinator and Professor of Endocrinology & Anti-Aging at University of UniAmericas, Brazil
- Past Official Latin American Delegate and Coordinator for the World Anti-Aging Academy of Medicine (WAAAM)
- Past Founder and Coordinator of A4M Brazil Society and Medical Congress.
- Past Personal Representative for Latin America to Dr. Robert Goldman, MD, PhD, DO, FAASP- hairman of A4M
- Past Adjunct Professor of Surgery. OCPM, Cleveland, Ohio
- Past Faculty member, lecturer, workshop, author - American Academy of Anti Aging Medicine (A4M)
- Chairman & President of Brasil American Academy of Aging & Regenerative Medicine (BARM)
- Chairman & President of I International A4M Brasil Anti Aging & Regenerative Medicine Conference, Sao Paulo, Brazil
- Chairman & President of I International Stem Cell & Genetics Conference, Sao Paulo, Brazil
- Chairman & President of II International A4M Brasil Anti Aging & Regenerative Medicine Conference, Sao Paulo, Brazil

- Chairman & President of III A4M International Brasil Anti Aging & Regenerative Medicine Conference, Sao Paulo, Brazil
- Chairman & President of IV International Brasil Anti Aging & Regenerative Medicine Conference, Sao Paulo, Brazil
- Chairman & President of V International Congress on Cellular Aging & Regenerative Medicine, Sao Paulo, Brazil
- Head Research Coordinator of a Multi-Center Clinical correlation Study on Endocrinology & Saliva Test – A Co-Project with University Americas, Brazil
- Chairman & Coordinator of VI International Congress on Cellular Aging & Regenerative Medicine, Sao Paulo, Brazil

MEDICAL BOARD CERTIFICATION

- Fellow – FACFS - American College of Foot & Ankle Surgeons
- Diplomate – ABPS - American Board of Podiatric Surgeons
- Diplomate - American Board of Anti-Aging & Regenerative Medicine (ABAARM): Written Exam (A4M)
- Board Certified Physician - American Board of Anti-Aging & Regenerative Medicine (ABAARM): Written & Oral Exam
- The Grand Physician General – The Supreme Council of the Sovereign Medical Order of Knights Hospitaller
- Past Professor, Dean of Endocrinology Dept. University of Natural Medicine, Quito, Ecuador.
- Member - Royal College of Papal Knights in Americas. Granted by Vatican H.H. Pope Benedict XVI, and signed by Vatican Secretary of State Cardinal Bertone.
- Diplomate & Certified Clinical Nutritionist of the American Clinical Board of Nutrition

MEDICAL PUBLICATIONS

Mesomorphic Cholesteric Crystals - A Thermographic Study, JAPA 1972
Acupuncture - A Clinical Study, JAPA 1973

American Academy of Anti-Aging Medicine, Anti-Aging Therapeutics Volume 8 –
"Clinical Applications & New Technology of Saliva Hormone Testing for Anti-Aging". August 2005.

American Academy of Anti-Aging Medicine, Anti-Aging Therapeutics Volume 9 –
"21st Century Technologies for Skincare – Research & Clinical Data".   December 2006.

American Academy of Anti-Aging Medicine, Anti-Aging Therapeutics Volume 10 –
"Avoid Common Pitfalls, Mistakes, and 87% Failure of Anti-Aging Saliva Hormone Testing". April, 2007.

American Academy of Anti-Aging Medicine, Anti-Aging Therapeutics Volume 10 –
"Avoid Common Pitfalls, Mistakes, and 87% Failure of Anti-Aging Saliva Hormone Testing". December, 2007.

American Academy of Anti-Aging Medicine, Anti-Aging Therapeutics Volume 10 –
"Innovative Natural Anti-Wrinkle Plant Extract, In Vitro & Controlled Clinical Studies". August, 2007.

Health Science Institute (HSI) Special Research Report –
"Underground Cures: Natural Ways to Beat Skin Disease". 2003.

Therapeia Natura, Natural Medicine International Scientific Magazine.
"Saliva vs. Serum Hormone Testing, Accuracy, Pitfalls & Clinical Data".
July – September 2008 Publication.

American Journal of Bariatric Medicine, The Bariatrician, Volume 23, No.2.
"Bauhinia: A New Herbal Substance for Weight Loss?" Summer 2008.

A4M Anti-Aging Medical News.
"Saliva Hormone Testing for Anti-Aging." Summer 2008.

Healthy Aging.
"Serum vs. Saliva Testing". July/Aug 2008.

American Journal of Bariatric Medicine, The Bariatrician, Volume 23, No.3.
"Follow up Report: Trial with Bauhinia Forficata" Fall 2008.

Anti-aging Conference Book, Las Vegas, Nevada.
"From the Amazon, an effective new plant for weight loss – Double blind study" 2008.

Journal of the Council on Nutrition of the American Chiropractic Association. Nutritional Perspectives, Vol. 36 No.1. P.16-18.
"New Science of Fat Metabolism for Weight Loss". Jan 2013.

AUTHOR

Book Publication: **Cordyceps Miracles, 2005**
Book Publication: **8 Powerful Secrets to Anti Aging, 2007**
Newsletter: **Healthy Lifestyle, 2008**
Medical Journal: **The Bariatrician, 2008**
Book Publication: **Fabulously Beautiful You! 2009**
Book Publication: **Thin Factor, 2010**
Medical Textbook: **Non-Invasive Plastic Surgery and Anti-aging 2010**
Book Publication: **The "Gold Book of Anti-Aging & Regenerative Medicine", Volume I, 2011**
Book Publication: **The "Gold Book of Anti-Aging & Regenerative Medicine", Volume II, 2012**
Book Publication: **Encyclopedia of Natural Products, Volume I, 2015**

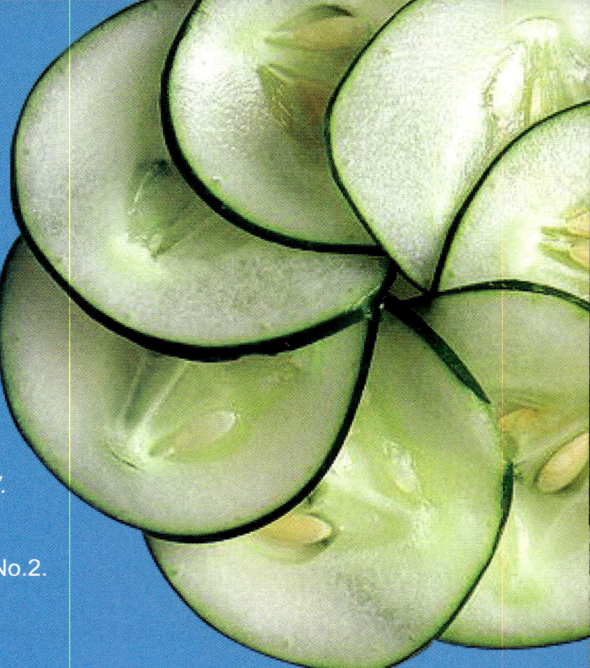

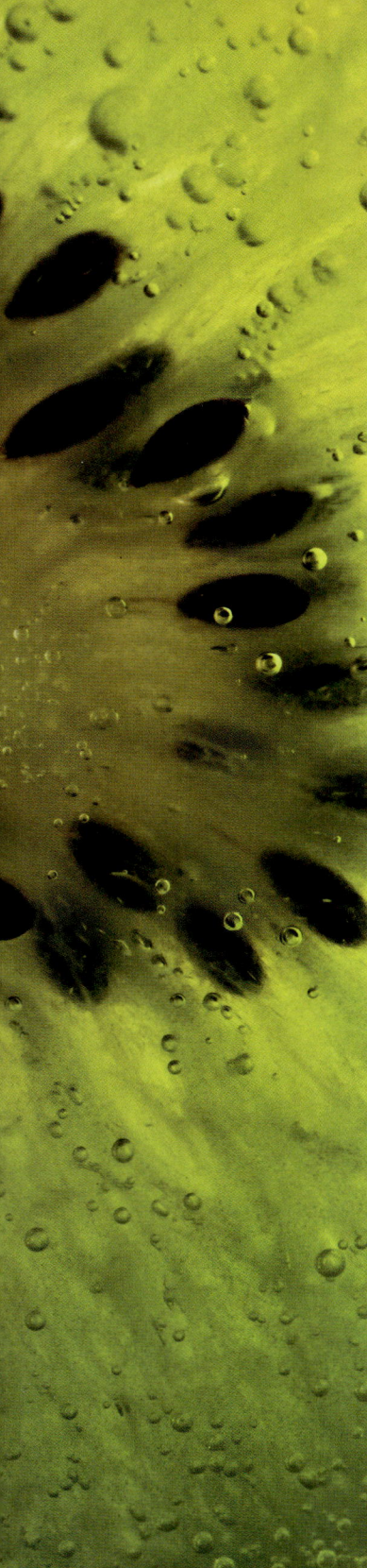

Contents

Disclaimer
About the Author
Table of Contents
Acknowledgments 1
Foreword – Prof. Dr. Paul Ling Tai 2
Bio-Liquid pH 3
Botanicillin 5
Cellular Energy Support 7
ChoLesstrol Specialist 11
Clot Buster 15
Craving Factor 19
Daily Energy 23
Daily Wellness 27
DHEA Lyposome 31
Essential Factors 35
Eye Specialist 37
Force C 39
Glutathione Specialist 41
Gum & Tooth Specialist 43
Hyperactive Support 45
Immune C Spray 47
Immune Gold 49
Ionic Micro Minerals 55
Lady Specialist 57
Liver Cleanse 59
Love Factor 65
Max Adrenal Specialist 67
Max Arthro 69
Max Bio Cell 71
Max Bone Specialist 73
Max Brain Specialist 75
Max Cellular & Immune Specialist 77

Max DeTox	79
Max Digestion Specialist	81
Max Enzybiotic Specialist	85
Max Feminine	87
Max Hot Flash Specialist & Women Anti-Aging	89
Max Intestine Specialist	93
Max Man & Max Woman	97
Max Menopause Specialist	99
Max Mitochondria Specialist	101
Max Pain Specialist	107
Max Performance Specialist	111
Max Prostate Liquid	115
Max Prostate Specialist	119
Max Receptor E Defense	123
Max Receptor E DeTox	125
Max Sea	129
Max Sinus	131
Melatonin Transdermal	133
Memory Specialist	137
Mineral Pak	147
The Molecular Therapy (TMT)	149
Muscle Specialist	151
Neural Specialist	153
Pregnenolone PleoLyposome	155
Progesterone PleoLyposome	157
Relax Pressure Specialist	161
Royal Ling Zhi Matrix	163
S.O.D & Catalase Specialist	167
Skin Hair Nail Specialist	169
Skin Specialist	175
Slimming Fat Burner	177
Stress Specialist	179
Stress & Anxiety Specialist	181

Super B12 Sublingual	183
Super Charge Specialist	185
Thin Factors & Thin Factor Liquid (Homeopathic)	187
Total Circulation Specialist	189
Ultra Charge	191
Ultra Inflammation Specialist	199
Ultra Intense	201
Ultra Masculine	203
Dr. 911 Ultra Skin Gel	205
Uplift Mood	207
Vitamin D3-K2 Specialist	209
Water Specialist	215
Weight & Inches Specialist	219
AcneDERM Urgent Care	221
Anti-Wrinkle Nano-Eye Serum	223
Body Sculpting Anti-Cellulite Cream	225
Chiffon Body Souffle	227
Diamond Microdermabrasion	231
Essence Flash Toner	233
Nano-Moist Renewing Day Cream	235
Nano-Restoring Night Caviar	239
Nattoyant Cleansing Gel	243
Refine Ice Mask	247
Skin Renew	249
SkinTox	251
Smart Skin	253
Testing	257
Resources	261
Index	262

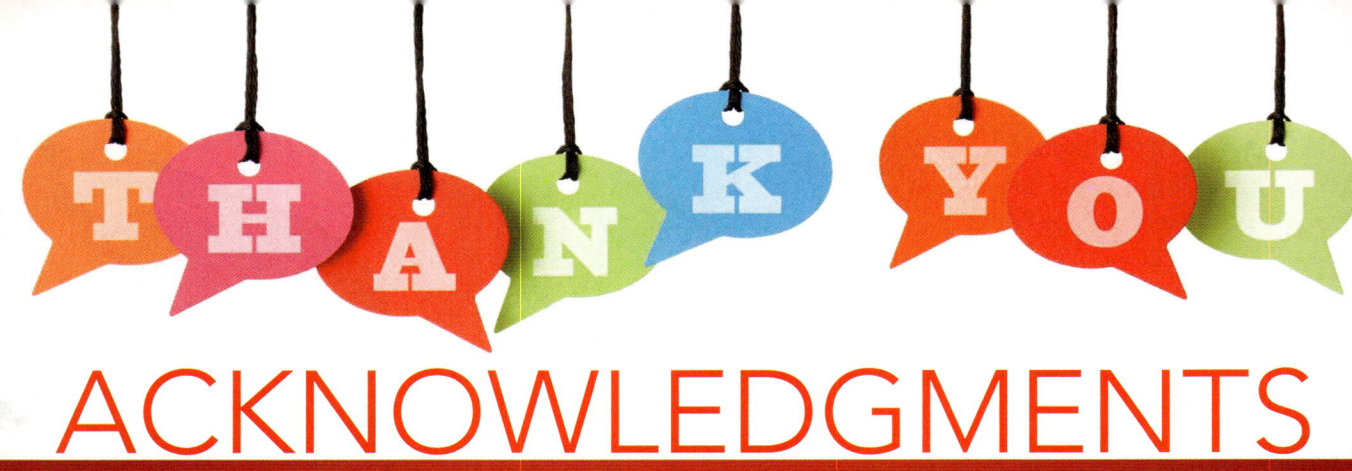

ACKNOWLEDGMENTS

Profound thanks go to **Katherine M. Lee.**
To **Yhasmin Wilder** for their enormous help preparing the book.
To **Dr. Kelly Miller** for review of the manuscript.
To my Extraordinary Staff — **Elaine Daniels, Cynthia Perrine, Jim Krupa & Kayo Assen.**
I am extremely grateful to the thousands of patients worldwide who have shared their experiences with me - they were my primary inspiration for the writing of this book.

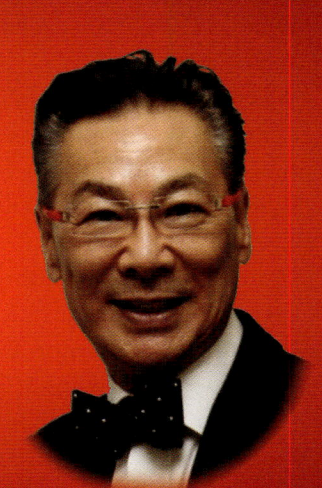

SECOND EDITION
By Popular Demand!

In this **Second Edition** of the **Encyclopedia of Natural Products**, you will find wonderful new products with even more References, Pearls and Clinical Cases for you to review. We worked earnestly to bring you the collective knowledge of thousands of years of **Chinese Herbals, the latest in Western Medicine, Medical & Scientific Journals and Real World Assessments**. With this information at your fingertips, I am certain that everyone will be able to navigate this book and find information that may be beneficial to them.

Stop buying supplements because slick, fast-talking marketing programs! This is Evidenced Based Research with backing information on not only the supplements, but ingredients along with efficient ways to use them.

Wishing you and your loved ones excellent health and long life!

Foreword

DOCTOR TAI'S ENCYCLOPEDIA OF NATURAL PRODUCTS

> **Have you ever wondered** what would be like to spend your whole life strapped into a 17 inch wide seat? Well, I can give you a glimpse into this unseemly world of torture... that's right, after spending nearly 2,000,000 miles on airlines in the last 10 years, I feel like I wear the airplane seat belt as a proud expensive designer belt holding my pants up.

As I crisscross the skies over continental USA, South America or the great vast oceans, you can always find me strapped into those tiny seats going to speak at yet another major medical conference in some far away exotic sounding city around the world.

The type of conferences are as diverse as the continents or capitals from the Great Wall of China, Beijing or Shanghai to Istanbul, Turkey, to the distant smallest villages in tropical Indonesia; how about Uzbekistan, Mongolia or a Farm town like Cedar Rapids, Iowa. They come in all "flavors" like the variety of medical specialty of the conferences I am invited to speak, like Homeopathic medicine, Anti-Aging, Geriatric, Clinical Nutrition, Orthopedic Surgery, Dermatology or Plastic Surgery. I have, as they say, "Done 'em All"!

There is one special "thread" of constant question from all the doctors in the audience – "We see a lot of conditions that prescription drugs don't seem to help, are there any alternatives?" "How do we treat all those conditions we see in our clinics using only Natural medicine?" "Can we "Really" help our patients without using synthetic pharmaceutical drugs that cause all those unwanted side effects, or worse, addiction?" "Can we use only Clinical Nutrition with therapeutic diets, vitamins, micro and macro minerals, herbs and extracts? Is it "doable"?"

The answer is a resounding "Yes!" and we lay it out for you in the following pages of treatment protocols backed up with very strong "Evidence Based" medical journal publications.

This is a book born from repetitive requests emanating from Medical Doctors, Naturopaths, Chiropractors, Nutritionist, Nurses, etc. A book of answers, solutions, protocols and hopes; a book of supplements to just about every health problem common to all humans in every country of the world.

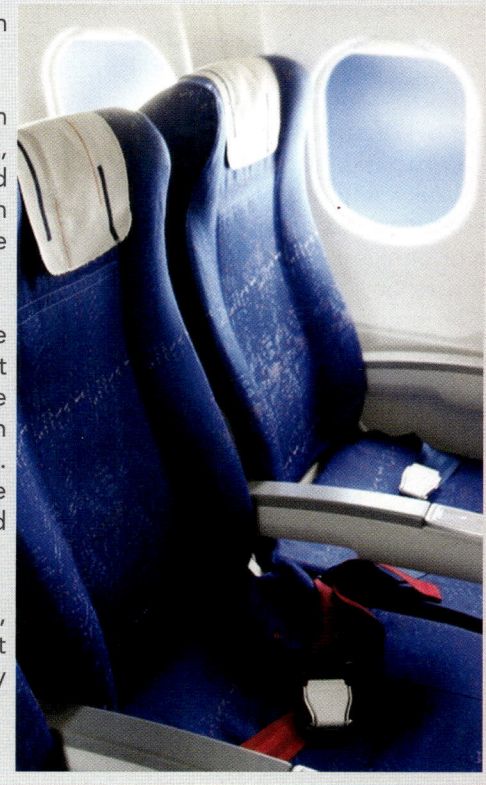

These products have been clinically used worldwide and time tested by thousands of doctors with great success, so that one could say that every products and ingredients are backed by thousands of family anecdotal stories filled with pain, fatigue, tears, as well as hope, relief and happiness. With the assistance of their loving physicians, patients are experiencing again renewed vigor, energy, laughter and Good Health.

It is our "Work of Love" to offer you this magnificent book, practical, resourceful and concise. Our whole team that worked on this book's completion wishes you and your family the Best of Health for the rest of your life! Cheers!

Prof. Dr. Paul Ling Tai & Team

2

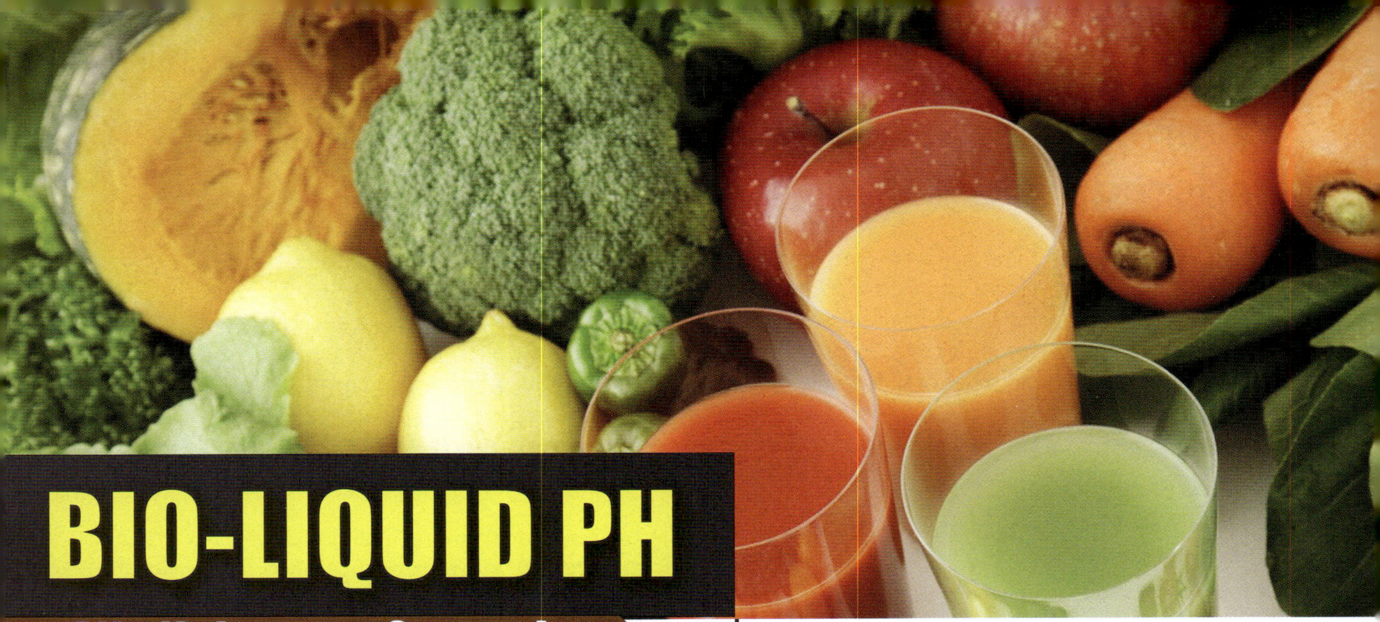

BIO-LIQUID PH
Alkalinize your System!

Guyton's Textbook of Physiology, a standard "Bible" of medical, osteopathic, and chiropractic schools determined that optimum blood and serum pH should be 7.3 as a healthy and imperative pH of the human body for normal cell reproduction, strong immunity, and healthy metabolism. Many physicians and researchers have written countless books and published health articles on the importance and proper balance of pH to sustain and achieve a healthy metabolism. We are often able to monitor the proper pH of our blood and serum by measuring the pH with a pH paper strip using saliva or urine. The saliva test is a quick and simple test. It can be taken first thing in the morning upon rising, before brushing your teeth, eating or drinking. It can also be checked anytime during the day, as long as nothing was eaten or drank for at least half an hour. Normal ranges of 6.8 to 7.4 are desirable for humans in good health. Many scientists and physicians consider saliva or urine pH from 5.0 to 6.5 to be a possible indication of abnormal physiology and an early warning of impending health problems.

What causes abnormal acidity in our body?

It is caused by an excessive acid production and accumulation of lactic acid or uric acid. It can also be caused by abnormal accumulation within the body from ineffective acid waste removal, a condition that causes the corrosion of the cell membrane, and abnormal metabolic pathway development within the cellular mitochondria.

Many individuals that suffer from Autoimmun Disease, i.e. Multiple Sclerosis, Lupus, Bowel Inflam mation Disease, Arthritis, Psoriasis, Metabolic Diseas es (Diabetes,) and many different kinds of cancer an leukemia, have a severely acidic pH of their saliva c urine.

One doctor explains that a highly acidic saliva pH like a Warning Sign similar to the red light on the dash board of your car to "Check Engine". This physicia considers an acidic saliva pH a warning mechanism. highly effective way of preventing unhealthy sever diseases is by quickly neutralizing the acidity level.

However, it is this doctor's personal experience that t reverse this acidic condition is very difficult. It ofte times takes several months or several years to achiev the return of neutral pH of saliva using only juicing c the avoidance of sugar. Liquid pH is made from simple and all natural process. The calcium cluster heated to very high temperatures, burning off ar impurities, leaving highly active clusters calcium ior when dissolved in water.

You can readily see the evidence that it is highly activ by adding 10-15 drops of Bio-Liquid pH in a glass c water. Taking this dosage 3 to 4 times daily ma support a balanced pH and help the body to achieve neutral 7.0 level of pH.

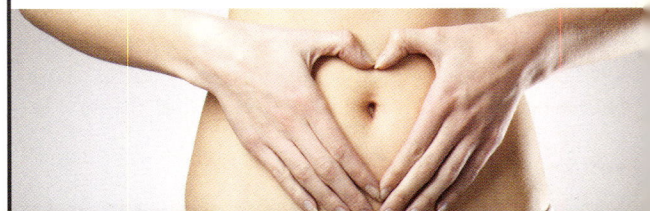

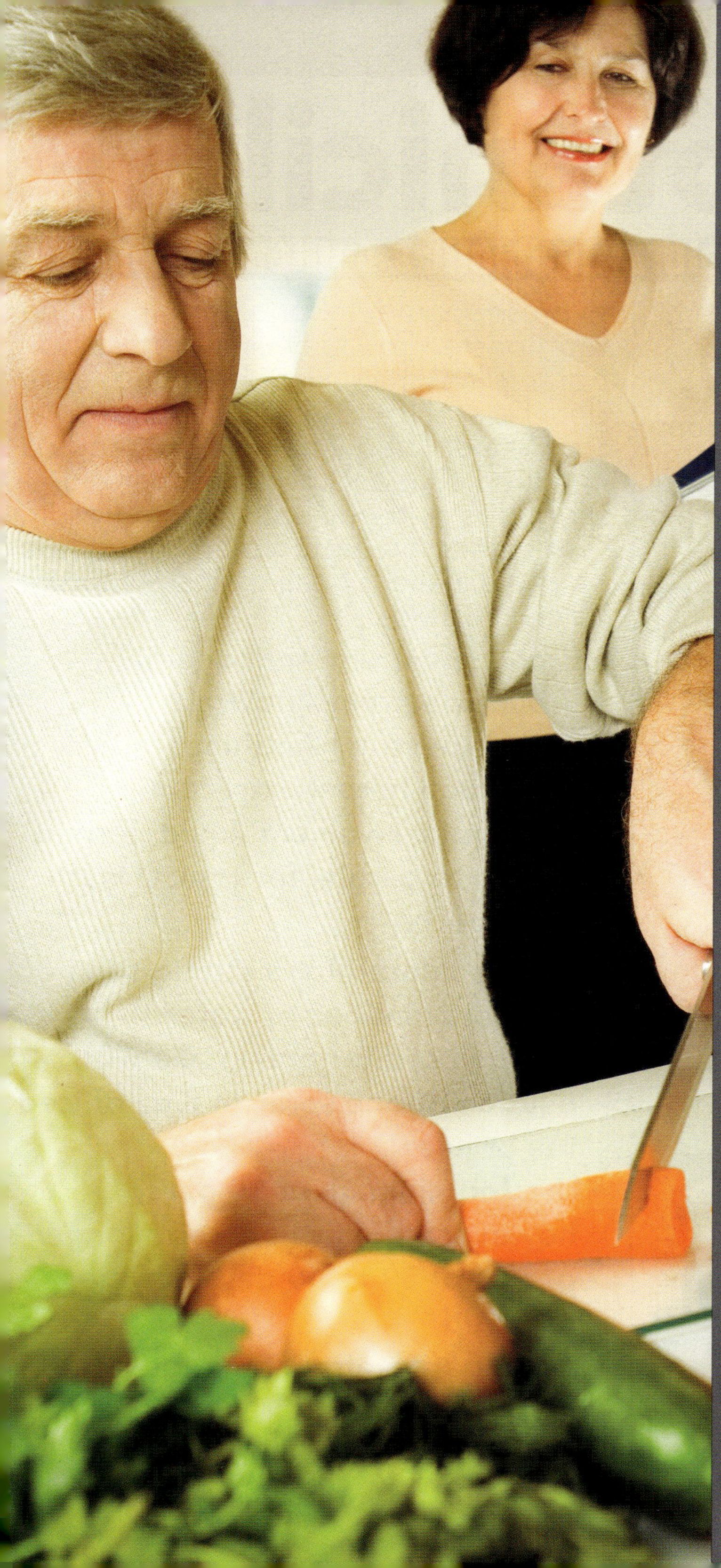

DIRECTIONS

Add 10-15 drops in water and drink 3 times daily or as instructed by your health professional. MUST BE TAKEN ON AN EMPTY STOMACH.

INGREDIENTS

Water, Oxygen-Ozone Modified Silicate
These statements have not been reviewed by the FDA. This product is not intended to diagnose, treat, cure, or prevent any disease.

Dr. Tai's Pearls

Avoiding Metabolic Acidity is one of the big debates within the medical profession. Although the pH in our blood is constantly being monitored by multiple systems to keep it exactly at 7.4 (or slightly basic), the tissues and cellular environment often become acidic due to fermentation and poor metabolic utilization of glucose with a lack of oxygen. This can occur to Super Athletes or even a regular man or woman on the street. Bio-Liquid pH is a short and easy way of which to achieve a more balanced pH within our tissues.

Side Effects: None

Contraindications:
Do not take if you are allergic to any of the ingredients.

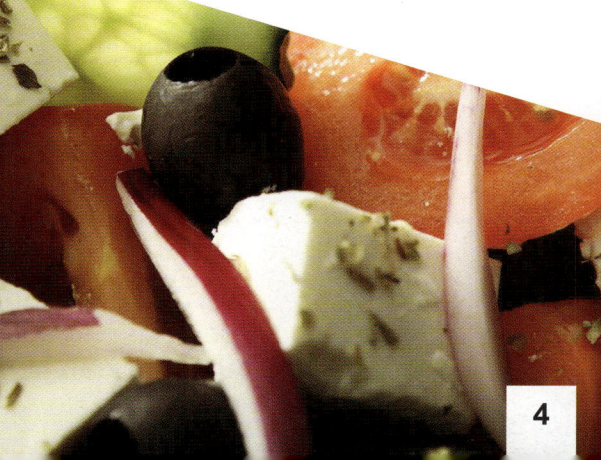

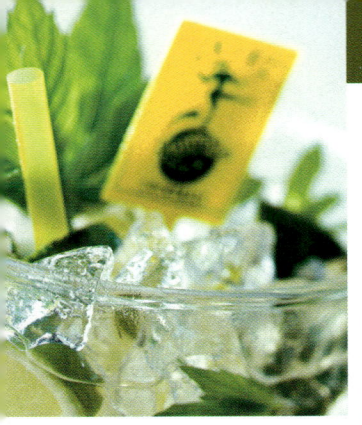

Botanicillin
Natural Antibiotic & Antifungal Remedy

Botanicillin is an extraordinary combination of natural herbal extracts with broad spectrum antibiotics covering both the Gram + and Gram- bacteria. It has been used successfully even in the most difficult methicillin resistance staphylococcus Aureas bacteria. Botanicillin is an effective broad antifungal. These kind of infections are the most difficult to control due to the superimposed infection with other fungal and bacteria colonies. Botanicillin is also a powerful antiviral. Many different kinds of viral infections are very difficult to address because there are no prescription drugs available as antiviral.

Research Doctors from the University of British Columbia Ethno Botany department performed several excellent studies of culture and sensitivity in the antiviral, anti bacteria, and antifungal effects of these natural herbal extracts.

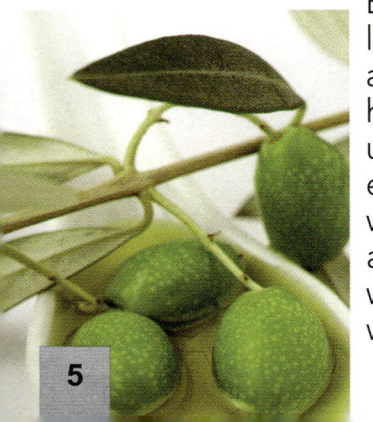

Botanicillin is in a liquid form for easy application and is highly effective. The ultraconcentrated extracts dissolve in water for gargling and swallowing, as well as for topical wash. It can be used to brush your teeth for gingivitis with no toothpaste. You may use it topically. Botanicillin may also be used as a douche and for Candida infections.

Dr. K said: "Very effective on Candida infection. Patient tried all sorts of prescriptions without satisfactory result. Two weeks on Botanicillin, patient is having excellent healing and symptom have vanished..."

- **Broad spectrum Antibacterial**
- **Broad spectrum Antiviral**
- **Broad spectrum Antifungal**
- **All natural herbal extracts**
- **Easy and convenient liquid format**
- **Usable to gargle, for topical wash and douche**
- **Can be diluted for a strong solution, one spray in 3 oz of water**
- **Can be used for oral intake with dilution of one spray in 8 oz of iced tea or juice**
- **Use for minmum of 10 days, however, in difficult cases a longer period of 30 to 40 days may be required.**
- **No negative effect on good bacteria in the GI Tract**

Directions: Shake well before use. Take 1 spray in a 10 oz glass of water or juice. Two to three times a day for 10 days or longer as needed. May also be used to wash cuts, gargle, brush teeth and gums.

Ingredients
L. Dissectum, M. Aquifolium, Usnea, T. Plicata, H. Perforation, Oplopanax Horridus, R. Nuticana, A. Alnifolia, Citrus Oil Extract

These statements have not been reviewed by the FDA. This product is not intended to diagnose, treat, cure, or prevent any disease.

Dr. Tai's Pearl
This is an extraordinary formulation with some of the best secrets in medicine. Use only a small amount to be effective. Don't waste, as this is precious.

Side Effects: None

Contraindications:
Do not take with Statins or AntiCholesterol medications. You may wash & Use externally however with these medications. Do not take if you are allergic to Grapefruit. Do not take if you are allergic to any of the ingredients.

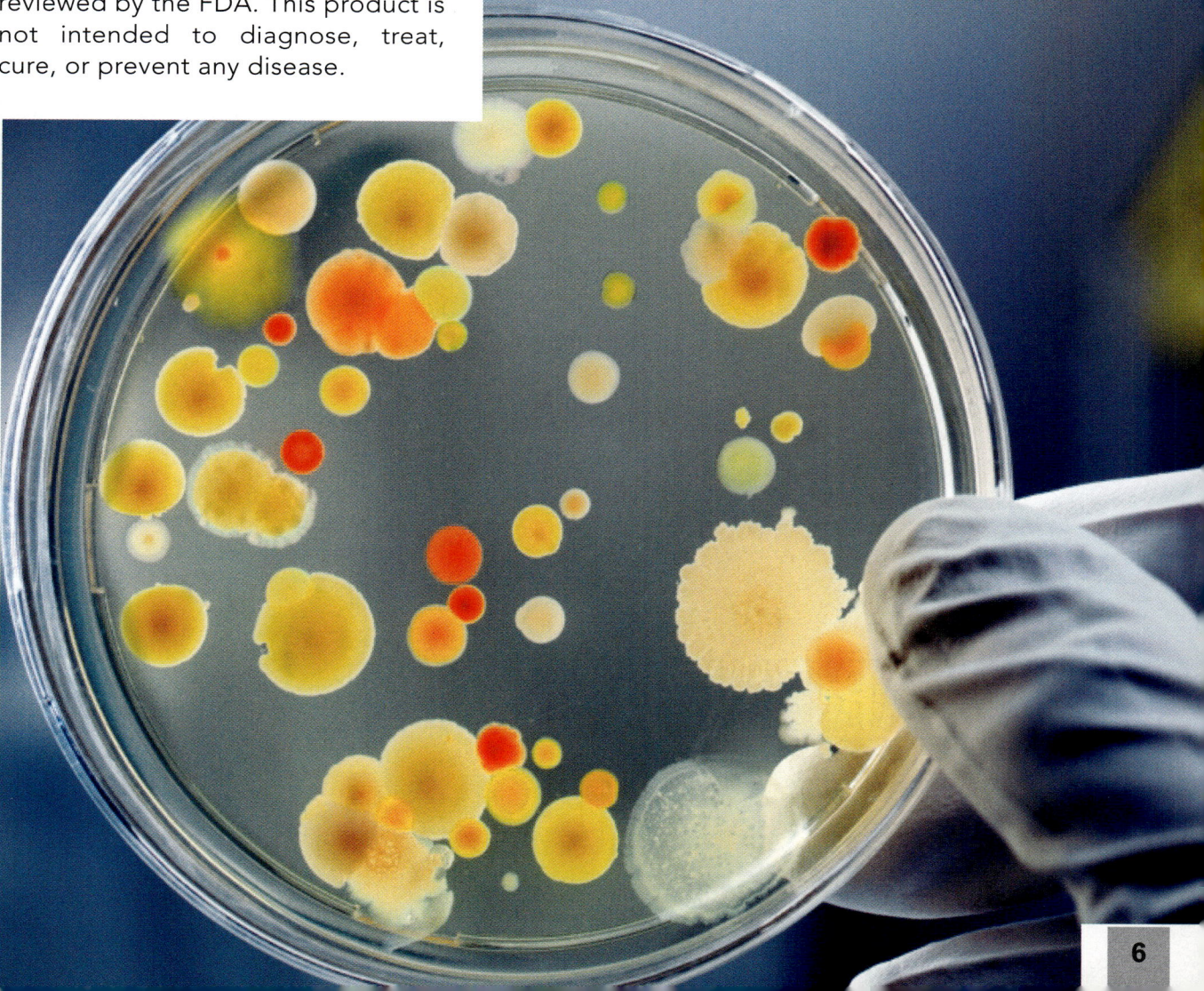

6

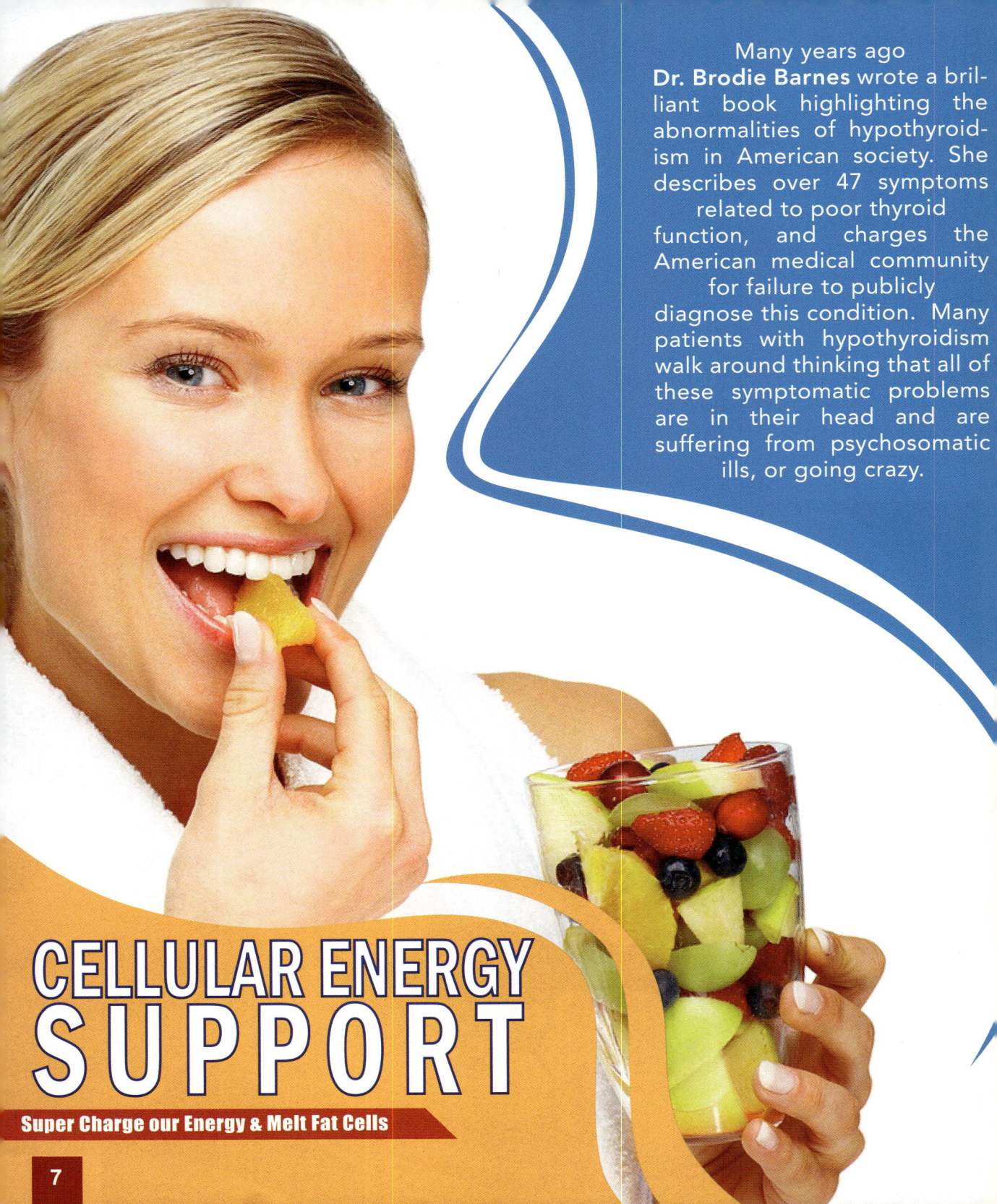

Many years ago **Dr. Brodie Barnes** wrote a brilliant book highlighting the abnormalities of hypothyroidism in American society. She describes over 47 symptoms related to poor thyroid function, and charges the American medical community for failure to publicly diagnose this condition. Many patients with hypothyroidism walk around thinking that all of these symptomatic problems are in their head and are suffering from psychosomatic ills, or going crazy.

CELLULAR ENERGY SUPPORT

Super Charge our Energy & Melt Fat Cells

Most health conditions today are related, one way or another, to functional hypothyroid conditions. Books and medical journals describe an epidemic problem of variety of diseases, metabolic abnormalities, overweight syndrome with obesity all rooted from a functional low hypothyroid. Laboratory studies and blood analysis test often do not shed any light into this horrible condition because the thyroid is not sick or diseased, but rather it is functioning at a very low capacity. Many individuals are walking around with low thyroid function and have symptoms of physical and mental components such as general loss of energy, weaknesses, susceptibility to cold, respiratory infections, recurrent sickness due to low immunity, difficulty breathing, suffering from muscle cramping, low back pain, easily bruising, mental sluggishness, very poor memory, inability to rationalize or think, transient headaches, emotional stability, and mood swings with anxieties.

Individuals with hypothyroid may also report feeling horribly cold even though it is warm outside, sensation of frozen hands, fingers, feet and toes. They wake up cold, they have hair loss, brittle nails, no appetite, joint stiffness with arthritis and no interest in sex.

Start by taking a simple underarm temperature test using an ordinary mercury thermometer upon awaking in the morning before getting out of bed. A range of below 97.8 degrees shows clinical hypothyroidism according to Dr. Barnes. Commence treatment even if the patients are borderline hypothyroid with the benefit of nutrition and increase of natural Iodine and Iodide from such products as Thyroid Specialist.

A new exciting product called Cellular Energy Support is a special formulation containing essential amino acids crucially needed for the production of the thyroid hormone. Thyroid hormone is a combination of amino acid L-Thyrosine. Oftentimes, because of poor diet, the amount of Thyrosine availability in the bodies is below those necessary for the proper production of Thyroid hormone. The second most important component for the manufacturing and production of Thyroid hormone and Thyroxine is Selenium.

The US Military Service shows in their report that individuals with low thyroid have a decline in performance and oftentimes suffer from stressful events which lowers their brain function and leads to depression, mood disorders and even affects an individual's memory, learning ability and thinking ability. Selenium produces at least 30 Selenol Enzymes important in the conversion of T4 to T3 which is the active portion of thyroid hormone. Furthermore, selenium is also important in the immune response system of patients with Hashimoto Thyroiditis where the individual's own immune system turns against their own thyroid gland.

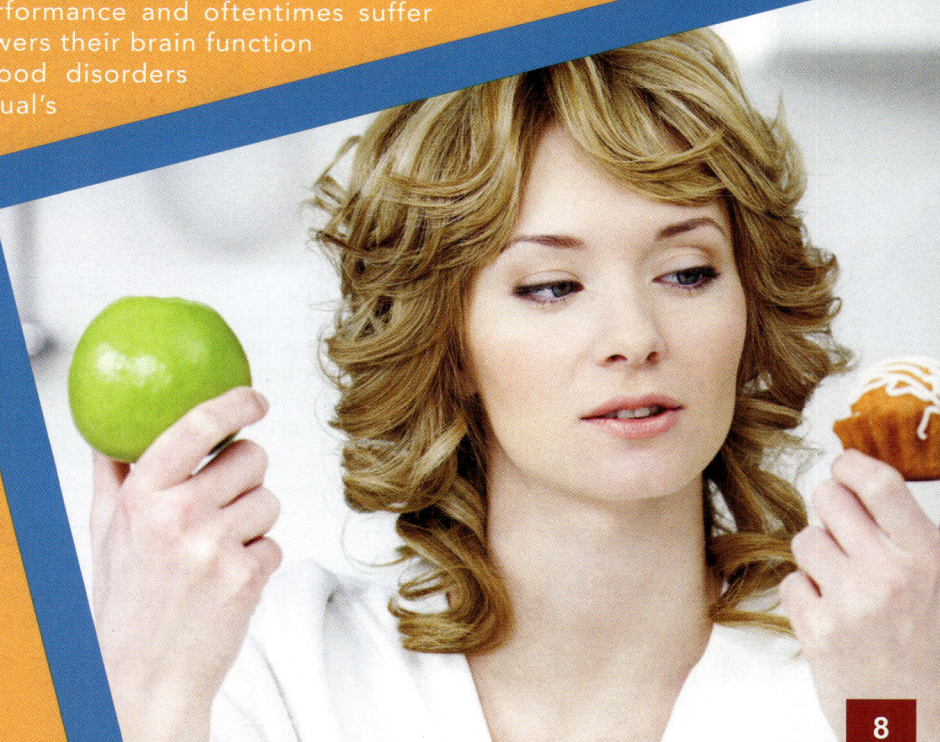

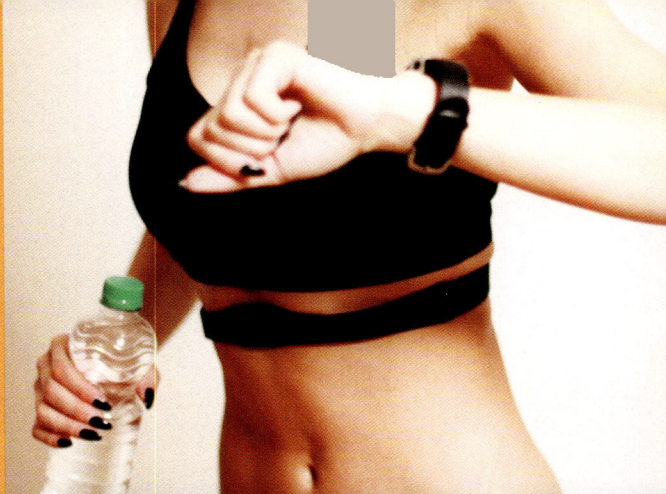

Cellular Energy Support contains the world renowned Ashwanganda. This herb from India is one of the highly prized Adaptogen from the Indian Ayurvedic medicine to balance life forces when encountering stress and slow down the aging process. The super extract of Ashwangandha with high levels of critical Withanolids, produces the extraordinary calming effect that is a tonic during stressful situations as well as calming when you are in a "fight" or "flight" situation. It also contains the world famous Rhodiola Rhosea which comes from the artic mountains of Siberia, Russia and has been known for centuries by the locals as the "Golden Root" with special extracts of Crenulin. Traditionally, it is used in these high mountain regions for the treatment of flu, cold and viruses, to improve longevity and increase the body's resistance to physical and mental stress.

In many clinical studies, Rhodiola has been used to improve the symptoms of depression. Over 65% of the patients studied, that is 26 out of 35 men, showed improvement. In another study, physicians using Rhodiola, were able to witness significant improvements in short term memory, concentration and critical thinking after 2 weeks. Even students undergoing very stressful long-term exams showed the use of Rhodiola improved their mental fatigue and improved their sensation of greater well-being.

Cellular Energy Support contains 80 critical micro elements of fulvic acid and Humate extract to support normal production of thyroid hormone. Finally, it contains the homeopathic Thyroidinum 3C, which is a powerful support of the thyroid gland in the recuperation and production of thyroid hormone.

Directions: Take 1 capsule AM and 1 capsule at Bedtime with a large glass of water. You may take higher dosage after consultation and supervision of a health professional.

Keep out of reach of children.

Ingredients: Manganese, Zinc, Selenium, Fulvic/Humate, L-Thyrosine, Homeopathic Thyroidinum 3c, Ashwanganda, Rhodiola Rosea
These statements have not been reviewed by the FDA. This product is not intended to diagnose, treat, cure, or prevent any disease.

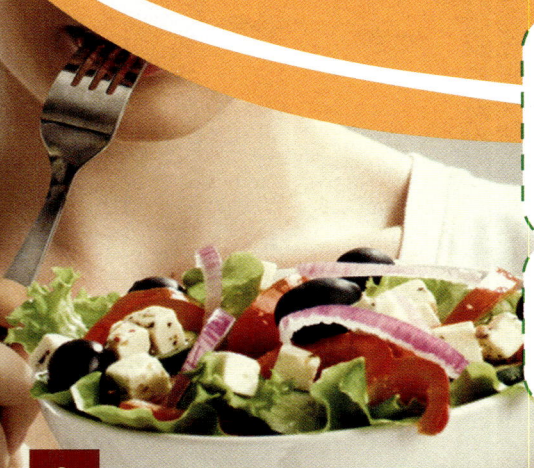

Side Effects:
Dosage is key to Max Metabolism. The side effects only occur when you have either too high of a dosage or you have increased the dosage too quickly or if you have problems with adrenal fatigue. There is no way of which to increase the Max Metabolism dosage when you have adrenal fatigue. The symptoms of too high a dosage are anxiety, palpitation, and shortness of breath.

Contraindications:
Do not take in case of hypothyroidism, unwanted weight loss, or in cases of high strung or hyperactive individuals. Do not take Product if you are allergic to any of its ingredients.

Dr. Tai's Pearl

The function and purpose of Cellular Energy Specialist is to increase the basal metabolic rate of individuals. The metabolic rate is the rate of calories burned while at rest. This increase is the center piece for cellular metabolism which is controlled by the mitochondria of the cells. Cellular Energy increases the numbers and quantities of mitochondria in each cellular structure as well as improving the quality of the mitochondria. Extremely useful in cases of overweight/obesity due to lack of mitochondria and cellular metabolism as well as severe fatigue, lack of energy, and very slow metabolic rate from hypothyroidism. However, the controlling aspect of the metabolic rate beyond the mitochrondria is the availability of cortisol which provides for the sugar fuel for the mitochondria to go to work. Without the cortisol availability and optimum adrenal activity, a person having a high metabolic rate cannot sustain due to lack of constant glucose energy when needed. As a complication and side effect to this lack of glucose, the body will overreact and create tachycardia and fast racing of the heart rhythm to make up for the lack of sugar. This often times is removed by bringing the adrenal fatigue to improved activity. So before you can treat or help anyone with their metabolic rate or their hypothyroidism, one must first address the complications of malfunctioning adrenal fatigue.

Clinical Cases:

Marilyn, 62-year-old grandmother and health worker complaining of problems with arthritis of both knees and other joints of her arms and hands. With muscle pain and cold hands and feet. She saw her hair falling out in the previous 30 days with horror as she screamed every day when faced with hands full of locks of hair. She said to herself that she will not be having much of her blonde curly locks left if this continues at the same pace. She sought help from her physician which promptly ran blood tests and complete laboratory urinalysis and x-rays. She was pronounced by the family physician to be within normal limits. He did not feel this constituted any abnormality – just aging and the symptoms should pass over time. She went to get a second opinion from her friend's doctor who specializes in integrative medicine. Upon careful review of her laboratory blood work found her TSA to be in the high range of normal and her T3 and T4 to be on the low range of normal. The thyroid antibodies were within normal limits. Even though they were within normal limits, the integrative physician chose to give a clinical trial of 30 days for treatment of hypothyroidism. This is often the case when dealing with hypothyroidism type 2, which has low-normal ranges of the thyroid blood test, but patient symptoms are indicating possible malfunction. She was placed on Synthroid, which is a synthetic medication with T4 for a trial of 30 days. It did seem to improve her status in terms of fatigue and energy, as well as general improvement. But still she was complaining of the symptoms and the clinical progress was not at the level of her expectations. She obtained some supplements from a friend, including the Max Sea Extract and Max Metabolism. Within 30 days, she saw major improvement, which gave her a sign she was going about in the right direction. She adjusted the dosage during the next 60 days and found the perfect dosage for her body and most of her symptoms have now disappeared – her arthritis has improved, her hands and feet are warm, she has no fatigue, and her energy levels have improved.

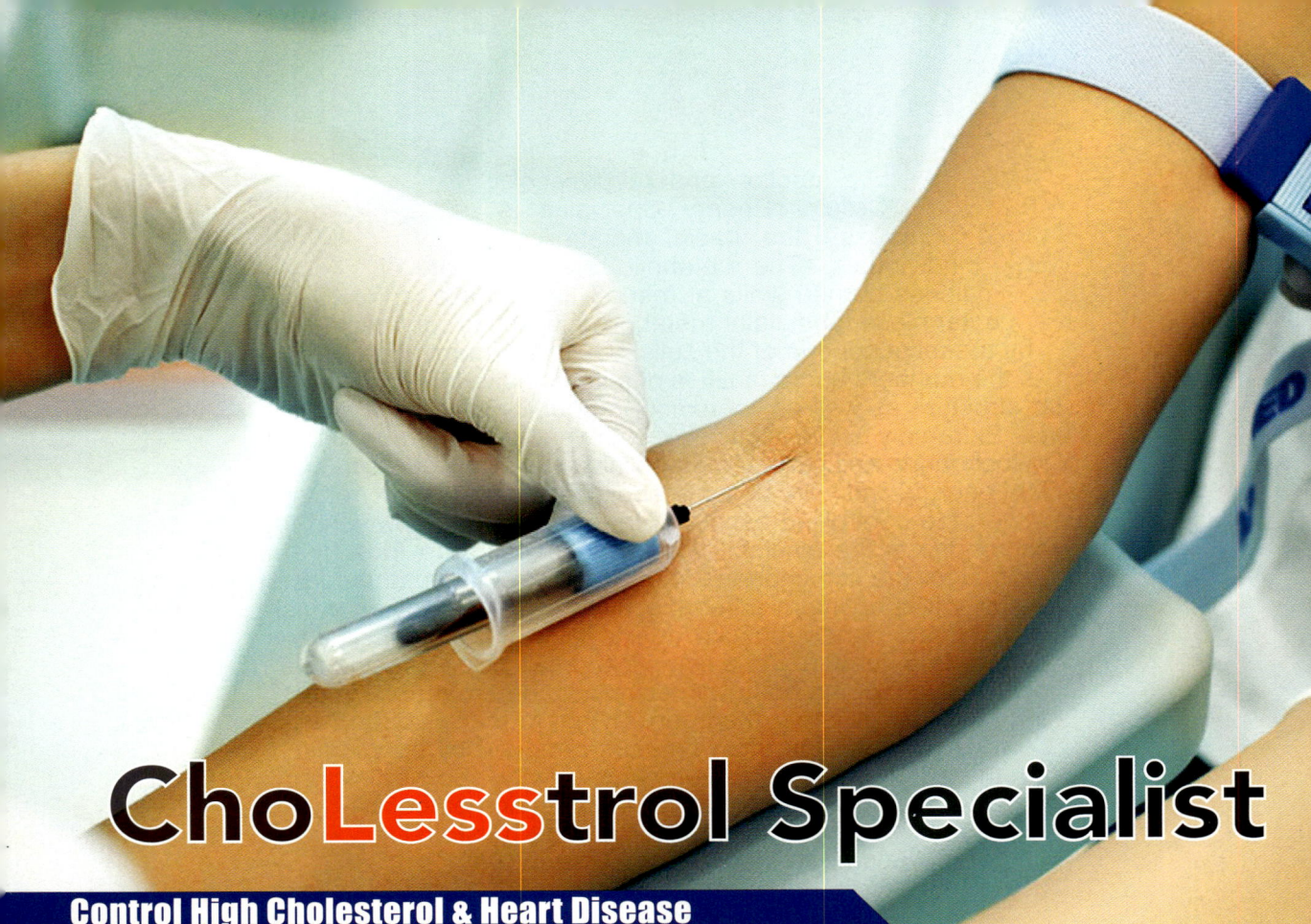

CHoLesstrol Specialist

Control High Cholesterol & Heart Disease

THIS IS A LIFE SAVING FORMULA! THIS EXTRAORDINARY NEW, All Natural Herbal Breakthrough may RADICALLY CHANGE THE FUTURE COURSE of Alternative MEDICAL HEART SUPPLEMENTATION. This Amazing COMPREHENSIVE Formula will thrill you with results. It is Backed by Proven Research and has been CLINICALLY TESTED, containing an ingredient that goes to work immediately to REPAIR, PROTECT, and RESTORE YOUR HEART TO ITS HEALTHIEST AND STRONGEST CONDITION.

#1 DEADLY HEART BLOCKER– CHOLESTEROL

Octacosanol is a natural compound made from Sugarcane. A medical study by Dr. Gourini-Berticold states that Policosanol reduces LDL (bad) up to 29% and raises HDL (good) by up to 15%. (Am. Heart. J. 2002) It was confirmed by Dr. Castano G that Policosanol in postmenopausal women LDL (bad) dropped up to 25%, Total Cholesterol dropped 16.7%, and raised HDL (good) by 27%. (Gynecol Endocr 2000). Further safety studies of Policosanol by Dr. Fernandez J.C. on nearly 28,000 participants concluded that Policosanol is effective safe and well-tolerated. (Curr. Ther. Research 1998 & J. of Geron. March 2000)

Pleorotus – Dr. Solomon Wasser reports an edible mushroom containing a high content of natural cholesterol lowering statin in the fruiting body of Pleorotus Ostreatus. (Int. J. of Med. March 1999). A number of laboratory studies by Dr Bobek, et al. show that Pleorotus Ostreatus effectively prevented accumulation of cholesterol in blood and liver of animals studied.

Inositol Hexanicotinate – Vitamin B3 niacin is well accepted by the traditional mainstream medical community to

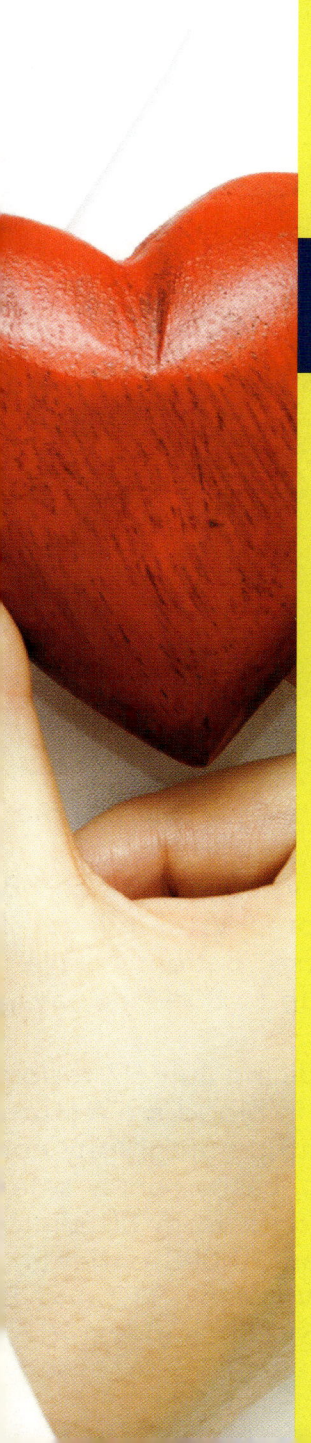

lower cholesterol but unfortunately niacin, when taken in quantities to lower cholesterol, can cause severe flushing, headaches and occasional liver inflammation. Now you can have a more powerful alternative. Inositol Hexanicotinate is an extensively studied, super potent, safer alternative to niacin without side effects according to Dr. Head K.A. (Alt. Med. Rev. 1996). Dr. Welsh A.L. says Inositol Hexanicotinate is improved, powerful and more effective than Niacin. (Int. Record Med. 1961).

#2 DEADLY HEART BLOCKER - INFLAMMATION

It is obvious that mainstream medicine's opinion of cholesterol as the culprit of heart disease missed a great deal of the total picture. While millions of people continue to suffer heart disease and die, research has shocking proof that doctors are complacent and ignoring the main culprit: INFLAMMATION.

QUESTION:

What is invisible and silent, but deadly?
Dr. Stephen Prescott of the University of Utah told SCIENCE NEWS that clinical data suggests that Inflammation is "Central to the Pathogenesis" of blocked arteries. The chemicals from inflammation further harm the blood vessel walls. White cells congregate at the site of this injury and become engorged with fat molecules, forming the FIRST sign of atherosclerosis (Science News 1/20/90).
Dr. Paul Ridker, MD, a cardiologist with the Harvard Medical School did an extensive study of more than 22,000 male physicians over a 14 year period. Doctors with the highest CRP scores ended up over the next 10 years with a 300% increase in heart attacks and 200% strokes. Dr. Ridker did another Monumental study with nearly 30,000 healthy post-menopausal women revealing those with the highest CRP test had 700% increase in heart attacks or strokes. (NEJM Nov 2003)

DOUBLE HERBAL HEART BYPASS! - THOUSAND YEAR OLD HERB TO THE RESCUE. Turmeric has a strong active ingredient called Curcumin. It is known for its powerful anti-inflammatory properties worldwide.
Reuther's Health reports: A study in a recent issue of the Journal CANCER links curcumin to be a potent anti-inflammatory agent with health benefits.

Researchers at the University of Illinois found that Curcumin helps prevent plaque formation and that Turmeric reduced the number of plaques by half. Studies at Vanderbilt University suggest that Curcumin may block progression of Multiple Sclerosis and Alzheimer's. Turmeric has significant
anti-inflammatory and additional cancer protection benefits. Dr. Motterlini R. reports that in laboratory studies, the use of the anti-inflammatory properties of Curcumin protected the inner lining cells of the bovine aorta resulting in "enhanced cellular resistance to Oxidative Damage" (Free Radic Biol Med, April 2000.)

#3 DEADLY HEART BLOCKER – HOMOCYSTEINE

Homocysteine is a toxic Amino Acid. It accelerates the aging of your circulation by attacking the inner lining of your blood vessels, causing premature heart disease.

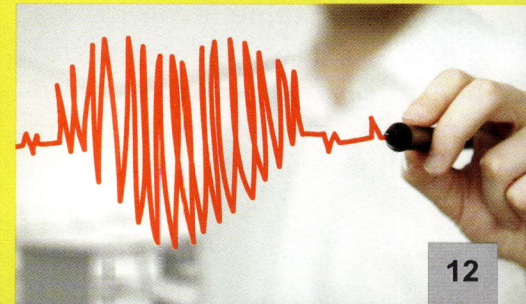

INGREDIENTS

Homocysteine is dangerous because it can cause blood vessel blockage or clots even if your cholesterol and triglycerides are not significantly elevated. Researchers believe that excess levels of homocysteine may set the stage for cholesterol to penetrate the blood vessel walls and start the plaque formation. Detoxify the excess homocysteine by "methylating" homocysteine into a non-toxic amino acid methionine by supplementing Folic acid, vitamin B12, and B6. Men and women younger than 60 years old have a 220% increased overall risk of coronary and other vascular diseases in those with highest homocysteine blood levels.

Dr. Donald Jacobsen, Ph.D. Director for Homocysteine research at Cleveland Clinic says that patients with elevated homocysteine levels have a 800% greater incidence of heart disease, strokes and clogged arteries of the legs than the general population.

TRIPLE HERBAL HEART BYPASS! - SCIENTISTS "BREAK THE SILENCE"

Scientists from all over the world "Break the Silence" by revealing secrets that revolutionize the All Natural Heart supplement.

Dr. Xavier Pi-Sanyer, MD, professor of Medicine at Columbia University, reveals that people consuming higher Folic Acid and Vitamins B12 and B have a significant reduction of Homocysteine levels i their blood. "We estimate these patients have reduced risk of heart disease by up to 80%" he says.

The New England Journal of Medicine July 97 report that "High Homocysteine" levels in blood are a stron prediction of death in patients with angiography con firmed coronary artery disease". Lastly, on a safet issue worth noting, a review of data from 80 clinica studies, which included more than 10,000 patients, was concluded that Folic Acid, Vitamins B12 and B are an efficient and safe means to reduce elevated homocysteine.

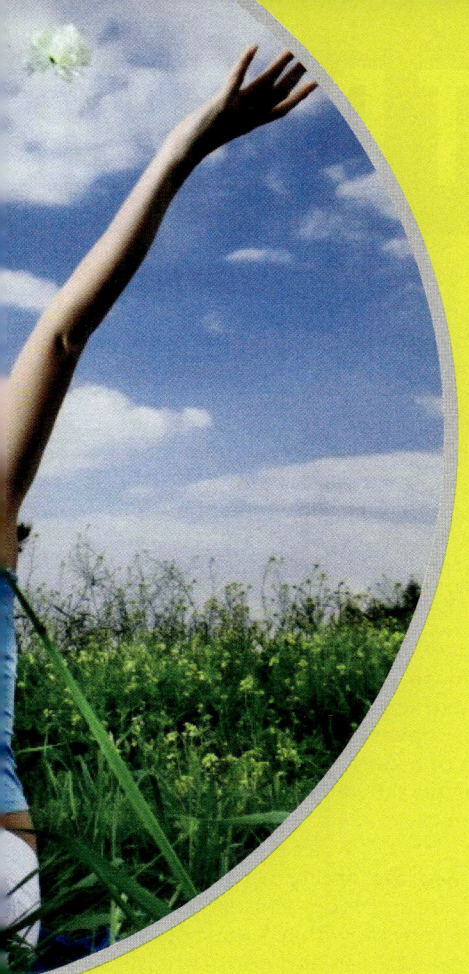

Dr. Tai's Pearl

I do not believe as many doctors do that cholesterol levels need to be as low as they are presently claiming as a clinical objective. I believe that a total cholesterol level of 200 is appropriate and not excessive to the general public. Levels that physicians are now claiming as the goal, down to 100 total cholesterol, I think is potentially detrimental to the many different cell materials and tissues of the body. The cellular membranes are made from lipids and the brain and neurological tissues are made from cholesterol. Hormones that sustain men and women's characteristics are made from cholesterol and having levels excessively low can injure the production of essential hormones that are essential for healthy living, as well as a young body.

Directions:
Take 1 capsule two times a day or a higher dosage as needed and recommended by your physician or health practitioner.

Ingredients
Inositol Hexanicotinate, Pleurotus Ostreatus, L-Arginine, Curcumin Longa, Policosanol, Tetracosanol, Hexacosanol, Heptacosanol, Octacosanol, Nonacosanol, Triacosanol, Docosanol, Piperine Longa

These statements have not been reviewed by the FDA. This product is not intended to diagnose, treat, cure, or prevent any disease.

Side Effects:
Much diminished from the prescription drugs of anti-cholesterol. However, still precaution must be taken for possible numbness or weakness of muscle. Precaution of utilization with CoQ10 supplementation with this supplement of anti-cholesterol is recommended and may help in achieving overall general health.

Contraindications:
This supplement should not be taken together with prescription anti-cholesterol medications as it will have tentative as well as synergistic effect that may cause complications. Do not take if you are allergic to any of the ingredients.

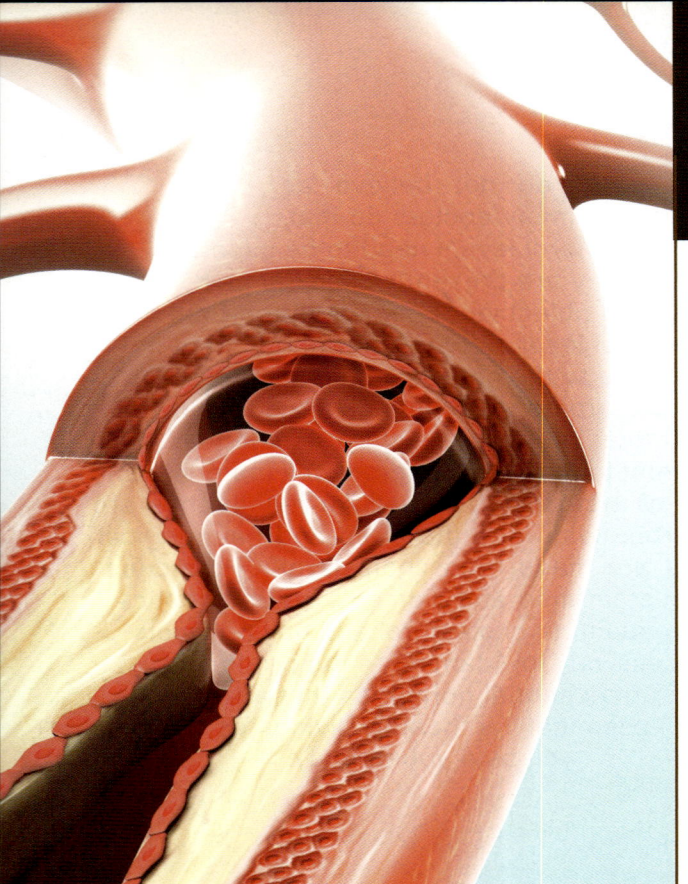

CLOT BUSTER

Prevention of MicroClots in Blood & Tissues

Any inflammation, bacteria, fungus or virus can trigger blood clotting abnormalities thru excess cross linked Fibrin and Fibrinogen circulating through the blood vessels and sticking to the walls. This contributes to the formation of excess blood clots and atherosclerosis which slows the blood flow, increasing blood viscosity and resulting in increased blood pressure. Blood clots block blood flow to the muscles, brain, heart and organs, cutting off vital nutrients and oxygen, leading to ischemia such as angina, heart attacks or total tissue necrosis and death.

ClotBuster is a "new, unique, one of a kind proprietary blend" (1. nattokinase, 2. serriopeptidase, 3. lumbrokinase) of natural extracted anti-Fibrinogen & anti-plasminogen enzymes never available before in a single formula. This one of a kind natural formula exhibits a powerful fibrinolytic activity and antiplatelet aggregation factors.

ClotBuster may have the ability to prevent, as well as dissolve, thrombi from blood vessels and capillaries. ClotBuster may go to work within 1 hour of taking it and lasts 4-6 hours to re-establish and normalize blood circulation. Researchers from Biotechnology Research lab of Japan tested Nattokinase's ability to dissolve a thrombus in carotid arteries of rats who regained 62% of blood flow. (Enzyme Wave, vol. 3, June 2002)

1. Nattokinase was discovered by Dr. Hiroyuki Sumi M.D. at the blood laboratory of the University of Chicago. It now has over 17 published chemical studies. Dr. Sumi induced blood clots in male dogs, gave them 4 capsules of Nattokinase (250mg per capsule) and gave them an angiogram. The dogs with Nattokinase were able to regain normal blood circulation within five hours of oral treatment. (Sumi, H et al JTTAS, 1995)

ClotBuster contains a Standardized Nattokinase of 20.000 FU made from fermented soybean with beneficial bacillus, Natto producing enzymatic peptidases, to be absorbed in the intestine duodenum. Therefore, it must be Enteric Coated. Most commercial enzymes in the market are not enteric coated and are destroyed by the stomach making them ineffective. See published Nattokinase references.

Question:

What do Heart attacks, Strokes, Atherosclerosis, Thrombophlebitis, Angina, Deep Vein Thrombosis, Ischemia, Cancer, Fibromyalgia, Chronic Fatigue, Lyme Disease, Crohn's Disease, Diabetes, Gulf War Syndrome, Heavy Metal Toxification, Inflammation, Infections, Vascular Dementia, Intermittent Claudication, Autism-ADD-ADHD, Ulcerative colitis, Hypertension, Spasm, Sinusitis, Laryngitis, Retinopathy, Fibrocystic Breast, Ovarian Cysts and Uterine Fibroids have in Common?

Answer:

Blood clots, thrombus and fibrin in large, medium and small blood vessels virtually anywhere in the body cause or exacerbate the above conditions.

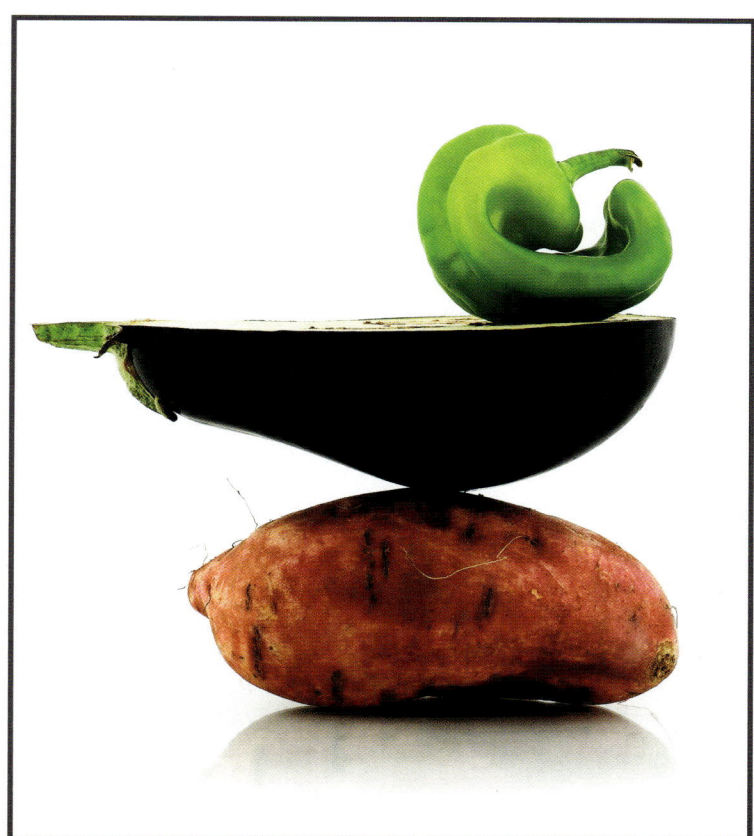

3. Lumbrokinase (100.000fu) is a potent fibrinolytic enzyme purified from the digestive track of the earthworm, Lumbricus Rubellus. In China, lumbrokinase won the Science and Technology Advances Award.

The active ingredient in the Earthworm Plasminogen Activator (e-PA) is similar to the famous Tissue Plasminogen Activator (t-PA) which is used worldwide to save lives in Sudden Death and coronary thrombosis in heart attacks. Earthworm Plasminogen Activator (e-PA) can convert plasminogen into plasmin to carry out fibrinolysis and dissolve fibrin from thrombus.

A PubMed search revealed 29 citations related to this research. Lumbrokinase is non-toxic, free of negative side effects, and convenient to use, showing no abnormal bleeding time and clotting time in in vivo studies.

Clinical studies showed oral Lumbrokinase is very effective in ischemic cerebrovascular diseases with an overall therapeutic efficacy of 93.73%, and 73.60% patients demonstrating marked improvement.

See published Lumbrokinase references

2. Serrapeptase (100.000 unit) is a proteolytic enzyme extracted and purified from the intestine of silk worms. This vitally important enzyme allows the newborn silkworm to dissolve the surrounding fibrous cocoon.

Serrapeptase must be absorbed from the intestines into the bloodstream as an enzyme active form (Moriya N et al, Biotech Appl Biochem Aug 20, 1994). A clinical study involving the treatment of inflammation of breast engorgement with oral serrapeptase oral patients showed a "marked" improvement of breast pain, breast swelling and indurations in 85.7% of patients taking serrapeptase with no negative side effects (Kee WH et al. Sing Med. J. Feb 30, 1989)

Another prospective study on postoperative swelling and pain of the ankle showed the serrapeptase group had 50% decreased swelling by the third day over placebo group (esch PM et al. Fortschr. Med. Feb 10, 1989)

Serrapeptase succeeds in cleaning airway passages by mucolytic effect on sputum viscosity, elasticity, viscosity of nasal mucus and powerful fibrinolytic, anti-inflammatory, mucolytic expectorant and blood vessel anti-inflammatory.

See published Serrapeptase references.

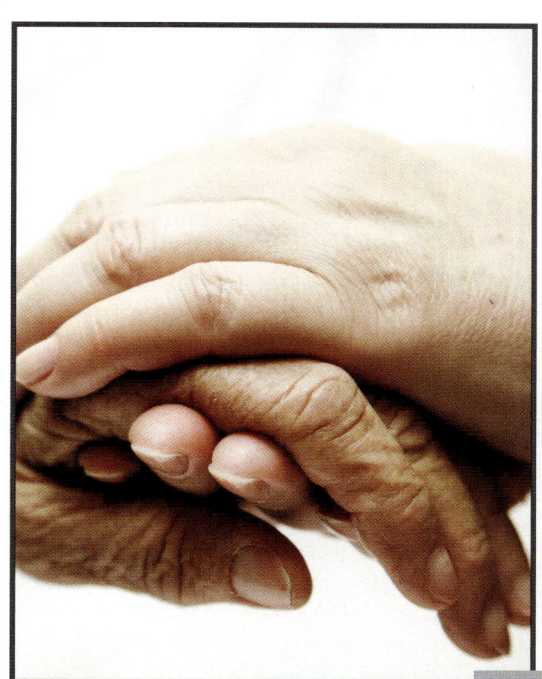

FREQUENTLY ASKED QUESTIONS
ClotBuster

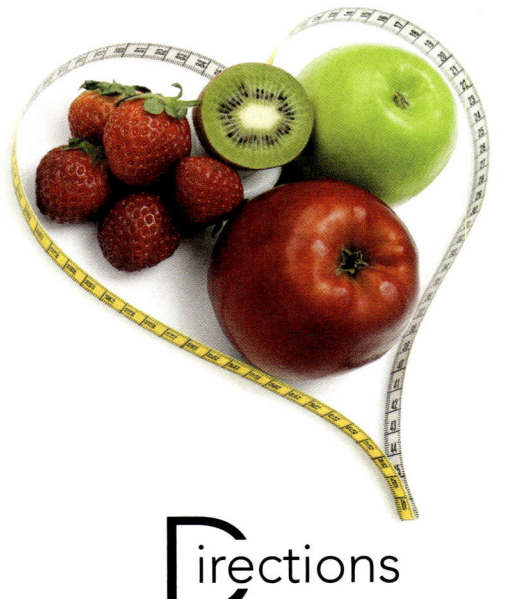

Are there any side effects with ClotBuster?
ClotBuster uses all natural enzymes of botanical origin with no known side effects. No bleeding or clotting abnormality has been reported. If you experience negative side effects, discontinue the product.

Can I take ClotBuster after surgery?
There is no known bleeding or clotting side effects but as a precaution we recommend a waiting period of 5 days after surgery before starting on ClotBuster.

Can ClotBuster be taken with blood thinners or antiplatelet aggregation?
ClotBuster does not significantly alter blood tests, such as Prothrombin Time (PT), activated Thromboplastin Time (aPTT) and International Normalized Ratio (INR). Patients should discuss this with their Health Practitioner and monitor blood work closely as usual.

How should I take ClotBuster?
ClotBuster should be taken on an empty stomach (nothing eaten for at least 3 hours) and do not eat for at least one hour afterwards. Drink water only with Clot Buster.

Directions
Take 1 capsule daily on an empty stomach and do not eat for one hour after. You may increase dosage up to 4 capsules daily or as recommended by your health care practitioner. Keep out of reach of children.

Ingredients
Proprietary Formulation: 450mg Nattokinase (Nattoseb) 20,000 Iu/G Serratiopeptidase (Peptizyme Sp-En) 100,000 Iu/G Lumbrikinase 100,000 Iu/Mg Bromelain 2400 Gdu, Allicin

These statements have not been reviewed by the FDA. This product is not intended to diagnose, treat, cure, or prevent any disease.

Nattokinase Published References
1. Sumi H. Healthy Microbe "Bacillus natto". Japan Bio Science Laboratory Co. Ltd.
2. Fujita M et al (December 1993). "Purification and characterization of a strong fibrinolytic enzyme (nattokinase) in the vegetable cheese natto, a popular soybean fermented food in Japan". Biochemical and Biophysical Research Communications 197 (3): 1340-1347.
3. Sumi H, et al. "A novel fibrinolytic enzyme (nattokinase) in the vegetable cheese Natto; a typical and popular soybean food in the Japanese diet." Experientia 1987, Oct 15;43(10):1110-1.
4. Sumi H, Hamada H, Nakanishi K, Hiratani H. "Enhancement of the fibrinolytic activity in plasma by oral administration of nattokinase." Acta Haematol 1990;84(3):139-43.
5. Sumi H et al (November 2000). "Determination and Properties of the Fibrinolysis Accelerating Substance (FAS) in Japanese Fermented Soybean "Natto".". Nippon Nogeikagaku Kaishi (Japanese). 74 (11): 1259-1264.

Serrapeptase Published References

1. Moriya N, Nakata M, et al. Intestinal absorption of serrapeptase in rats. Biotechnol Appl Biochem. 1994 Aug;20 (Pt 1):101-8.
2. Guyton, A. Function of the Human Body. WB Saunders pp. 83-84
3. Malshe PC. "A preliminary trial of serratiopeptidase in patients with carpal tunnel Syndrome." J Assoc Physicians India, 2000, 48(11):1130
4. Bracale G, Selvetella L. "Clinical study of the efficacy of and tolerance to seaprose S in inflammatory venous disease. Controlled study versus serratio-peptidase." Minerva Cardioangiol. 1996 Oct;44(10):515-24.
5. Kee WH, Tan SL, Lee V, Salmon YM. "The treatment of breast engorgement with Serrapeptase (Danzen): a randomised double-blind controlled trial." Singapore Med J. 1989 Feb;30(1):48-54.

Lumbrokinase Published References

1. Fan Q, Wu C, et al. Some features of intestinal absorption of intact fibrinolytic enzyme III-l from Lumbricus rubellus. Biochem Biophys Acta, 2001; 1526(3): 286-92
2. Gao Y, Qin MZ. Lumbrokinase in treatment of patients with hyperfibrinogenemia of coronary atherogenesis disease. Journal of Capital University of Medical Sciences, 1999; 4(20)
3. Gong B, Wu XY. Observation of using Baiao lumbrokinase capsules to treat ischemic cerebrovascular accident with hyperlipidemia. Capital Medicine, 2000; 7(12): 39
4. Quo ZF, Liu XX. Observation of treating ischemic cerebrovascular accident with Baiao lumbrokinase capsules. Capital Medicine, 2000; 7(11): 45
5. Huang ZO, Li ZW, Zhang WX. Lumbrokinase in treating cerebral infarction. Chinese Journal of New Drugs and Clinical Remedies, 2000; 6(19): 453-455

Dr. Tai's Pearl

Most of the nasty conditions that we experience that cause severe illness such as cancer and infections, severe inflammation, all have one thing in common. The pathology deals with small micro-clotting of the tissues in order to defend the nutrients as well as the blood and immune system to combat the pathology in the site of injury. The bacteria in cancer, as well as inflammation, create these blockages to the tumor and infectious area in order to grow and create the optimum environment for the propagation and perpetuation of the condition. We think that by using the enzymes, effectively breaking up the congestion and the walls of cell protection, can be vital to the beginnings of its demise of the pathology, and healing can commence. By having open capillaries and blood vessels, bringing nutrients, antibiotics, immune system into the healing process, is critical to improvement and healing of many conditions.

Side Effects: None

Contraindications:
Although it is generally accepted that the enzymes used as ingredients in Clot Buster are not normally interfering with bleeding and clotting time as well as anti-coagulant therapy, I personally feel that one must be careful when taking the enzymes just in case there are individuals who see synergistic or additive effect on their bleeding/clotting time. Care and evaluation should still be taken; however, after 20 years of using this supplement and ingredients I have never seen any complications. Do not take if you are allergic to any of the ingredients.

Craving Factor

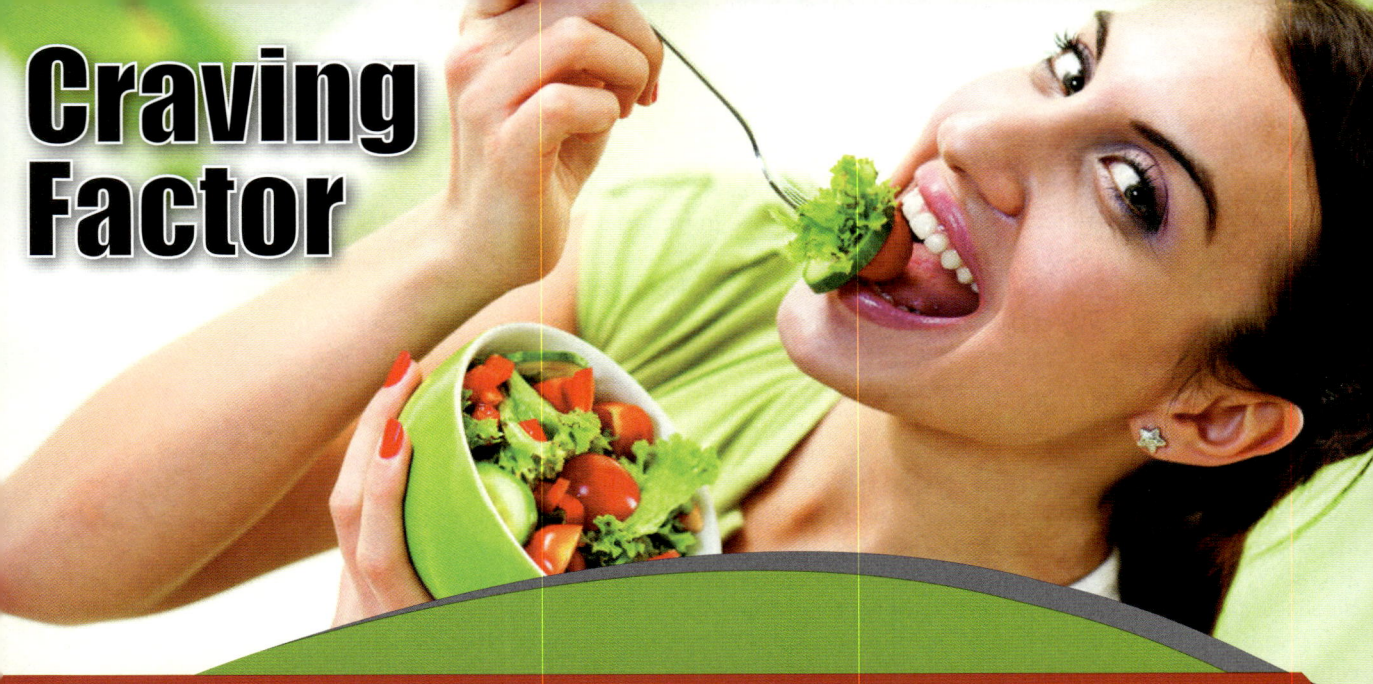

Fat Burning Diet Turn the Thermostat UP and the Craving DOWN

Calcium, one of the most researched minerals, is the key to optimum metabolism and fat burning. Calcium is a powerful messenger to your metabolism, to keep you lean and satisfied. This is based on new scientific research on the lipolytic (fat burning) action of calcium in moderately increased doses that just hasn't gone public yet. This information is also based on twenty years of personal experience of Dr. Stephen Levine, who is a renowned nutrition researcher, the experience of many of his colleagues, doctors and thousands of patients in the realm of environmental medicine. It's time that this important message gets out to you.

What if I were to tell you that a simple nutrient, in the right amounts and in the right form, could help you lose a significant amount of weight without even changing your diet or exercise routine? And not only would it help you lose weight, but combined with some other simple nutrients, in the right form, can make your cravings go away.

You would probably think that this sounds too good to be true. But it's not. In the last 5 or 6 years, scientific researchers have discovered that calcium, one of the most common minerals; can actually help you lose weight without changing diet or exercise because of its effect on the body's fat burning mechanism. In addition, calcium, combined with the right nutrients, can be used to reduce or eliminate cravings.

The newly discovered role of calcium's profound effect on fat metabolism and energy production has become clear within very recent years, through the compelling results of animal and human scientific studies. No one yet, to our knowledge, has announced these findings to the public. Clearly, this calcium research is a critically important discovery in relationship to dieting and weight control, as well as health and longevity. The implications are far reaching, to say the least.

Herein, we have integrated the recent calcium research, along with some of our own research in the area of allergic and addictive dietary phenomenon to present a truly unique and transforming dietary plan.

The buffering (neutralization of acid) action of this high calcium is very important and critical to neutralize food cravings and even cravings for drugs. This buffering effect, especially with calcium, can change your life dramatically and instantly. The buffering effect and how it reverses adverse reactions to foods, has been known in limited circles for decades. In fact, a study done at the Haight Ashbury Free Clinic in San Francisco in 1984, demonstrated that a modified calcium formula could reduce withdrawal symptoms in seriously addicted patients by 90%, with only 1 to 1 1/2 teaspoons a day. These patients were withdrawing from alcohol and stimulant drug abuse.

If high calcium buffered minerals and vitamin C can accomplish these dramatic effects on seriously addicted individuals, there's a very good chance that it can help you.

If there were an award for the most important fat burning nutrient of the decade, First Place would go to calcium. Second Place would also go to calcium and Third Place, well, you know. The benefits that may be achieved by increasing calcium intake goes way beyond the temporary benefits of imbalanced super high protein diets or extreme low-fat diets. There are individual biochemical factors involved. The benefits can be immediate as described above, but are also for long term health and longevity by maximizing fat burning, which converts into extra energy for enjoying your life. Calcium may melt your adipose tissue and keep you warm from the inside out. The approach we present is balanced, the doses are reasonable and has many other benefits. It also makes sense from an evolutionary perspective. It is based on good scientific evidence, mostly published within the last 5 or 6 years.

When you read this material you're going to be amazed. Why hasn't anyone told you this before? Why hasn't the government put out this information through the National Institute of Health or some other governmental institution? It is because some scientists and physicians would like to see twenty more years of research to confirm what has already become clear. It's up to you. You can wait twenty years for more research or you can explore the possibilities yourself right now.

Directions: Dissolve 1 teaspoon in 16oz of water. Drink 2 bottles of Craving Factor per day, A.M. & Noon. May be used 3 – 5 times a day for additional weight loss. You may add non-caloric sweeteners, i.e. Stevia or flavorings to your taste preference.

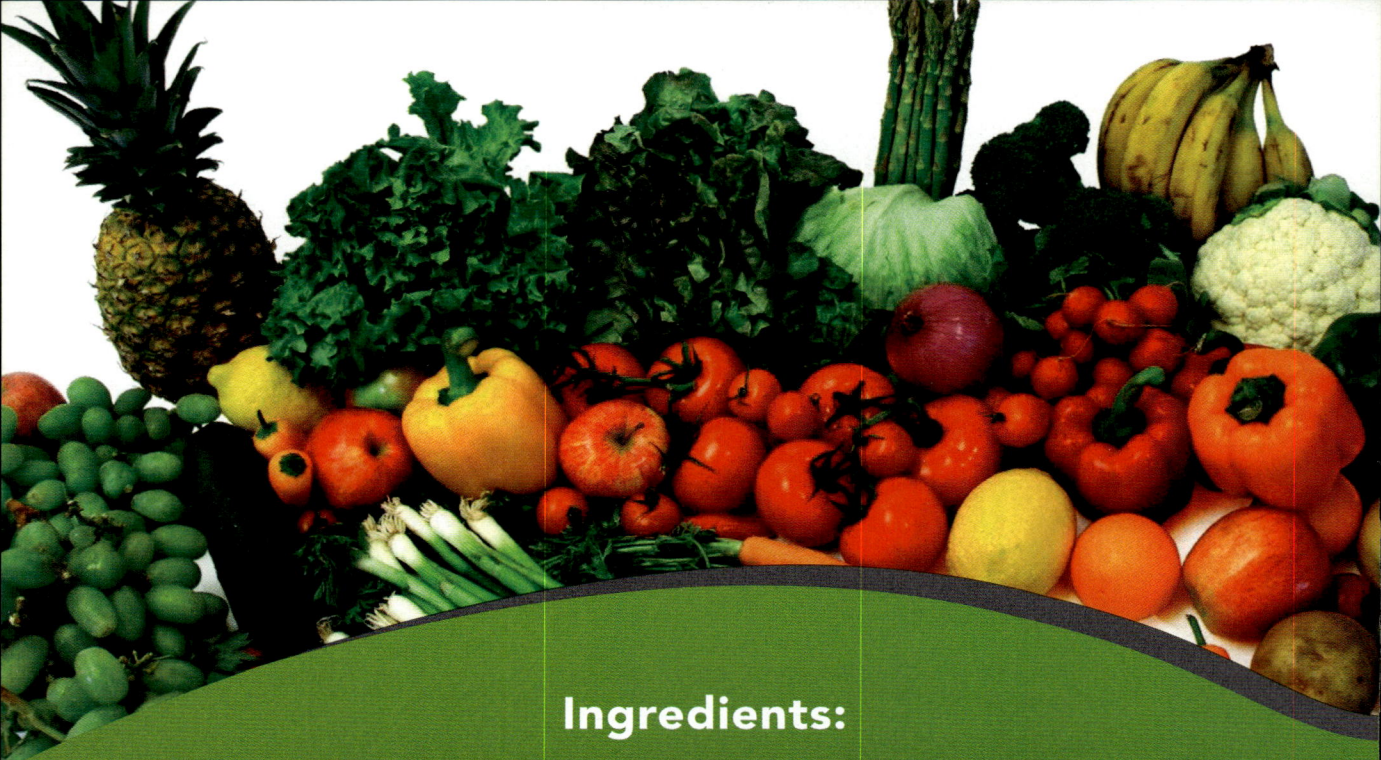

Ingredients:

Vitamin C, Vitamin D3, Vitamin B6, Calcium (Calcium Carbonate, Fossilized Coral Calcium), Magnesium (Magnesium Carbonate), Potassium (Potassium Carbonate), Proprietary Blend (L-Glutamine, Boron Citrate), Natural Orange Flavoring, Natural Vanilla Flavoring, Natural Beet

These statements have not been reviewed by the FDA. This product is not intended to diagnose, treat, cure, or prevent any disease.

Quality Assurance:

This is a patented product by Dr. Tai because of a special binding of vitamin C with glutamine which creates a compound that is extremely bio-available and will regenerate the anatomically important cilia fingers that are present in the inner lining of the stomach and intestines. The presence of cilia provides for protection from inflammation and leaky gut. Craving Factor was designed for those who have those abnormalities generating the cilia. Craving Factor is very effective in the treatment of IBS and constipation. This is a very useful protocol for treatment of leaky gut syndrome.

Clinical Case:

46-year-old Alicia – Nurse in an orthopedic surgery hospital. Suffered from migraine headaches for 12 years. Was taking two prescription medications for conditions but at least twice a month would be under such severe pain of migraine attacks that she could not leave the bed or face the light. Even wearing sunglasses in the house did not seem to control pounding headaches. Would not be able to go to work for 2 – 3 days until after powerful narcotic and analgesics would control symptoms. As a mother of 3 with a working husband, she sometimes felt extreme guilt for not being able to take care of her family and the basic needs of housekeeping. In many of the years in the past, she would have exhausted all her medical leave for the entire year by the time May or June came around. Thus, many times she was put in employment probation due to missing work from migraine episodes. She started to take the Craving Factor as part of a regimen to control her weight gain. She was trying to lose some weight principally as she was approaching peri-menopausal years and had recently gained 12 pounds. As a special bonus, as she lost weight, approximately 5 pounds, she started to notice she did not have the symptoms of migraine headache. Six weeks of treatment using Craving Factor, she did not take any more of her migraine medication, as she no longer felt as though she needed it. She was placed on a diet avoiding gluten and dairy, which was a very important part of her clinical improvement. This patient was followed for 1 ½ years. She was still using the Craving Factor daily and still asymptomatic.

Side Effects:

One must monitor the intake of the size of teaspoons in 16 ounces of water to avoid GI tract irritation. Many individuals report loose stool if intake of the Craving Factor powder was higher than the body needed. They would simply lower the amount of Craving Factor powder in the 16 ounces of water, continuing to use a very small teaspoon in 16 ounces of water five times a day, sipping rather than guzzling.

Contraindications:

Individuals with kidney stones should be careful with the presence of calcium in Craving Factor which may irritate the kidney stones. Normally not an issue, but still precaution should be taken. Do not take if you are allergic to any of the ingredients.

Dr. Tai's Pearl

Craving Factor is extraordinary for treatment of migraine headaches. As you know, migraine headache is extraordinarily difficult to treat, with very powerful medications for even minor relief. Drinking one small teaspoon in 16 ounces, five times per day has shown to be extraordinary for control and relief of migraine headache. The success rate is extremely high and treatment itself is very easy, without side effects or complications. Most importantly, you are going to the root cause of the problem with the vascular migraines.

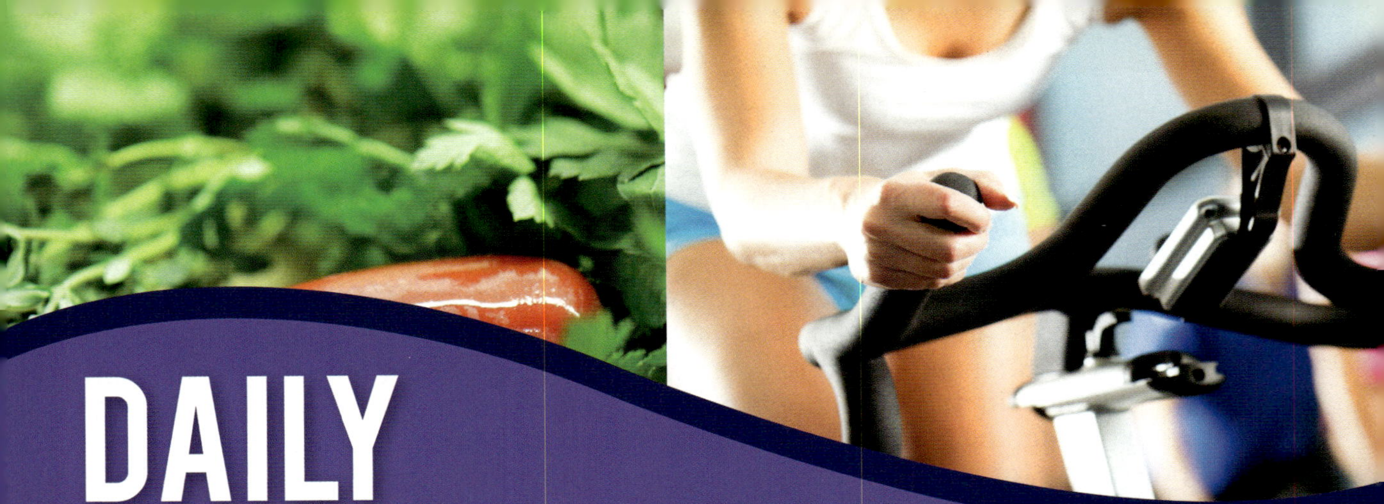

DAILY ENERGY

ESSENTIAL BASE VITAMIN COMPLEX

This is a powerful essential vitamin group that helps protect your eyes from Glaucoma giving them support so you have optimum night vision.
- Vitamin A sharpens your vision and prevents blindness by protecting your eyes from the damage of ultraviolet light.
- Vitamin C prevents capillary fragility, stopping those bruises that you get easily and prevents bleeding gums.
- Vitamin D for absorption of calcium and phosphorus for strong bones
- Vitamin E, which according to the medical journal, shows a possible 40% reduction in heart disease. If you happen to have a heart attack, it will improve your survival rate by making it non-fatal in approximately 75% of individuals.

THE COMPLETE B COMPLEX:

Your entire blood system depends on B complex. It helps with cell reproduction and growth. It flushes out all your toxins and it helps give your blood cells the hemoglobin and oxygen carrying capabilities, which is super important to provide the oxygen that is required in every cell of your body. The cholinergic complex is a powerful antioxidant protecting you from UV sun damage. This complex is the ever so important layer protecting your skin from cancer. It will also help fight against heart attack by controlling hemocysteine. This is a new and exciting development.

ALL PROTEIN CHELATED MINERALS COMPLEX:

These are what we call the soldiers in the field. They are all important minerals which fight diseases. Without them, life cannot take place. Most cheap vitamins use inorganic minerals that are ground into powder, which is kind of like eating rocks, and many times passes through your body completely unabsorbed, and useless. Dr. Tai's Millennium minerals are all amino acid chelated, which means your body can recognize them as a potential amino acid food source, the base unit of protein. These minerals may foster strong bones and joints, a strengthened heart muscle and help your kidneys to work more efficiently. Additional benefits include keeping your prostate healthy and invigorating your skin's capability of immediate wound healing. Powerful, yet gentle!

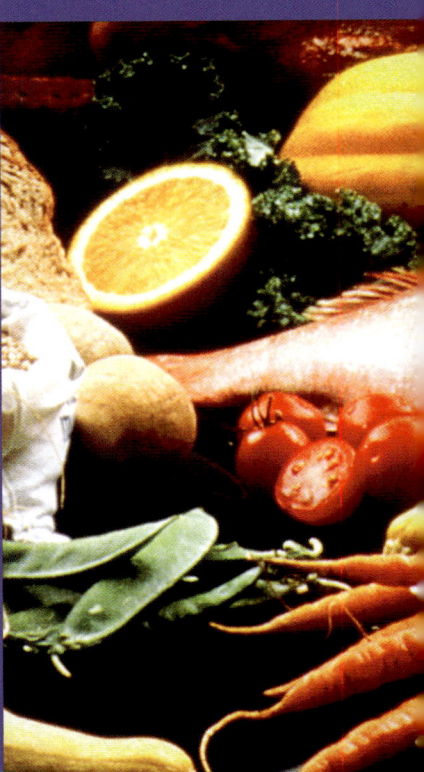

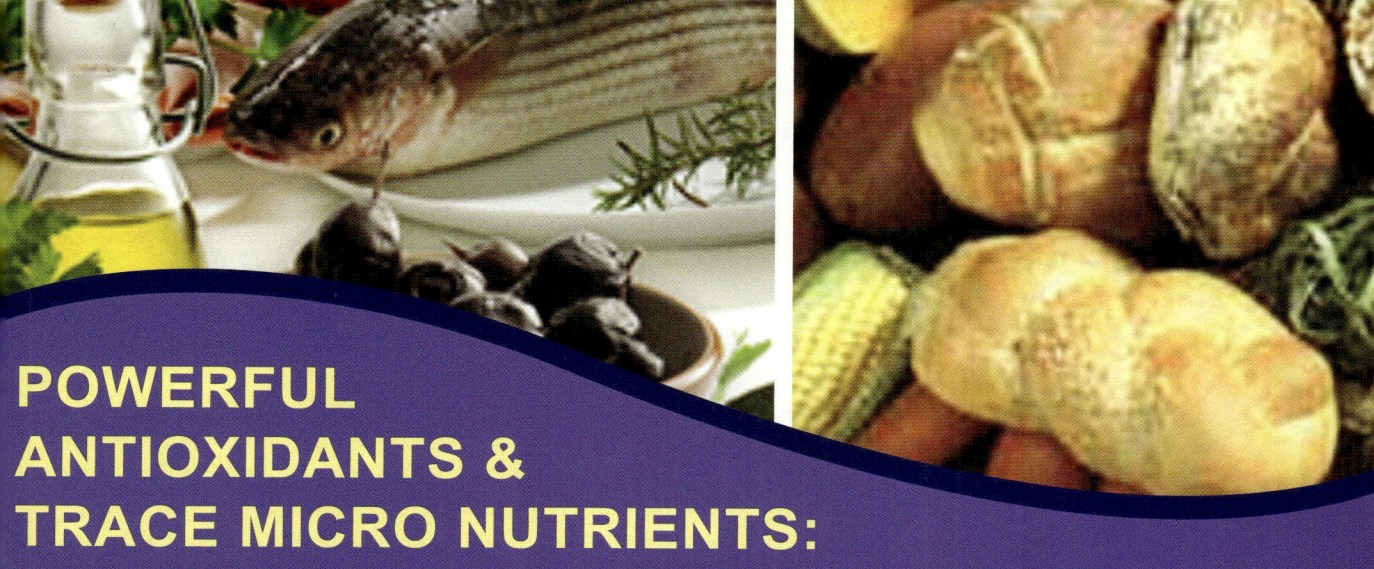

POWERFUL ANTIOXIDANTS & TRACE MICRO NUTRIENTS:

These are powerful protectors and tireless fighters of Free Radicals. Free Radicals are crazy cancer producing by-products of your own body's metabolism. They also help to maintain your muscle strength and support the carbohydrate and fat metabolism. Your entire aging process is a result of the free radicals attacking your body. Recent research shows that the aging process can be halted, even reversed, if we are able to counteract the free radicals with powerful antioxidants to neutralize these poisons within our body. Maximize anti-aging by fortifying your immune system to promote a longer and healthier life.

ANTI-CHOLESTEROL:

Omega 3 and Omega 6 are the essential fatty acids that produce the EPA and DHA. Both of these important fats are present in deep marine fish and will protect your heart and help support your circulation. By controlling your total cholesterol and specifically lowering LDH, the bad cholesterol, you will reduce plaquing of the arteries to your heart.

ANTI-GAS ENZYME:

You may NOT be getting all the healthy nutrients from the food you eat!
Do you feel bloated or suffer from gas because of poor digestion? This complete complex will help you to digest your carbohydrate, fats and protein, keeping your entire digestive enzyme in order. Furthermore, it provides you with all the beneficial lacto-bacteria necessary for fast, easy and smooth digestion just as if you were eating yogurt daily.

POWER ENERGY SOURCE:

SPIRULINA - The exclusive green food protector. Spirulina (crystalline water) comes directly from the northwest and is a refined algae, single cell animal, with the most complete DNA, RNA and micro-nutrients ever found in nature. It will give you unparalleled energy and help give you wonderful, soft skin and beautiful, strong hair growth.
YOU CAN ACTUALLY FEEL THE SURGE OF ENERGY!

VITAL ESSENTIAL AMINO ACID:

This is a complete Amino Acid Pak. All 8 essential amino acids are present in this package. Your body cannot make these amino acids and they are only available when taken by mouth. They are called essential because they support your muscles and life. Don't be without them. If you are not eating properly, the Amino Acid Pak will assure you have all of the 17 Cardinal Amino Acids your body needs, therefore, never lacking a single amino acid for proper muscle replenishment. Powerful insurance if you are on the go and not eating properly.

HEART PROTECTOR:

This proprietary formulation artfully combines COQ10 with the essential L-Carnitine which increases the efficiency and regeneration of antioxidants, helping to invigorate and strengthen the heart cells. Selenium empowers the muscle to contract and work more efficiently. Safeguard your heart!

FAT & CARBOHYDRATE METABOLISM:

Loaded with Inositol, Betaine and Chromium Proteinate – the triple Fat Burners work to efficiently re-route your calories away from Fat deposits into a readily usable Glycogen for immediate energy. It fine tunes your Carbohydrate Metabolism through a more efficient Glucose Tolerance Factor and builds more muscle while burning and mobilizing fat.

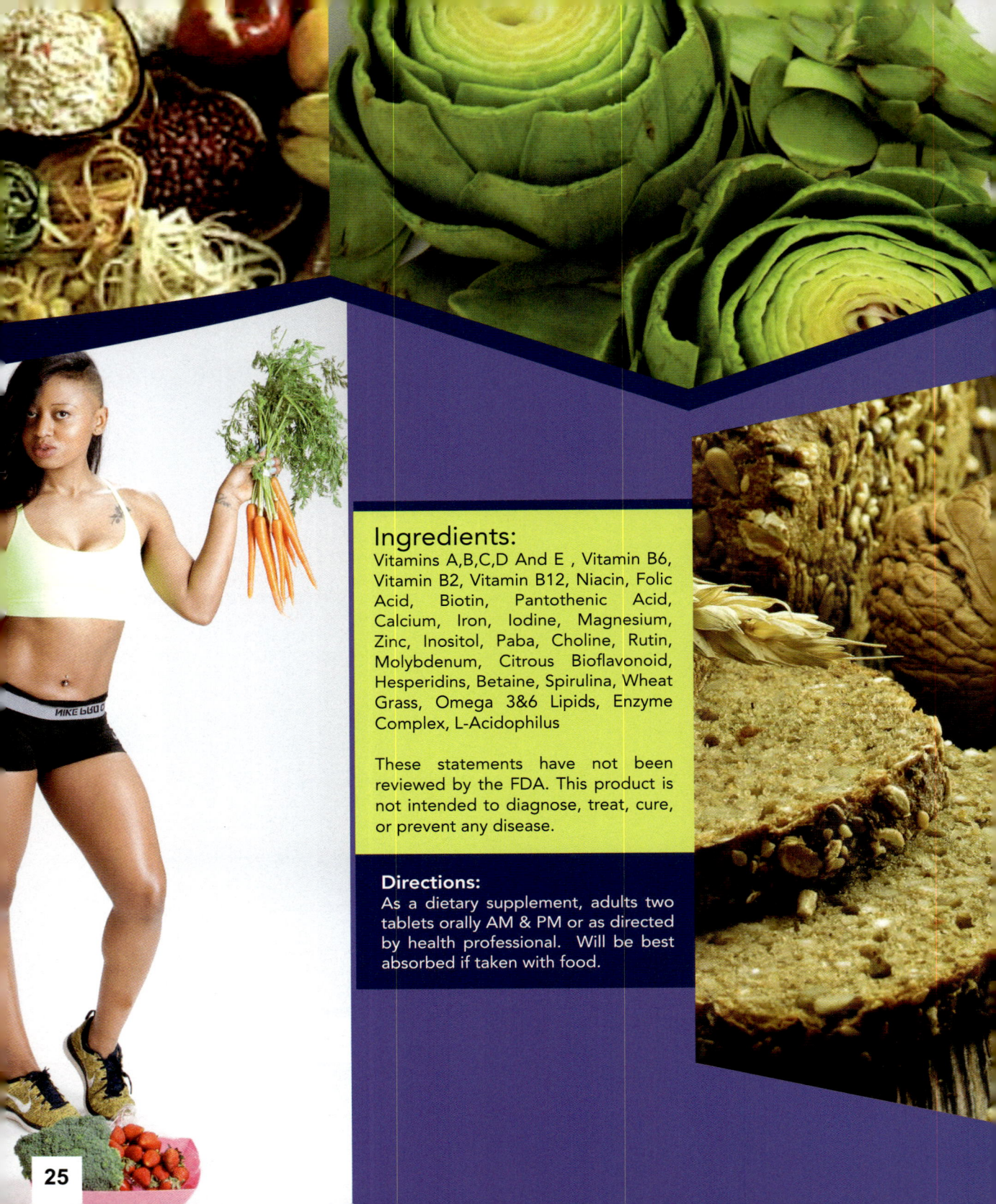

Ingredients:
Vitamins A,B,C,D And E , Vitamin B6, Vitamin B2, Vitamin B12, Niacin, Folic Acid, Biotin, Pantothenic Acid, Calcium, Iron, Iodine, Magnesium, Zinc, Inositol, Paba, Choline, Rutin, Molybdenum, Citrus Bioflavonoid, Hesperidins, Betaine, Spirulina, Wheat Grass, Omega 3&6 Lipids, Enzyme Complex, L-Acidophilus

These statements have not been reviewed by the FDA. This product is not intended to diagnose, treat, cure, or prevent any disease.

Directions:
As a dietary supplement, adults two tablets orally AM & PM or as directed by health professional. Will be best absorbed if taken with food.

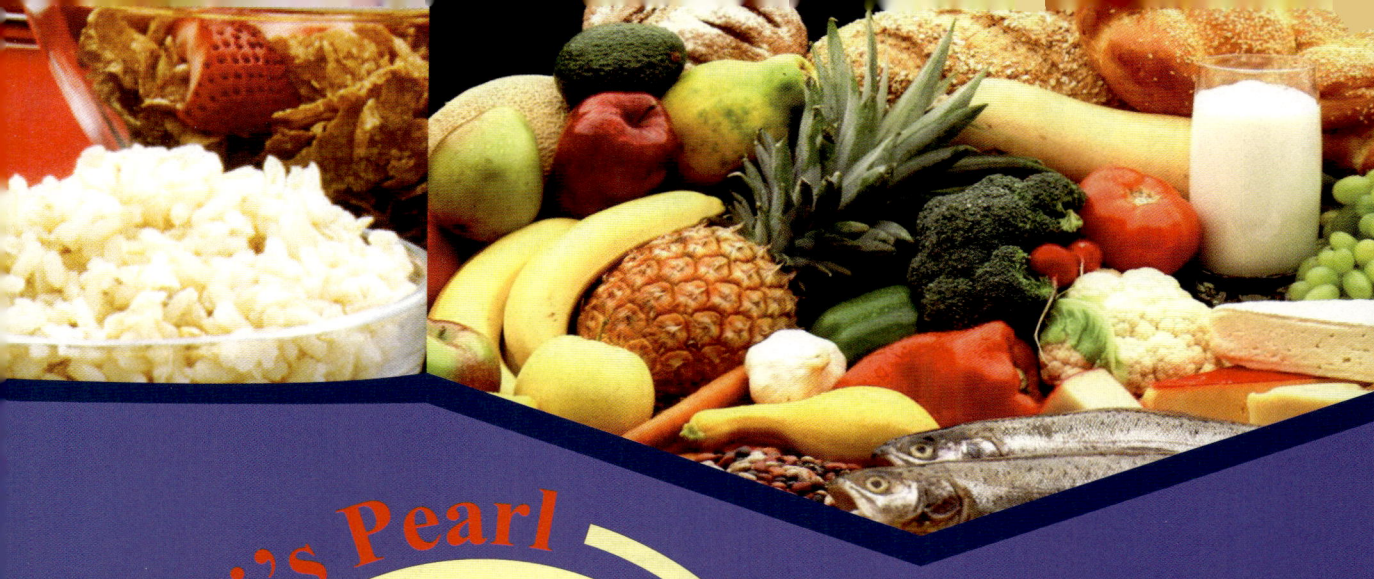

Dr. Tai's Pearl

I always wanted a food based vitamin. This Daily Energy has all of the essential vitamin complexes with greens from all natural foods. Therefore it is very effective and easy to digest. Take Daily Energy along with food because it IS food!

Side Effects: None

Contraindications:
Do not take if you are allergic to any of the ingredients.

DAILY WELLNESS

ANCIENT CHINESE HERBALS

These Chinese herbs have been used for a thousand years. They have been used and time tested. These herbals support and help create balance in all the organs in your body, allowing for improvement of your circulation. They support and enhance your hormones that are necessary for vitality and that perfect balance of well-being. These ancient herbal secrets such as DONG QUAI, FO-TI, ASTRAGULUS ROOT, etc., have been passed on by generation after generation by the Chinese Traditional Herbalist.

ANTIOXIDANTS & BIOFLAVONOIDS:

This is like recharging the battery in your cells, the power that sparks life. It will help to "Bullet proof" your heart and help to improve your blood pressure. It is a tireless fighter of free radicals and anti-aging. These free radicals attack the cells in your body at the rate of 10,000 times a minute, trying to break through your cell immunity and the cell wall. Once the normal healthy cells lose this battle, they become tired, old and potentially ruptured. This is the most complete and powerful antioxidant formulation known on the market. It combines both the water and fat soluble antioxidants. No single antioxidant can do the entire job by itself; this calls for "Team Work". This is the most powerful combination of antioxidants. Glutathione is a remarkable Antioxidant rejuvenator and replenishment system.

ANTI-CHOLESTEROL:

The power of garlic! It is widely accepted, researched and promoted that the Allicin present

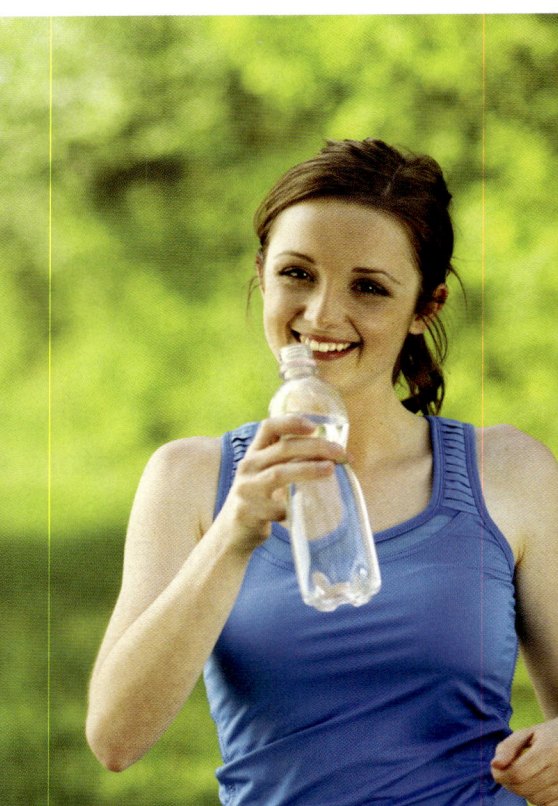

"BULLET PROOF" YOUR HEART
"POWERFUL CANCER PROTECTOR"
"MAXIMUM IMMUNITY BUILDER"

naturally in garlic is the key component to helping maintain a healthy heart and improve your circulation. Your blood pressure could use the help of this powerful natural substance that has been known by ancient cultures for thousands of years.

BOOST IMMUNITY:

To help you fight FLU & COLD through the winter and during stress times, Echinacea builds your immunity and resistance from infection of viruses and bacteria. Echinacea is made from a natural flower, collecting all of the goodness of the sun, to help your body fight infection. It is known for its help in the war against the common cold.

ANTI-CANCER:

Ancient Japanese research has long held the powers of special mushrooms as having natural potent substances called Beta Glucans to fight against cancer. We have combined many different kinds of exotic Asian mushrooms to give you one of the best and most powerful complexes available in the **market by artfully using extracts of mushroom complex to fortify and combining them with the famous South American Cat's Claw, all anti-cancer ingredients.** No formulation would be complete without the Chinese anti-cancer secret of Isoflavones which is in Tofu, long been used by the monks for good health. It is widely researched that Shark-Cartilage is a powerful component in the fight against cancer and arthritis.

GINGKO BILOBA BRAIN MEMORY:

In order to improve your memory, circulation through your brain is enhanced by this herbal extract called Gingko Biloba. Strong anti-coagulant properties prevent the cells from sticking to each other and clogging up the small blood vessels. This is not a powder. It is an extract, powerfully concentrated and effective in improving your mental alertness and clarity.

ATHLETE ENERGY POWER:

All athletes desire for not only a burst of power, but also the stamina to stay with it. We have brought you the Triple Crown winner of the herbal world. (1) Ginseng is well known and has been respected for thousands of years for its stamina building power. (2) Spirulina to provide you with TURBO charging instant power from the micro-crystalline seaweeds. We have added a 3rd little known ancient secret called (3) Cordyceps, heretofore not available in the U.S. until recently. This extremely expensive root is harvested in the high mountains of China and Asia for the benefit of the very few lucky individuals that can afford its wonderful benefit. Cordyceps works in helping the glucose metabolism through the ATP-ADP mitochondria complex.

MICRO BLUE GREEN ALGAE:

This comes in as one of the most perfect micro-organisms in the world. Blue green algae provides all the chlorophylls and micronutrients of the crystal clear water from lakes. Micro Blue Green Algae possesses important RNA and DNA constituents in its cell wall that are the most important key of life.

LIVER REGENERATION:

Milk Thistle Extract - There is no more important organ in the human body than the liver. It deals with all the toxins and elimination of all of the poisons within the body. We rely completely on its ability to keep us healthy through detoxification, and as a healthy processing center of our metabolism.

NATURE'S GARDEN:

Vegetable and Fruit Complex - We all know we need to eat a minimum of 5 to 9 servings of fruit and vegetables daily for our daily nutritional needs. When you are on the run or not getting your proper amount of vegetables for your daily nutrition, this vegetable/fruit complex will help you to meet some of the requirements that are necessary for a healthy diet. Imagine having the benefits of vegetables and fruits without actually having to eat them.

POLYPHENOL COMPLEX:

This is known as the "French factor". How could the French eat such rich food and still have one of the lowest heart disease rates in Europe. . There is well received research showing that a glass of red wine, due to its grape seeds and grape skin extract help fight the diseases of the heart. Now you can have all the benefits of a glass of wine without the dangerous side effects of the alcohol.

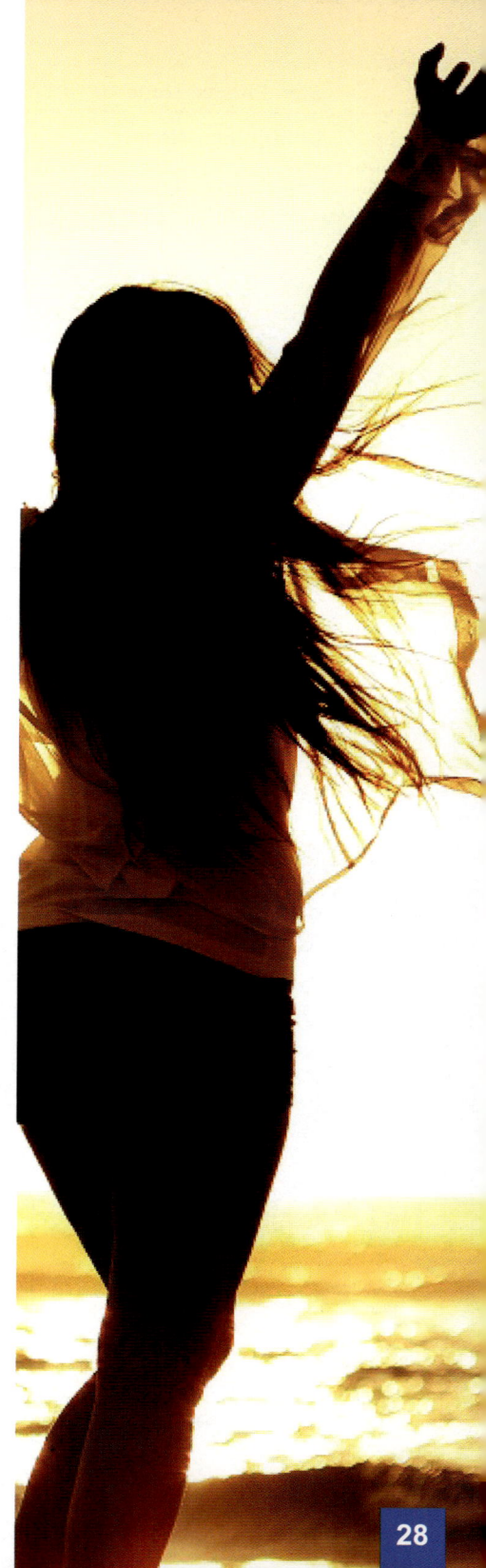

Side Effects: None
Contraindications: Do not take if you are allergic to any of the ingredients.

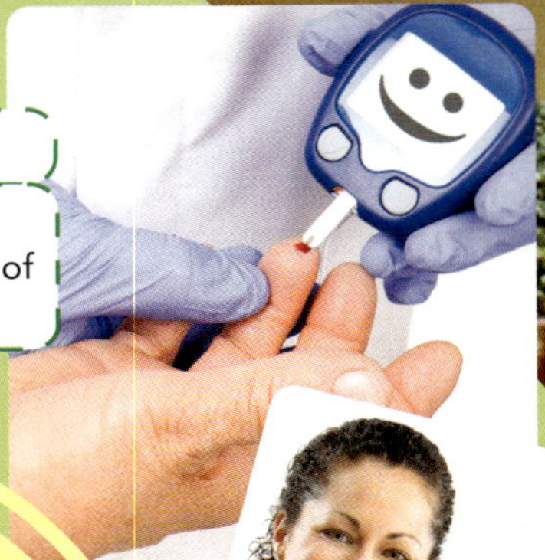

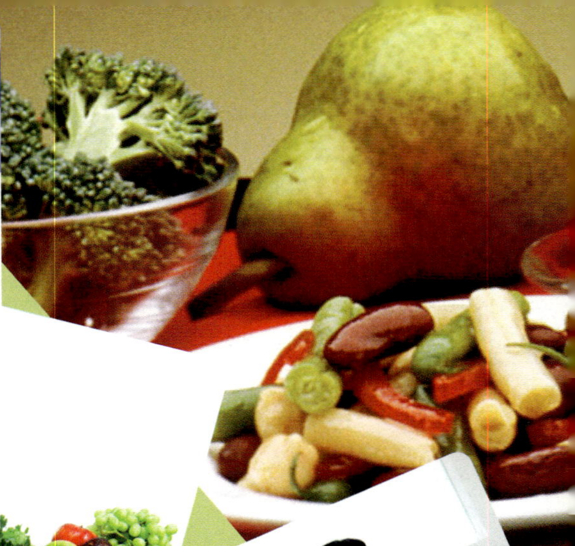

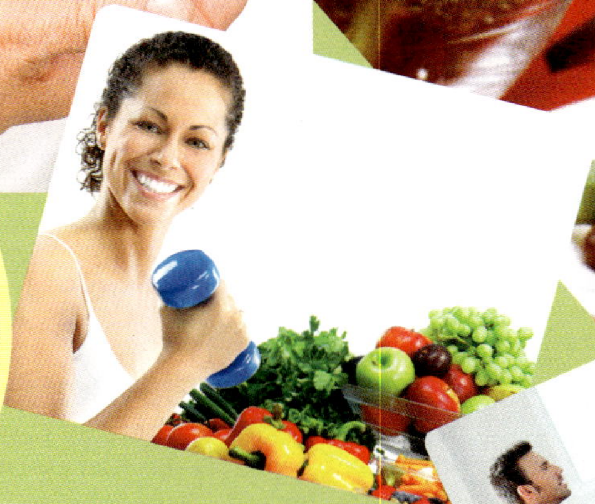

Dr. Tai's Pearl

I created Daily Energy and Daily Wellness as part of my daily supplement. I travel world-wide in my teaching assignments and often times I don't have the time to eat properly. It has in it, five recommended portions of fruit and vegetables. As you can tell, it is so green, I get all the natural bioflavonoids that I need to keep up the nourishment in my heavy work load. It is highly digestible. Nutrients are easily bio-available. On days that I am unable to eat regularly, I will take a double-dose of Daily Energy and Daily Wellness to make up for the nutrient losses.

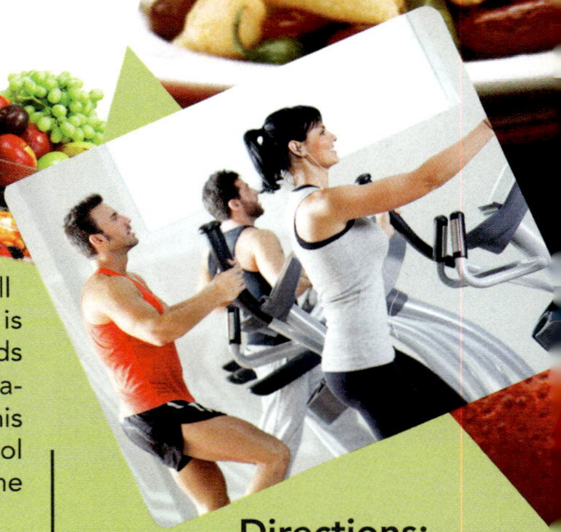

The "Chinese factor" is also well known for the green tea extract, it is well known for cutting greasy foods as well as providing a healthy elevation of the basal metabolic rate. This is one of the best polyphenol complex formulations available in the market.

ANTI-INFLAMMATION:

Turmeric Extract: An excellent anti-inflammatory in the fight against arthritis. It is well regarded in the ancient Middle East as a helpful herb for its fight against fat by blocking its absorption, and for its ability to cleanse the body.

NEW BREED ANTIOXIDANTS:

This is a masterful combination of the latest technological breakthrough of new antioxidants little known by the public, such as Elagic Acid (Pomegranate), N-Acetyl Cystene, Pine Bark extracts (shown to be 50 times more powerful than Vitamin E), Alpha-Lipoic-Acid, Co- Q10, S.O.D., and countless more. This army of SPECIAL FORCES fight tirelessly to keep you younger and healthier for an enjoyable life!

Directions:

As a dietary supplement, adults should take two tablets orally AM PM or as directed by health professional.

Ingredients:

Echinacea, Astragulus Root Extract Schisandra Ext., Ginko Extract, Citru Peel, Cordiceps Powder, Fo Ti Roo Extract, Dong Quai Root Extrac Ginseng Root Extract, Blue Gree Algae, Cat's Claw Bark Powder, B-Glucans, L-Carnatine, Soy-Isoflavone Shark Cartilage Powder, N-Acet Cystene, L-Methionine, L-Glutath one, Pine Bark Standard Extrac Alpha Lipoic Acid, CoQ10, S.O.D Lutein, Milk Thistle Extract, Turmer Extract, Elagic Acid, Garlic Extrac Polyphenol Complex, Vegetab Complex, Citrus Complex, Mushroo Complex, Spirulina, Calcium, Magne sium, Bee Pollen, Royal Jelly, Essenti Amino Acids

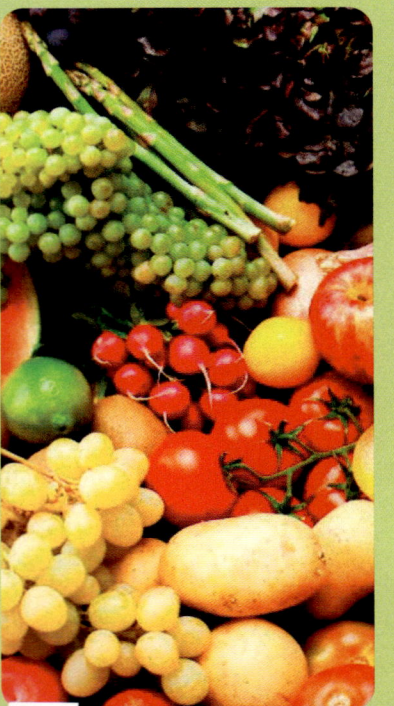

These statements have not been reviewed by the FDA. This product is not intended to diagnose, treat, cure, or prevent any disease.

Clinical Cases

"Dr. Tai's vitamins are miraculous! It is by far the best, most complete and balanced super vitamins I have ever had! It has none of those terrible vitamins smell that upset me. It is now going to be part of my diet forever!"-**K.L., CEO, Chemical Company**

"The vitamin and herbal combo changed my life! It gave me a new lease on life, recharged my batteries, I feel like a human DURACELL® battery. I can out last any of my employees. They can't keep up with me! I am forever grateful to Dr. Tai."-**J.S., Manager, Chain Store**

"Dr. Tai's vitamin and herbal formulations are the most powerful one/two punch vitamin and herbal combination on the market! I should know, I probably tried them all. I highly recommend to my patients. I can actually see their overall health improve before my very eyes. No one should be without it." -**Dr. A.L., Dental and maxillary Surgeon**

"Let me tell you straight! Dr. Tai's vitamin and herbal really work…WOW! I feel my body coming alive, Fantastic; I will never go without it." -**K.T., Manager, Physicians & Medical Clinic**

"I am generally under a lot of stress because of my demanding jobs internationally. Dr. Tai's vitamin and herbal combination made a great difference. I noticed I am not sick as often; when I am traveling, I double the dose. I don't feel the exhaustion and I am able to fight the colds I used to get. I am definitely impressed. Recommend it highly."-**L.A., President, Retail Chain**

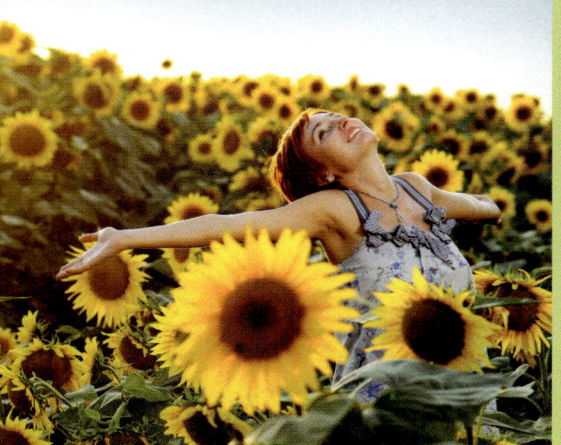

"I recently had a terrible accident and lost my big toe. Dr. Tai reattached the toe when I thought it was gone forever. He also put me on his vitamins and herbals. I am 75 years old, and I have never recuperated as fast from surgery as this time! I am so thankful to Dr. Tai for his surgical skills. But those vitamins are going to be a part of me and my daily habit from now on." -**J.A., Patient, retired worker**

"I am a University student on honors accelerated program in the doctoral program of Pharmacy. As with practically all my classmates, we don't eat regularly and stay stressed on all those tests, exams and term papers. Since I have been taking Dr. Tai's vitamin and herbal, my mind is clearer and I feel strong and full of vitality. I feel I am doing better in school." -**M.C., Honors student, doctoral program**

"I have recently undergone major bone and joint reconstruction surgery. I really dreaded it. But with Dr. Tai's surgery skills and putting me on his vitamins and herbal to help me heal up faster. I have to say that I went through surgery without a problem, and recuperation was great. I am already back to work in only 1 month. Thanks to Dr. Tai." -**R.M. Patient reconstructive foot surgery**

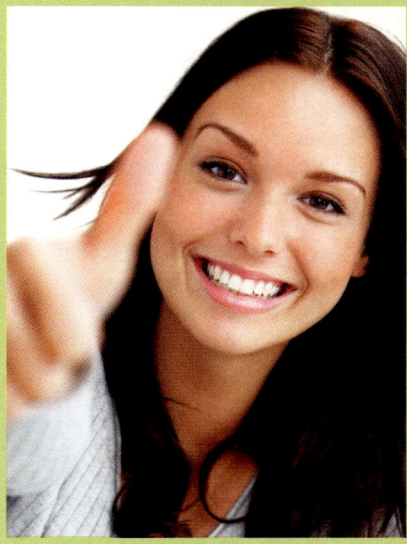

30

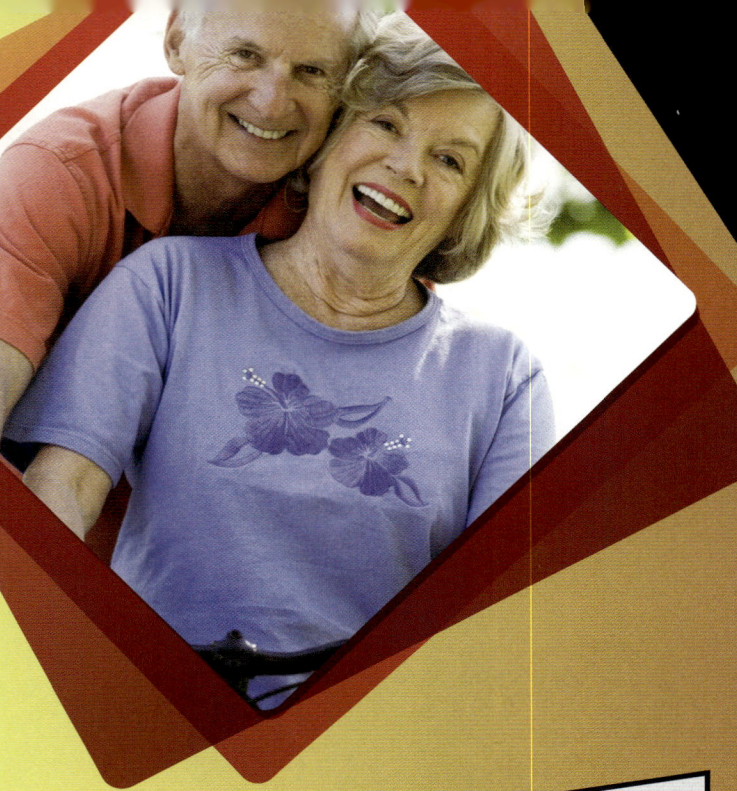

DHEA Specialist

Most ABUNDANT Youth Hormone

DHEA is an essential member of a reverse aging program.

1. Improves energy, vitality and youth
2. Fights osteoporosis
3. Improves depression & chronic fatigue syndrome
4. Improvement of adrenal fatigue & cortisol levels
5. Improvement of thyroid function
6. Healthy immunity – Enhance Immune System Efficiency
7. Stimulates and improves in preventing osteoporosis & cardiovascular diseases
8. Improvement of muscle mass.
9. Improves Alzheimer's diseases, mental memory and logical thinking.
10. Stress reduction, resistance to damages of stress
11. Energy improvement in menopause
12. Improvement in immunity and repair of the nervous tissues
13. Protection from Cancer
14. Protective from Cardiovascular Disease
15. Increases Thermogenesis & Burning Fat
16. Improves insulin receptor sensitivity & reduces diabetes risk

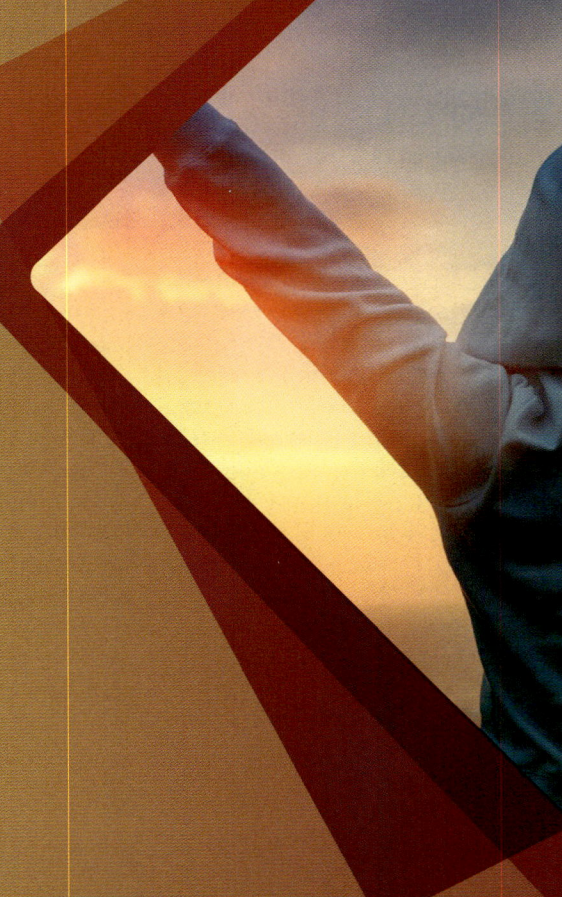

Did we find the Fountain of Youth?

According to Dr. Leo Wattana, in an article from the Journal of Medical Association, Thailand, October 2001, our DHEA (dehydroepiandrosterone) level is peak when we are approximately 25 years of age. It decreases rapidly when we age, and by the time we are 85 years old, we may have lost up to 95% of it. DHEA is considered one of the "Grandparents of Hormones", plus it is through DHEA and Pregnenolone that we get all of our progesterone, testosterone, and estrogen. Dr. Wattana goes on to say in his publication that DHEA plays an important role in longevity and in the body's ability to produce energy and burn fat. In addition, DHEA also plays an important role in anti-inflammatory properties and is critical in the prevention of chronic diseases of aging such as heart disease, Alzheimer's, as well as certain types of cancer.

How can DHEA help me with the fat and the "middle bulge" growing around my waistline?

A recent article in the Journal of American Medical Association (JAMA) November 2004, Dr. T. Villarreal reveals the effects of DHEA on abdominal fat in elderly men and women. He found that supplementing DHEA can significantly reduce visceral fat, so called "abdominal fat". DHEA replacement can also play a significant role in the prevention and treatment of metabolic symptoms associated with Syndrome X.

DHEA Rescues Adrenal Fatigue & Fibromyalgia

According to Dr. Elmer M. Crantin, M.D., author of "Setting the Clock", DHEA is a "Master Hormone". He tells a story of a 67 year old woman named Amy who could hardly muster enough energy to get out of bed in the morning. "I've gotten used to feeling bad" she said "it became a way of life". Amy was a mild diabetic and diagnosed with chronic fatigue syndrome. She has tried everything with no avail, but when she tried supplementing DHEA, in less than 30 days she came back to tell Dr. Crantin, "I have never felt so much energy in my life, I feel like I am 25 again!"

In a clinical study at the University of California in San Diego, 50mg of DHEA daily, over 6 months increased lean body mass and muscle strength as well as the physical and psychological well-being of both men and women.

What has science showed us about DHEA?

Multiple published research studies as well as human clinical studies shows additionally that DHEA makes tremendous improvement in memory, striking psychological improvement, osteoporosis and fatigue.

32

What makes DHEA Specialist different?

The latest technology advancement in anti-aging is a new delivery pathway called the "First Pass Technology". It is a Transdermal Lyposome protected delivery through the skin or sublingual mucosa, much faster and much more effective, a direct route to the blood stream without overworking or damaging the liver. Common "store bought" tablets of DHEA are over 95% metabolized and excreted by the liver, making it almost completely obsolete with very little benefit to the user. This newer Lyposome technology delivers DHEA directly to the blood stream with lower dosage, faster results and less side effects.

The Natural Advantage: What is the youth hormone? What makes you feel young? What gives you a young body? Youthful energy and stamina? The answer is DHEA – the Quintessential Youth Hormone!

Directions:
Apply to Pelvic Area.
<u>Females:</u> Apply 3 pumps daily (AM).
<u>Males:</u> Apply 5 pumps daily (AM).
4 mg of DHEA per pump.
Adjust dosage to your individual needs.

Ingredients:
Fulvic Ext., Essential Phospholipids, Evening Primrose Oil, Shea Butter, Aloe Vera, Lavender Oil, Dehydroepiandrosterone, Resveratrol, Almond Oil, Hemp Oil

These statements have not been reviewed by the FDA. This product is not intended to diagnose, treat, cure, or prevent any disease.

DHEA - Clinical Applications:

- Aging (Hormone Marker) Bellino F.L. Ann. NY Acad Sci 1995; Belancer A et al.
- Immune Deficiency Synd. Regelson W. et al. Ann NY Acad. Sci 1994; Khorram, D. et al.
- Obesity Jakubowicz, DJ, et al. J. Clin Endoc Met. 1995; Porter J. et al. Ann NY Acad. Sci 1995
- Memory Loss, Majewska M. Ann NY Acad. Sci 1995; Melanoir CL et al. Neuroscience Abs. 1992
- Depression Wolkowitz O. Ann NY Acad. Sci 1995
- Lupus Erythematosus V. Vollenhoven et al. Arthri Rheum 1994
- Cancer Prevention Boone CW et al. Cancer Res. 1990
- Osteoporosis Spector TD et al. Clin Endoc 1991
- Chronic Fatigue Synd. Galabrese VP et al. Lancet 1989; Lebihuber FE et al. AM. J. Psych 1992
- Atherosclerosis Inhibition Eich D.M. Circulations 1993

Dr. Tai's Pearl

Many Men and Woman ask me, "What is the Secret Potion for Love? Not only love and sexuality, but what drives the desire of Men and Women?" DHEA, being the youth hormone, fits this description perfectly. Use copious amounts of DHEA to add more spice to your love life and discover your sexuality.

Clinical Cases:
Jason, 42-year-old supplement salesman. Was feeling really fat and tired, days were long and dragging. Used transdermal DHEA Specialist and what a difference. He now feels stronger, peppier, even lost 2 inches off his waist. His best friend started taking DHEA tablets by mouth around the same time and didn't feel anything. Seeing Jason's results, his friend has now also switched to DHEA Specialist.

Side Effects:
Watch out for signs of masculinization – signs of facial hair, discontinue usage or balance with topical pueraria in the areas where masculinization may occur.

Contraindications:
Do not take if you have PCOS. Do not take oral DHEA. If you have cancer or other health conditions, check with your health practitioner before using DHEA. Do not take if you are allergic to any ingredients.

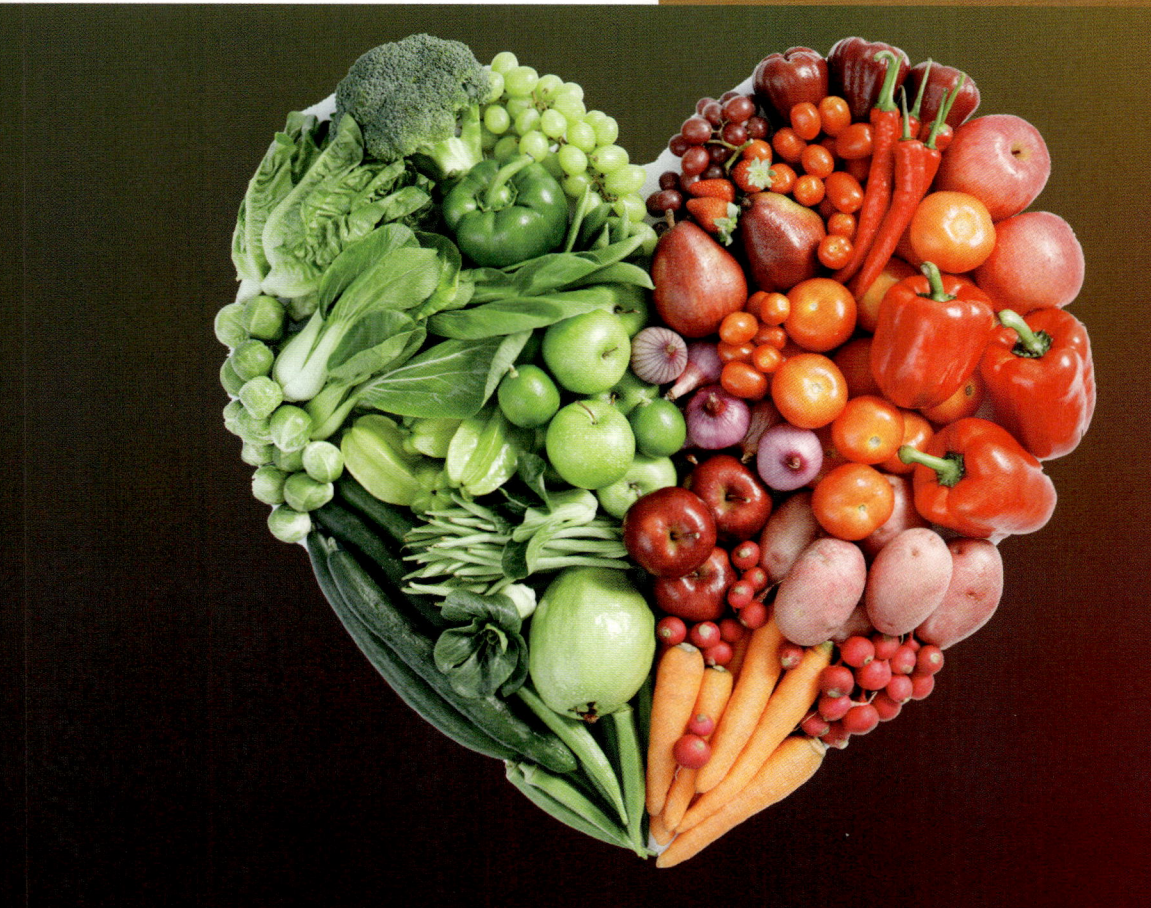

ESSENTIAL FACTOR

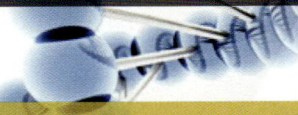

Improve Intrinsic Benefit of HGH

No single hormone is more publicized than Human Growth Hormones (HGH). For the last 20 years, books have been extolling its virtues as being the "Fountain of Youth", the Quintessential Youth Hormone of this century. It promotes vitality and reverses aging. Human Growth Hormone peaks at the age of 20 and by the age of 75 you have lost almost 90% of it.

HGH Test
The elasticity of your skin is a great indicator of the level of HGH in your body. Gently pinch the skin on the back of your hand and pull upward. The older you get the slower the return of the skin to its original position. With aging the skin becomes thinner and loses the elasticity, it is slower snapping back. In some older individuals, the skin actually stays in the position that was pulled and does not snap back at all! In children the pinch test will not allow the skin to be pulled up at all, it snaps back instantly!

Who needs HGH?
Anyone that can afford it! It is only administered by injection and it can cost up to $20,000 a year for treatment of HGH under a Doctor's supervision. Your pituitary gland (your body's master gland) is tired and old; therefore, not producing enough HGH. It is part of your biological aging process.

Do secretagogue amino acids make you young again?
It is very difficult to accomplish. Secretagogues are supposed to stimulate your pituitary by using external amino acid stimulants. It is like whipping an old horse which is biologically unable to run as fast as a young horse. The idea of beating an old horse for it to run faster is quite ridiculous! Most authorities and doctors don't believe secretagogues work anyway.

What is special about Essential Factor?
It is a little known scientific fact that Human Growth Hormone by itself does not do anything. It is only a pre-hormone. Human Growth Hormone has to go through the liver to be metabolized into functioning IGF-1, IGF-2 (Suttle1991, Sadighi 1994, and Elliot 1996) Epidermis Growth Factor (Koetal 1986), Nerve Growth Factor, Vascular Growth Factor, and Transfer Growth Factor.

Researches with Master Growth Matrix:

- Improvement in Strength & Muscle (Broeder 04)
- Improve the Elasticity of the Skin (KO 86)
- Improve Bone Quality & Osteoporosis (Zhou 99)
- Enhanced Immunity and Health (Suh 99)
- Enhance Energy, Vigor and Vitality (Shin 89)
- Anti-Inflammatory Activity (Chin 89)
- Improvement in Sugar Metabolism (Cho 94)
- Improves Arthritis and Joint Health (Zhao 92)
- Anti-Tumor Activity (Kim 94)
- Decrease Blood Pressure (Yudia 1974)
- Increase Blood Cells (Young 64)
- Liver Detoxification (Choi 1979)
- Boost Immune System & NK cells (KO 1986)
- Anti-Microbial & Anti-Inflammatory (Siu 2001)
- Anti-Aging (Wang 1988)
- Anti-Candida, Anti-Fungal (Dark 98)
- Protection to Liver Damage (Choi 79)
- Improve Sexual Function (Zhewg 97)
- Lower Cholesterol (Jai 64)
- Improve Endocrine & Adrenal Fatigue (Kim 85)

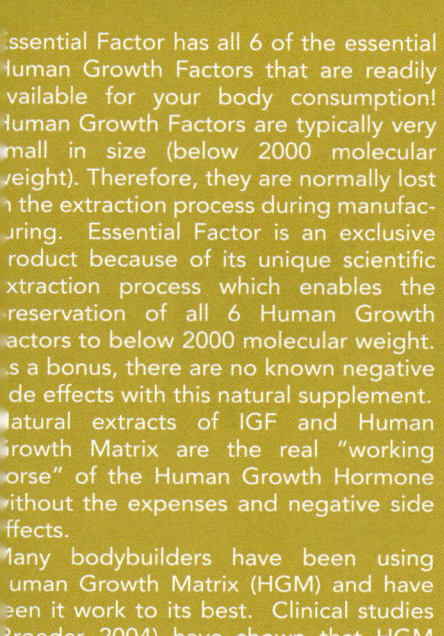

Essential Factor has all 6 of the essential Human Growth Factors that are readily available for your body consumption! Human Growth Factors are typically very small in size (below 2000 molecular weight). Therefore, they are normally lost in the extraction process during manufacturing. Essential Factor is an exclusive product because of its unique scientific extraction process which enables the preservation of all 6 Human Growth Factors to below 2000 molecular weight. As a bonus, there are no known negative side effects with this natural supplement. Natural extracts of IGF and Human Growth Matrix are the real "working horse" of the Human Growth Hormone without the expenses and negative side effects.

Many bodybuilders have been using Human Growth Matrix (HGM) and have seen it work to its best. Clinical studies (Broeder 2004) have shown that HGM increases exercise capacity and also increases muscle mass as well as reducing fat. HGM may also potentially improve diabetes (Glucose metabolism) and improves energy and vitality.

NEW! Lyposome Instant Absorption with Ultra Concentrated 5,000 mg IGF units per bottle

Dr. Tai's Pearl

Very few people know that human growth hormone has to be injected in order to do any good. This is a very expensive therapy and the pain of daily injections is unpalatable for most individuals to use. Most people also do not know that HGH does not work on the tissue directly. With a half-life of only 20 seconds, HGH produced in the middle of the night between 2 – 4 a.m., goes directly to the liver to make the six growth factors that actually are the work horses of hormones – called the growth factors, for the skin, the brain, the blood. And it cleanses the receptors of the body. So instead of paying astronomical prices to inject yourself daily with HGH, Essential Factor is a much smarter, natural oral supplement. This is the intellictual basis for the creation of Essential Factor.

Side Effects: None

Contraindications:
Active cancer.
Do not take product if you are allergic to any ingredients.

Directions:
Shake well. Take sublingual 2 pumps AM & PM hold for 1 minute before swallowing. Adjust dosage to individual athletic needs.

Ingredients:
Fulvic Extract, Humate Ext., Deer Antler Ext., Igf-1, Igf-2, Egf, Ngf, Tgf,Vgf, Cocoa, Stevia, Pituitary Ext., Eurycoma Extract
These statements have not been reviewed by the FDA. This product is not intended to diagnose, treat, cure, or prevent any disease.

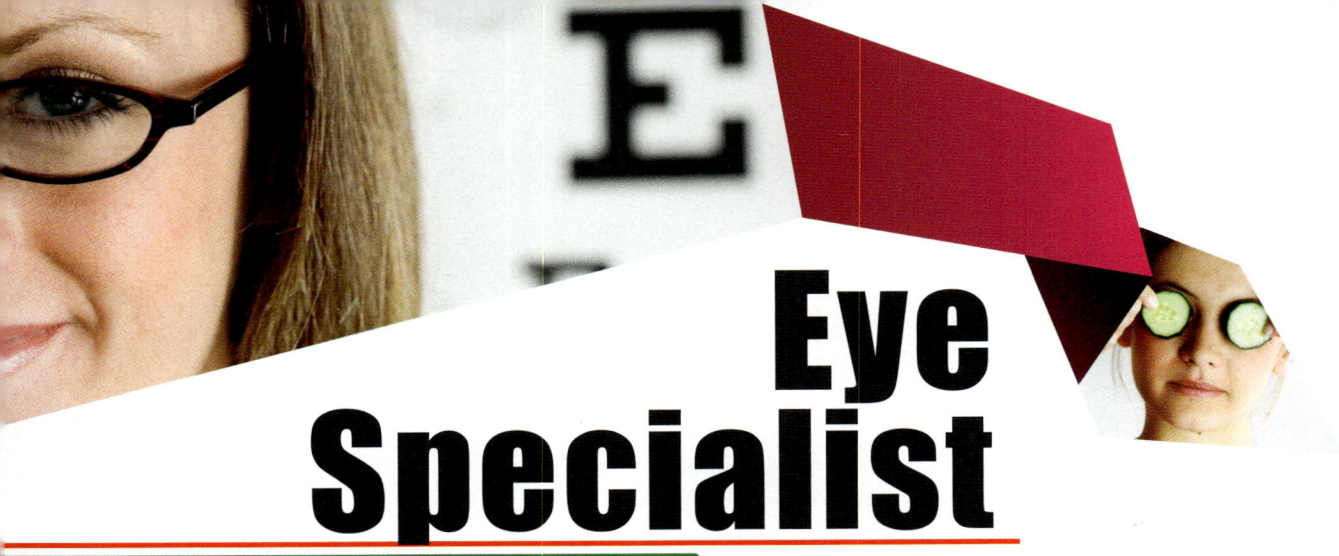

Eye Specialist

Protect Eyes and Prevent Cataracts

Preserving Your Eyesight

Young eyes contain high concentrations of natural antioxidants that protect against cataract, macular degeneration and other ocular disorders. In the aging eye, synthesis of the antioxidant glutathione is reduced, resulting in excessive free radical damage.

Antioxidant supplements have been shown to help protect against senile eye disorders. [3] Unfortunately, circulation is diminished to the aging eye, [4] thereby reducing the efficacy of orally ingested supplements.

The findings from a recent study conclude: [5]

"A need exists for development of therapeutic agents to slow age-related loss of antioxidant activity in the nucleus of the human lens to delay the onset of cataract."

Free radicals for the most part cause cataracts and other senile eye disorders. Oxidative stress is also a contributing factor in the development of macular degeneration. [6] According to a recent report, [7] "nutritional intervention to enhance the glutathione antioxidant capacity...may provide an effective way to prevent or treat age-related macular degeneration." Even glaucoma has been linked with reduced blood flow and increased levels of damaging free radicals. [8]

Another problem with aging eyes is protein degradation and the formation of advanced glycation end products. Aged eyes fail to break down and remove old proteins linked by sugar molecules, which results in the accumulation of non-functioning protein crosslinks. The resulting accumulation of damaged proteins leads to senile ocular diseases. [9]

Applying Nutrients Directly to the Eyes:

Degenerative changes in the eye often begin in middle age, resulting in macular degeneration, glaucoma, cataracts and other forms of retinopathy in later life. Scientific studies indicate that the topical application of certain nutrients may help to prevent common senile eye disorders. In response to these published reports, an eye drop solution called EYE SPECIALIST has been developed which contains specially designed antioxidants, lubricants and anti-glycating agents.

EYE SPECIALIST contains two lubricants (Hydroxymethylcellulose and glycerin) for ophthalmic use. These lubricants provide a synergistic effect in protecting against "dry eyes" and other forms of eye irritation. Additionally, EYE SPECIALIST contains potent concentrations of the following antioxidants:

L-Carnosine is a naturally occurring antioxidant and anti-glycation agent and has shown remarkable effects that protect the eyes in published studies. EYE SPECIALIST contains 1% N-Acetyl- L-Carnosine which acts as a time-release version of L-Carnosine. This form of carnosine has access to both the aqueous parts and lipid compartments of the eye. [11] After entering the lipid compartments of the eye, N-Acetyl-L-Carnosine degrades to L-Carnosine, thus protecting the lipid tissues of the eye from light damage. [10] A recent study showed that carnosine helped to prevent light-induced DNA strand breaks. Furthermore, carnosine application to the eye allowed significant repair of all DNA strands examined. [11] In Russia, carnosine eye drops are approved for corneal erosion, trophic keratitis, postherpetic epitheliopathy, primary and secondary corneal dystrophy and bullous keratopathy. [12]

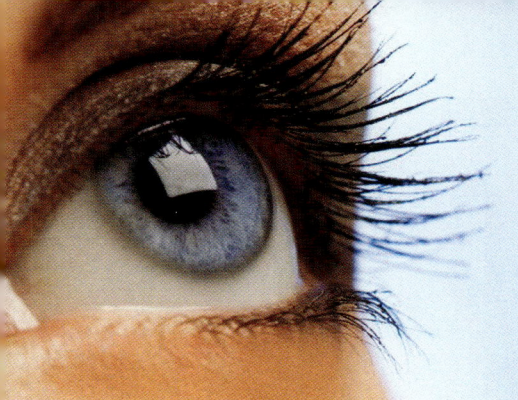

Eye Specialist

EYE SPECIALIST may offer protection above and beyond any other eye formula on the market. **The suggested use of EYE SPECIALIST is to apply 1-2 drops in each eye every day.** Those with any kind of eye problem may want to apply 1-2 drops several times a day. The 2 ml re-sealable tubes allow for a small amount of product to be exposed to oxygen and bacteria at a time. The unopened tubes can be stored in the dark in the refrigerator to extend shelf life.

Ingredients:

Active Ingredients: Glycerin & Hydroxypropylmethylcellulose – Inactive Ingredients: boric Acid, citric acid, N-acetyl-carnosine, potassium bicarbonate, purified benzyl alcohol and sterile water.

These statements have not been reviewed by the FDA. This product is not intended to diagnose, treat, cure, or prevent any disease.

1. Roy H. Rengstorff OD, PhD. Topical Treatment of External Eye Disorders with Preparations Containing Vitamin A. Published clinical studies.
2. Mark A. Babizhayev, Anatoly I. Deyev, Valentina N. Yermakova, Yuri A, Semiletov, Nina G. Davydova, Valerii S. Doroshenko, Alexander V. Zhukotskii and Ita M. Goldman. Efficacy of N-Acetylcarnosine in the Treatment of Cataracts. Original Research Article.
3. Arch Ophthalmol 2000 Nov; 118(11): pp. 1556-1563, Int J Vitam Nutr Res 1999 May; 69(3): pp. 198-205
4. Ophthalmology 1996 Mar; 103(3): pp. 529-534
5. J Ocul Pharmacol Ther 2000 Apr; 16(2): pp. 121-135
6. Mol Vis 1999 Nov 3; 5:3
7. Prog Retin Eye Res 2000 Mar; 19(2): pp. 205-221
8. Arch Ophthalmol 2000 Aug; 118(8): pp. 1076-1080, Vestn Oftalmol 1999 Sep; 115(5): pp. 3-4
9. Curr Eye Res 2000 Jul; 21(1): pp. 543-549, Free Radic Biol Med 1987; 3(6):pp. 371-377
10. Mol. Biol. Part B: (2000), 127B; (4): pp. 443-336, Clin. Chim. Acta., 1996; 254(1):pp. 1-21

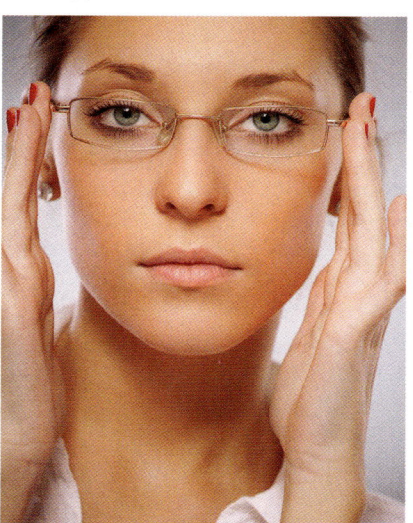

Dr. Tai's Pearl

I hate the thought of having my eyes undergo surgery to remove and vacuum my cornea. It gives me cold chills up and down my spine. Cataracts are nevertheless a common complication. As nutrients for the eye, I suggest supplementation of lutein and astaxanthin. For prevention of cataracts, Eye Specialist is head and shoulders above the rest. If you start early enough, before the clouding of the lenses of the eye, Eye Specialist can prevent and possibly reverse cataracts. Wearing UV protection over your eyes is very important.

Side Effects:

Slight irritation and burning sensation lasting for one minute may occur upon application of Eye Specialist to the eyes. This is natural, as the preservatives in the supplement causes minimal transient discomfort. Any sign of redness or continuation of discomfort, patient should stop using product and see health practitioner.

Contraindications:

Patients should not use this product in presence of open sores, redness, irritation, infection, or ulcerations anywhere in the eye. Do not use this product if you are allergic to any of the ingredients.

38

FORCE C

Herbal Protection & Treatment of Cancer Cells

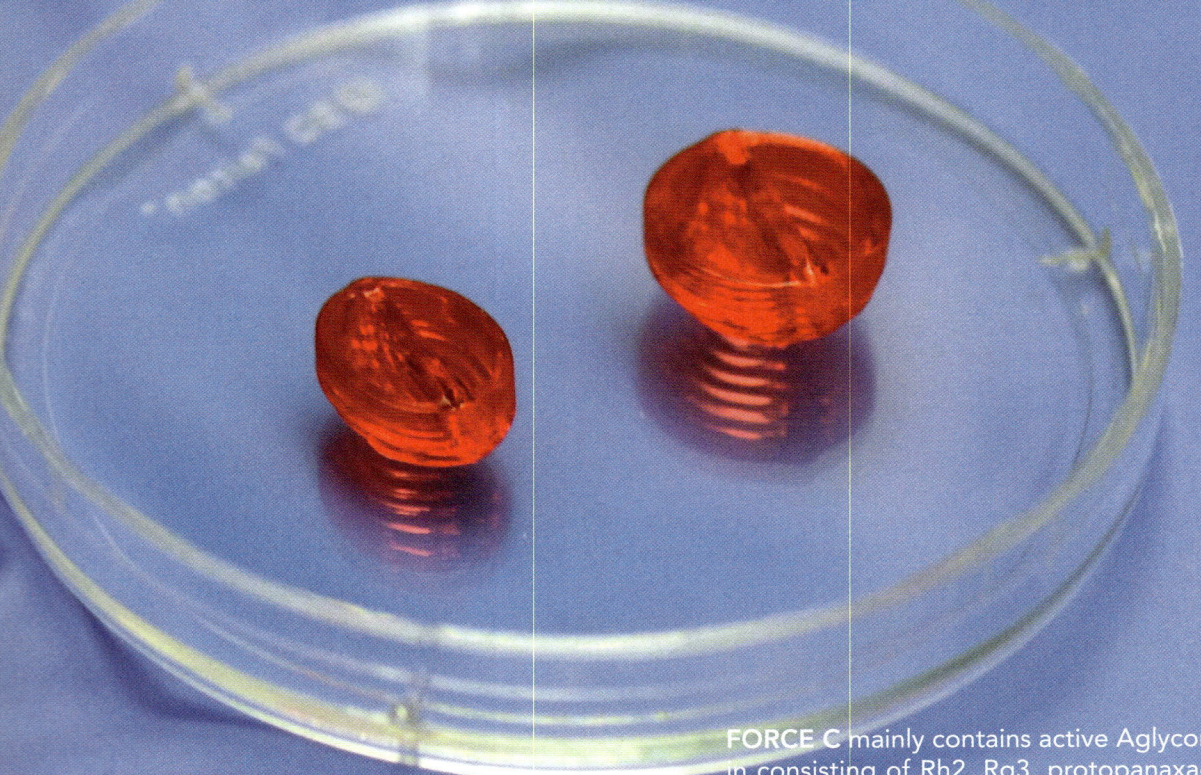

Force C is an all natural herbal extract product derived from PANAX GINSENG. The Patented extraction method removes all other ginsenosides, except Aglycon Sapogenin, which is reported in medical Journal to be active against multiple cancer cells. Conventional methods in the past producing 99% purity aglycon sapogenin took literally hundreds of pounds of raw ginseng root. Therefore, in the past, it was impossible to achieve therapeutic concentrations of this anti-cancer sapogenin compound from ordinary ginseng extract.

FORCE C mainly contains active Aglycon Sapogenin consisting of Rh2, Rg3, protopanaxadiol, protopanaxatriol and other Aglycon Sapogenins which published research have shown to be cancer cells specific. It does not affect normal cells. In vivo animal studies and human clinical studies it has shown near zero toxicity, so there are no side effects. Using this rare Aglycon Sapogenin, published laboratory studies in vitro and animal in vivo tests clearly show apoptosis, cancer cell death when used in higher doses. When Aglycon Sapogenin is used in very minute micron dose, it is able to inhibit cancer multiplication as well as reverse the DNA expression from cancer to normal cell.

Clinical Case: A rather famous movie star that lives in Manhattan contacted me once about her poodle that was dying of cancer. The veterinarian in charge of her care gave the poor dog only a month to live. Of course she was heartbroken as she was very attached to this dog – one of her favorite companions. She read about the ginseng – Force C – cellular normalizer and requested the proper dosage for her dog. Surprisingly, even though the poodle only weighed 12 lbs., animals actually take the same dosage as a human. The cancer was apparently in the stomach and had metastasized to the lung. Using the Force C along with other supplements, such as Max BioCell, Glutathione, and Cordyceps from Max Performance, she braved forward. The last time I spoke with her was two years after the dog commenced with the supplements. He was still doing extremely well, and according to my friend was more agile and younger in spirit that she was. All we can say is good for the pooch!

FORCE C is a "Cell Growth Normalizer" performing a unique task of policing our body of any abnormal DNA or cancer cell and may reverse the abnormality or cause apoptosis (natural death) to the abnormal behaving cells. It is a truly potent herbal supplement that will benefit humanity.

Dr. Tai's Pearl

There is still so much that we do not know about Panax Ginseng. At one point, early in the research, most people believed that ginseng was primarily to be used for energy. However, with very sophisticated liquid chromatography, they have discovered parts of the ginseng that is very active against cancer cells. Research is now quite advanced in isolating very specific active ingredients that focus only on the abnormal cancer replication and growth that occurs in cancer or tumors. Force C can help to restore normal apoptosis, natural cell death, and can be used with other supplements or chemotherapy.

Ingredients:
Panax Ginseng Root Extract (Aglycon Sapogenin), Cellulose.

These statements have not been reviewed by the FDA. This product is not intended to diagnose, treat, cure, or prevent any disease.

Directions: Take 1 to 8 capsules AM on an empty stomach. Do not eat for ½ hour.

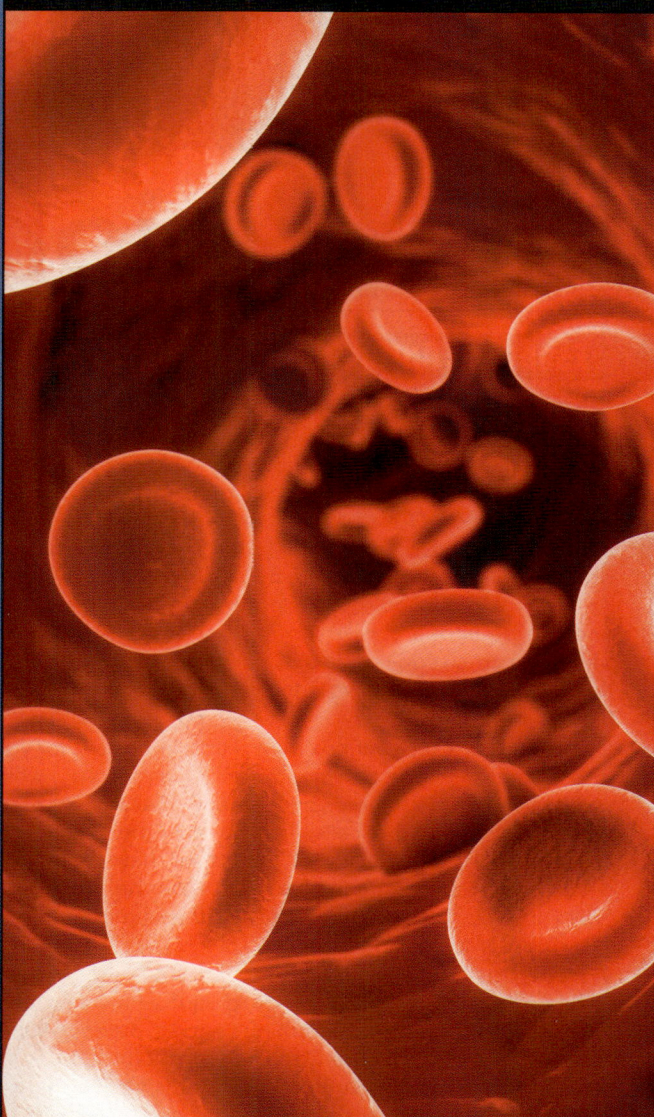

Side Effects: None

Contraindications:
Do not take with food. Do not take if you are allergic to any ingredients.

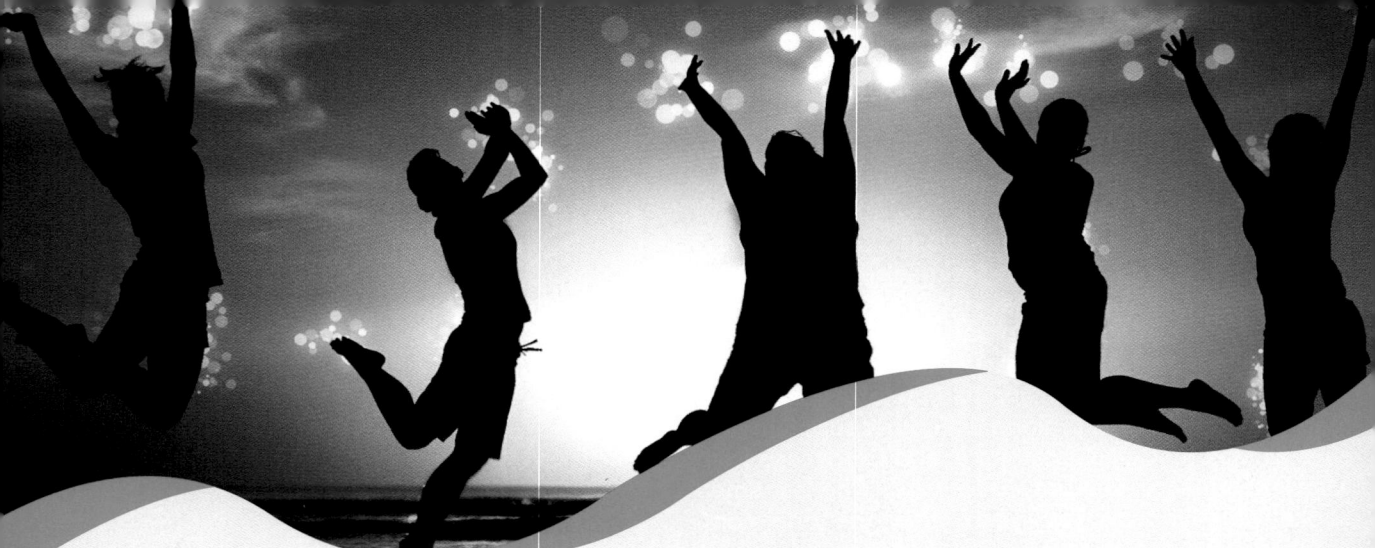

Glutathione Specialist

Essential Antioxidants for the Human Body

Glutathione:
The Super Supplement of the Decade
Who wouldn't like to have a naturally occurring substance that acts as a super antioxidant, an immune system booster and a detoxifier? As a bonus, it will help your body repair damages caused by stress, pollution, radiation, infection, drugs, poor diet, aging, injury, trauma and burns.

An army of advanced researchers are saying that glutathione can do all the above and maybe more. But can you believe such sweeping claims? What is the evidence to back them up? Here is what the experts have to say:

What is Glutathione?
Glutathione is a super antioxidant that is important for your good health because they neutralize "free radicals", which can build up in cells and cause damage. Because glutathione exists within the cells, it is in a prime position to neutralize "free radicals". It also has potentially widespread health benefits because it can be found in all types of cells, including the cells of the immune system, whose job is to fight disease.

What Does Glutathione Specialist Do?
The strong antioxidant effect of glutathione helps keep cells running smoothly. Glutathione expert, Jeremy Appleton, ND, Chairman of the Department of Nutrition at the National College of Naturopathic Medicine, say it also helps the liver remove chemicals that are foreign to the body, such as drugs and pollutants.

"IF you look in a hospital situation at people who have cancer, AIDS or other very serious disease, almost invariably they are depleted of glutathione," says Dr. Appleton. "The reasons for this are not completely understood, but we do know that glutathione is extremely important for maintaining intracellular health."

How should Glutathione be taken?
Glutathione is not absorbed into the body when taken by mouth. One way to get around that is to take it by injection in the vein. Another way is to take amino acids precursors, that is, the molecules the body needs to make glutathione, but there is no solid proof this works and most doctors doubt its validity.

Glutathione Specialist is a new major breakthrough because it uses the latest technology of micro-encapsulating reduced glutathione, methylcobolamine B12, Folinic acid into phosphatidylcholine, an essential phospholipids that is natural to the cell and brain, called Glutathione Lyposome to deliver it directly into the blood stream, even crossing the Brain Barrier in very high concentrations effectively and quickly.

Dr. Appleton says "Glutathione and other antioxidants, far from interfering with the activity of chemotherapy, appear to reduce side effects without decreasing efficacy and may, in fact, improve the efficacy of the chemotherapy in fighting cancer."

Glutathione is also used to prevent oxidative stress in most cells and helps to trap and neutralize "free radicals" that can damage DNA and RNA. There is a direct correlation with the speed of aging and the reduction of glutathione concentrations in intracellular fluids. As individuals grow older, glutathione levels drop, and the ability to detoxify free radicals decreases.

There is preliminary evidence that Glutathione might eventually prove to be useful in the management of some cancers, atherosclerosis, diabetes, lung disorders, noise-induced hearing loss, male infertility and to help prevent various heavy metal and chemical toxicities. Glutathione also has been researched for AIDS associated Cachexia, Cystic Fibrosis, Parkinson's, ADHD, Autism, Multiple Sclerosis, Cancer, Mercury Poisoning, Lupus, ALS and Liver Diseases.

A case history by Mr. Martin, a semi-retired researcher, experienced hands-on evidence of the power of raising his Glutathione level. For years, he suffered from Chronic Fatigue Syndrome and fibromyalgia that countless medical practitioners were not able to neither recognize nor treat. When by his early 50s he became so debilitated that he considered purchasing a walker or a wheel chair, he decided to take charge of his own health. After doing extensive research, then boosting his glutathione levels, he regained his mobility and natural high energy. "Within a week, I realized I didn't hurt anymore," says Mr. Martin. "I just got better and better. It was so simple and so astounding." He has never looked back. Today, he continues to maintain his glutathione level, which is vibrant and healthy, and he "rarely gets a cold." Research has shown increased Glutathione levels may help:

- Detoxify the liver
- Improve Lung Function
- Improve Heart Function
- Increased Energy, Endurance and Stamina
- Protect the Skin from UV sunlight
- Strengthen Immune Function
- Helping AIDS related symptoms
- Multiple Sclerosis, Lupus, ALS.
- ADHD & Autism
- Cancer & Chemotherapy side effects
- Alzheimer, Parkinson and Memory Deficits
- Diabetes & Sugar Metabolism
- Cardio Vascular Disease & Arthrosclerosis
- Adrenal Fatigue & Fibromyalgia

Directions:
Shake well. Take sublingual 1 pump AM & PM, hold for 1 minute before swallowing. Adjust dosage to individual needs.

Ingredients:
Essential Phospholipids, Reduced Glutathione, Methylcobalamine, Folic Acid, Water, Lecithin, Alcohol 12%, And Natural Flavor, Stevia These statements have not been reviewed by the FDA. This product is not intended to diagnose, treat, cure, or prevent any disease.

Dr. Tai's Pearl
Many doctors and patients ask me if Glutathione is the miracle supplement. My answer is, "I don't know, but it certainly comes close." Let me put it in a very practical way. If your body stops producing glutathione, you will most likely be dead within 20 minutes. It may not indicate whether glutathione is a miracle supplement, but certainly indicates the essential nature of supplementing your total health and longevity. There are actually four antioxidants that are essential to your blood, glutathione, superoxide dismutase, catalase, and melatonin. Without these, life would not exist.

Side Effects: None

Contraindications:
Do not take with food. Do not take if you are allergic to any ingredients.

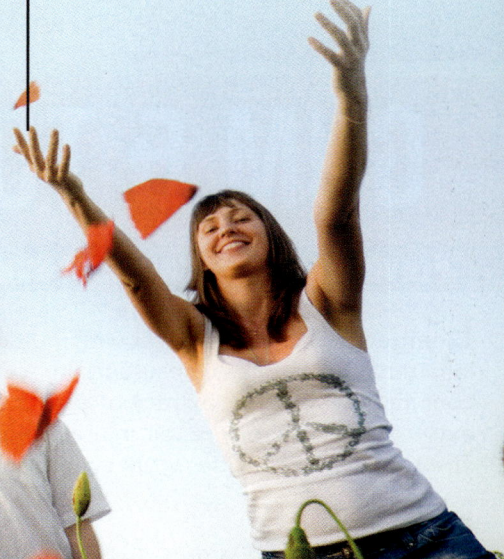

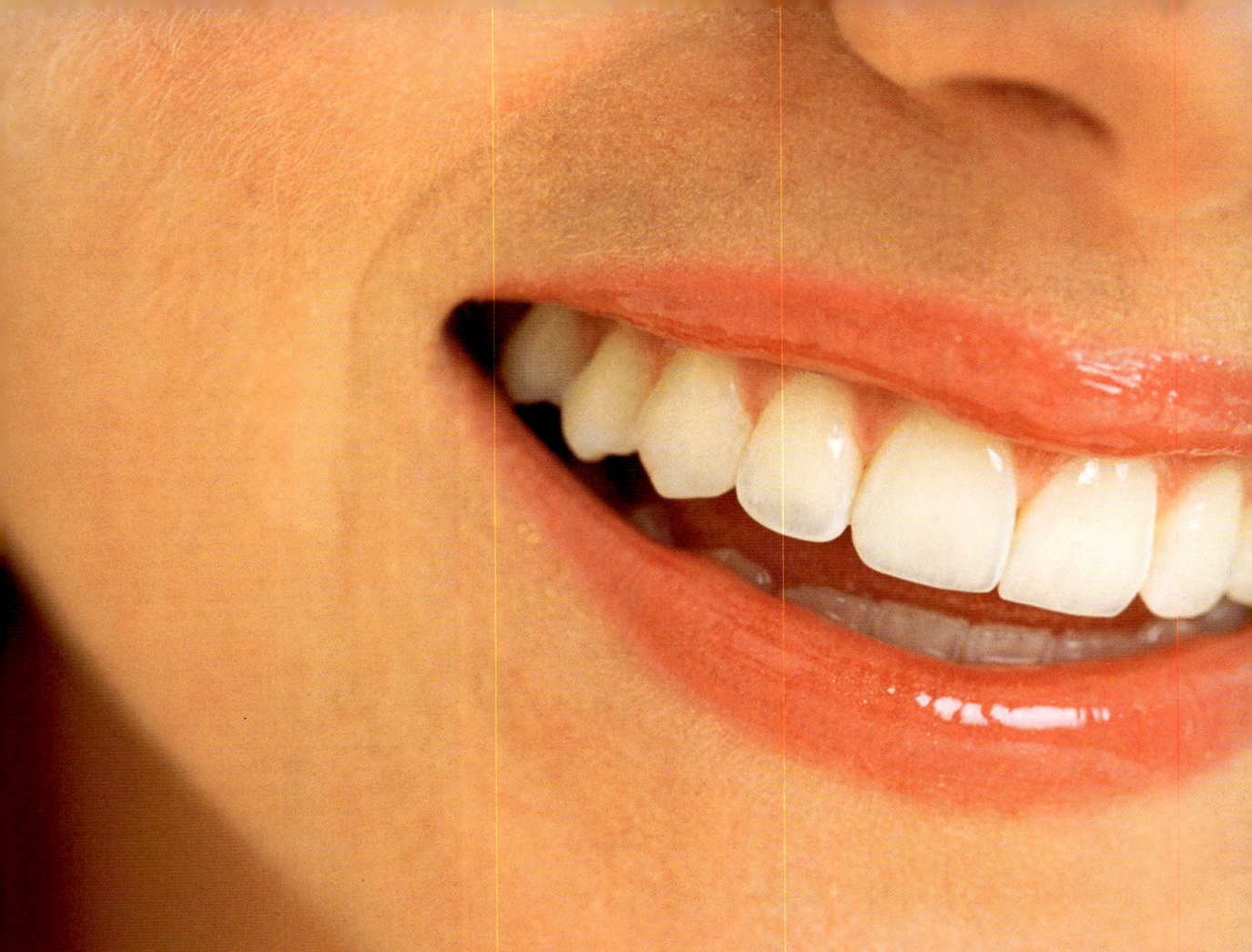

GUM & TOOTH SPECIALIST

Prevent & Protect against Gum Inflammation

Energetically charged water with multiple high frequencies to match the specific tissues of the body, regulate inflammatory process, resulting in reduction of pain and discomfort. Over 77 micro-minerals work in conjunction with the extract of plants as a natural anti-bacterial and antiviral activity. Homeopathic active extract of Arnica may repair injured and damaged tissues quickly and completely.
The triple level activities work synergistically to give you immediate results.

Directions:
Take 1-2 ounces by mouth. Swish or gargle, hold in mouth for 1 minute in area of discomfort. Safe to swallow. Repeat minimum 3 times daily.

Dr. Tai's Pearls:

It is not often in our profession that one comes across a supplement that is so effective in treating a very specific problem. Tooth pain and gingivitis, both among babies when they are teething, as well as youngsters during their tooth-bearing days. As we get older, problems with gingival infection as well as tooth ache plagues us, especially when the dentist's appointment book is full and he cannot see us for 2 to 3 weeks. Tooth ache can drive you crazy. Placing a mouthful of Gum & Tooth Specialist liquid on the side of the mouth as the toothache, holding there for 1 or 2, or even 3 minutes before swallowing, you will find relief is at your fingertips. This procedure can be repeated 2 – 3 times and just like magic, you start to feel better. You can see the relief expressed on the face when a smile starts to appear.

Clinical Case:

62-year-old architect was chewing away on his favorite snack of peanuts when all of a sudden, lightening sharp pain cut through his right jaw and sent excruciating pain through his face. One of the nut shells cut through the outer side of his gums causing it to bleed and resulting in severe discomfort. It was too late to call the dentist so he decided to tough it out through the night. Although he was able to stop the bleeding, the excruciating sharp pain started to envelop the entire right side of his face. First thing the next morning, he called his dentist who happened be vacationing in Israel with his family. Greatly disappointed and depressed, I offered him the Gum & Tooth Specialist to use for relief. He stated he didn't believe it would work, but was willing to give it a try. Eureka! Within 10 minutes, he was back in my office with light shining through his whole face, he pronounced, "Look! I have absolutely no pain! Can you believe it?" I knew with a certain confidence that I could overcome his pain, but I did not know that I could overcome his pessimism.

Side Effects: None

Contraindications:
Do not take product if you are allergic to any ingredients.

Ingredients:
Water, Grapeseed extract, Aloe, Microminerals, Arnica 30X
These statements have not been reviewed by the FDA. This product is not intended to diagnose, treat, cure, or prevent any disease.

Hyperactive Support

For care of Autism & Attention Deficit Hyperactivity Disorder

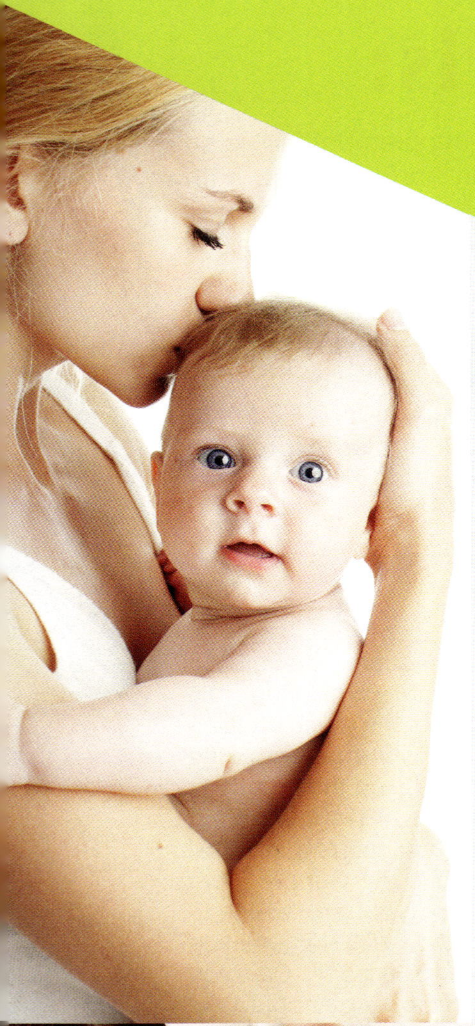

Attention deficit hyperactivity disorder is a serious illness involving imbalances of neurotransmitters in the brain. A neurotransmitter can essentially be classified as a chemical messenger, traveling through the brain to send messages from one neuron nerve cell to another. Different neurotransmitters produce different functions, ranging from feelings of pleasure to enhance our ability to manage stress. An imbalance in chemical neurotransmitters can cause anxiety, anger, impulsions, and ADHD.[1]

Depleted serotonin has been viewed as a major cause of ADHD.[2] When levels are low, symptoms may include inattention, impulsivity, hyperactivity, and fidgety behavior. The ratio of dopamine and serotonin activity is very important. Keeping them balanced is a key to relieving symptoms of ADHD.[2]

Serotonin modulates stabilizing actions in the brain, creating a balance in chemical activity. Proper Serotonin levels allows those suffering from ADHD to be mentally focused and alert. With sufficient amounts of serotonin, in balance with other neurotransmitters, our brain can approach intellectual endeavors and accomplish accurate calculations successfully and with ease.

An extract of very young grass leaves, which is a highly effective and natural, is a precursor to Serotonin. Dosage is the key! Dosage may need to be adjusted to individual needs. In the beginning, dosage may be increased given individual circumstances and beneficial effects for each individual.

List of some Neurotransmitters and Functions

- Dopamine – pleasure, attachment/love, and altruism.
- Norepinephrine – Arousal, energy, drive, stimulation, and fight or flight.
- Serotonin – Emotional stability reduces aggression, sensory input, sleep cycle, appetite control.
- GABA – Controls anxiety, arousal, and convulsions, and keeps brain activity balanced.

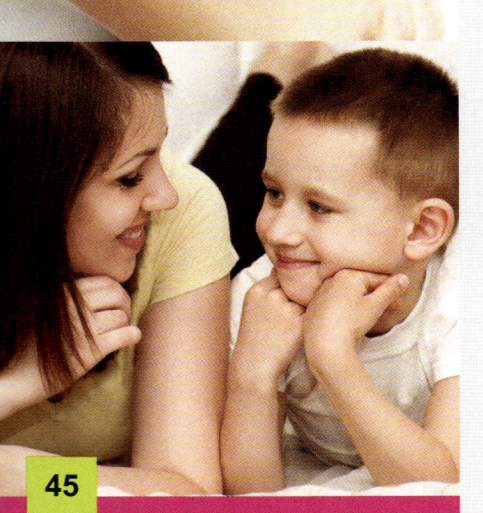

45

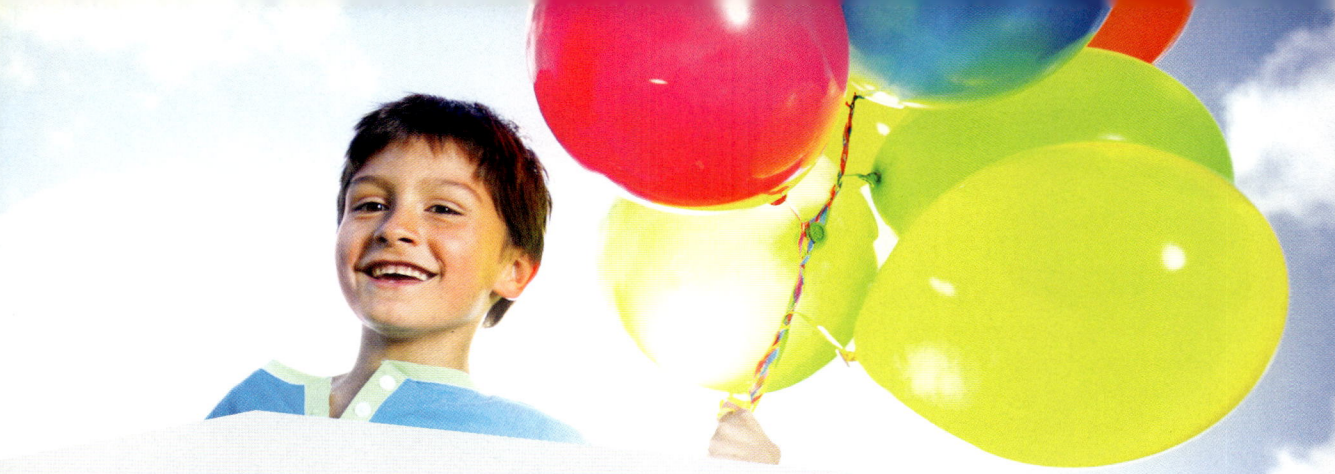

Serotonin Adaptogens are Reporting the Following Benefits:

- Heightened capacity for learning
- More attentive behavior
- Better mental focus
- Less erratic and irritable
- Better social skills
- Heightened self confidence
- Positive mood
- More constant mood
- More balanced mood
- Lessened anxiety
- Lessened anger
- Enhanced energy
- Improved sleeping patterns

Directions:
Take 1-2 full droppers twice daily.
Dosage must be adjusted for individual needs.

Ingredients:
Lingzhi Extract, Grass 10 Leaf Extract, Virgin Coconut Oil, Mint Flavors, Stevia

These statements have not been reviewed by the FDA. This product is not intended to diagnose, treat, cure, or prevent any disease.

1. Gainetdinov, R.R., Wetsel, W.C., Jones, S.R., Levin, E.D., Jaber, M. and Caron, M.G. (1999) Role of serotonin in the paradoxical calming effect of psychostimulants on hyperactivity. Science 283:397-401.
2. H. Soderstrom, K. Blennow, A-K Sjodin, and A. Forsman. New evidence for an association between the CSF HVA:5-HIAA ratio and psychopathic traits. Journal of Neurology, Neurosurgery and Psychiatry, Vol. 74, 2003, 918-21.

Dr. Tai's Pearl

Diet is extremely important – Most parents and children are not aware they are INTOLERANT and/or sensitive to a variety of foods. A blood test called LEAP/MRT is now the "gold standard" for discovery of foods and additives that may cause hyperactivity and worsen the symptoms of autistic and ADHD patients. These food restrictions are a "must" in the treatment and management of these conditions.

Side Effects: None

Contraindications:
Do not take if you are allergic to any of the ingredients.

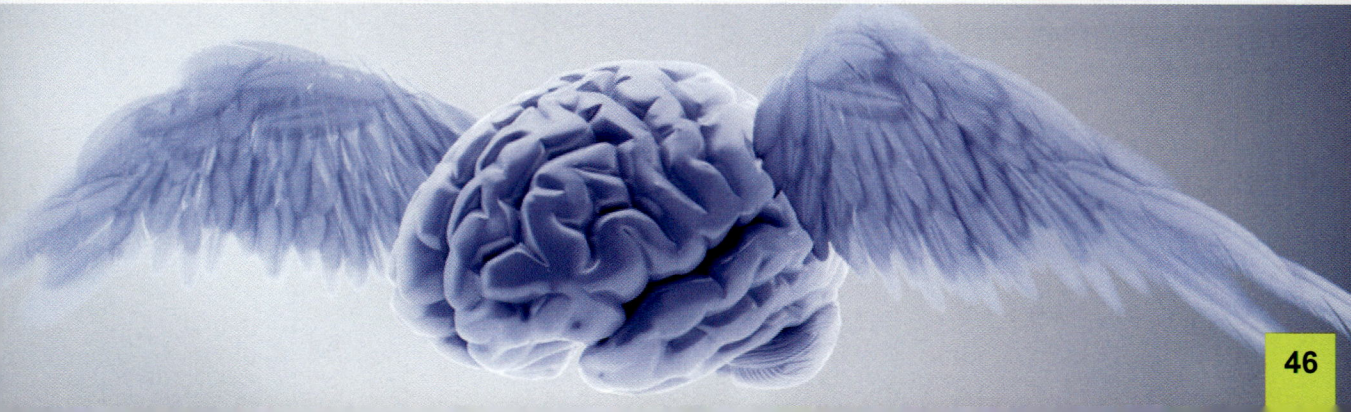

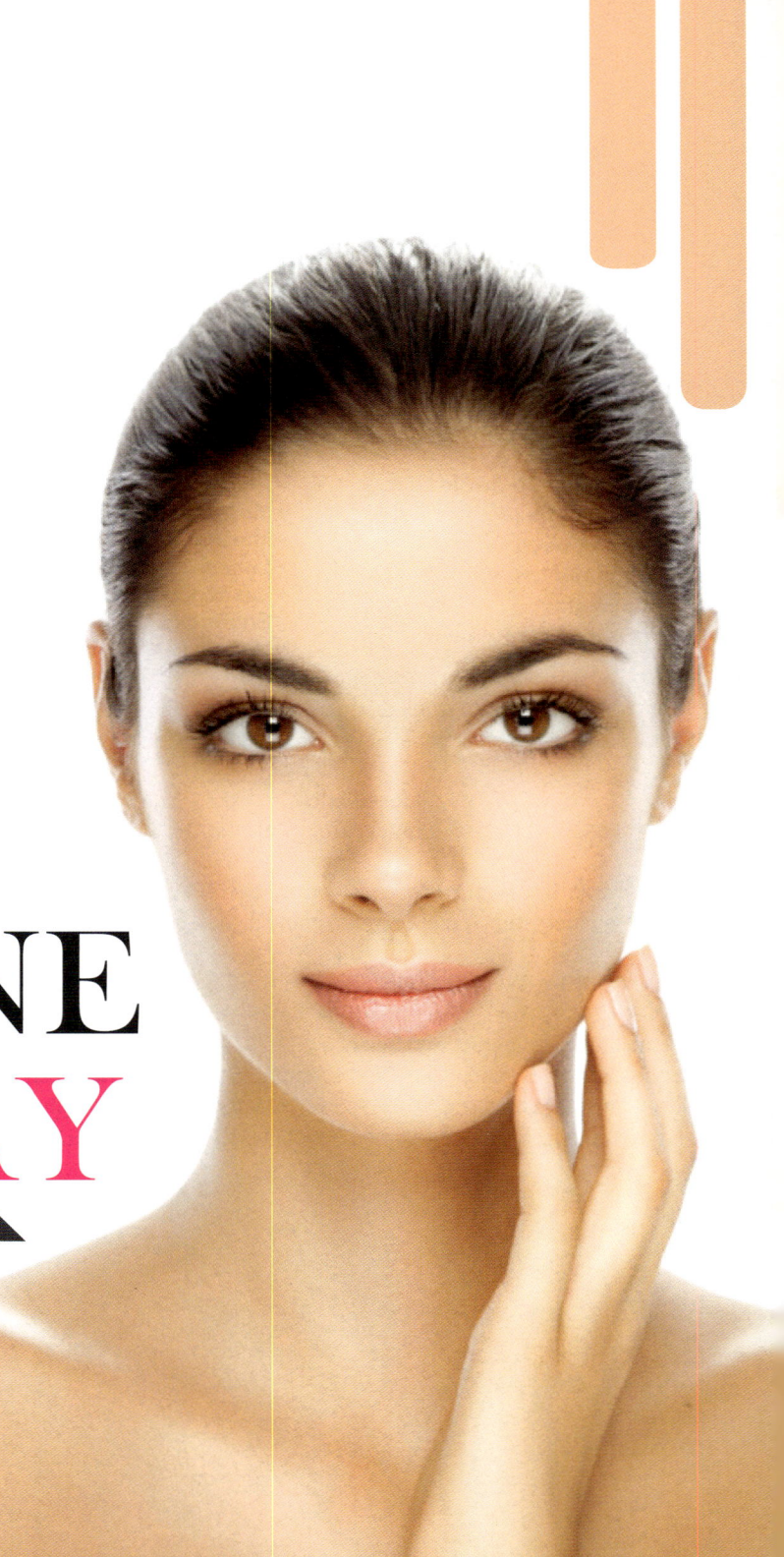

(Baccharis Trimera, Plantago Majora Extract, Rosmarinus Officinalis)

Immune C is a combination of several 100% natural herbal extracts carefully formulated to provide the best immune response from your own body. People using Immune C have reported that it is the best and the most natura supplement targeting blood and all tissue cells. Those that are discovering its efficacy say that it is indispensable and can be used as a complement to the traditional medication. A renowned oncologist reports excellent results in abnormal cell control as well as in the improvement of quality of life without side effects.

IMMUNE C SPRAY

Protection against Cancer Cells

USAGE AND CONTRAINDICATIONS

Immune C is not intended to diagnose, treat, cure or prevent any diseases. Patients should seek their physician for consultation, diagnosis and treatment.

It is not recommended for an individual who is pregnant, breast feeding, had transplanted organs or is sensitive or allergic to any of the components.

Patients should avoid eating too much red meat, fat, soft drinks, sugar, stimulants or alcoholic drinks.

Immune C is a liquid spray formulated for sublingual use and in your stomach. It must be taken on empty stomach and do not eat for 30 minutes. Dosages vary between 10-15 sprays per day, taken in divided dosages. Patients should use Immune C for a minimum period of 3 months before re-evaluation by your physician. With severe metastasis and late stage cancer, dosages may be increased to 25 sprays per day in divided dosages.

Ingredients: Panax Ginseng (Aglycon Sapogenin), Baccharis Trimera, Plantago Majora, Rosmarinus Officinalis, Extract

These statements have not been reviewed by the FDA. This product is not intended to diagnose, treat, cure, or prevent any disease.

DR. BERNARDO UDAQUIOLA

Chief Oncologist to the Oncology National Institute of Uruguay.

"It has been demonstrated to be safe for human use and does not interfere with any other treatment the patient may choose to carry on. In some occasions, it has been seen to minimize the secondary effects of radiotherapy and chemotherapy."

Dr. Tai's Pearl

This is a secret of the Patagonia in South America. The Research and resourcefulness coming from the Native Physicians that treated their entire village using Natural herbs to boost their immunity and fight the myriad of infections that tribal people suffered daily. This is an example of extraordinary power in a very small bottle.

Intelligent Usage:
Patients should avoid eating sugar, sweets, fats, alcohol, and too much meat or protein. Avoid gluten and dairy.

Side Effects: None

Contraindications:
Mothers who are pregnant or breastfeeding, indivuals with transplanted organs or those who are allergic to any ingredients should not take product.

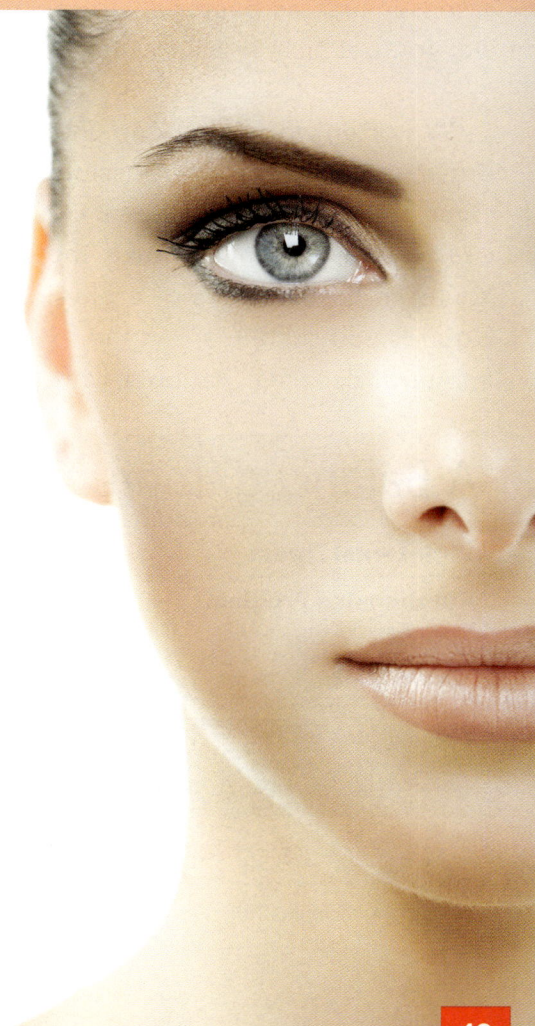

48

Immune Gold

Healing & Prevention of Diseases!

Doctor's and Scientists have been making remarkable strides when it comes to Immunity.

The Immune system is a marvelous and complex structure that all living things possess. It is the host defense that protects you from dangerous pathogens that cause illness and disease, such as bacteria, viruses and fungi. If the Immune System is compromised, not only will you get sick, it will result in severe complications.

We often worry about an underperforming Immune System and this is a very valid concern, but many overlook the possible consequences that wait at the other end of the spectrum. Over-active Immune Systems can cause just as much havoc! These overreactions to common, every day substances make the Immune System attack nearby cells and harm your body. You're in the trenches of a physiological WAR ZONE, being harmed by FRIENDLY FIRE. The wounds you sustain are in the form of allergies and inflammation that stems into full-on auto-immune diseases. Patients with autoimmune diseases often find themselves suffering from intense, life-altering conditions.

It takes perfect balance to properly regulate an Immune System.
Without that balance, we topple over from the inside out.

What is to be done when we are constantly torn between stimulating and suppressing our sick immune systems? There HAS to be a way to help calm and restore order to frenzied, over-active systems while helping to gently increase immunity for under-performing systems.

A Balanced Immune System

Internal Threat	External Threat
Autoimmune Problem (Hashimoto's Thyroiditis, Rheumatoid Arthritis, Inflammatory Bowel Disease, Type 1 Diabetes, Lupus)	**Allergic Reaction** (Food Sensitivities, Allergies, Eczema, Asthma, Sinusitis)

Immune Over-Reaction

Good Balanced Immune System = Optimal Effectiveness

Immune Under-Reaction

Cancer (Hepatitis, HIV, Shingles, TB)	**Infection** (Bacteria, Mold/Fungus, Parasites, Viruses)

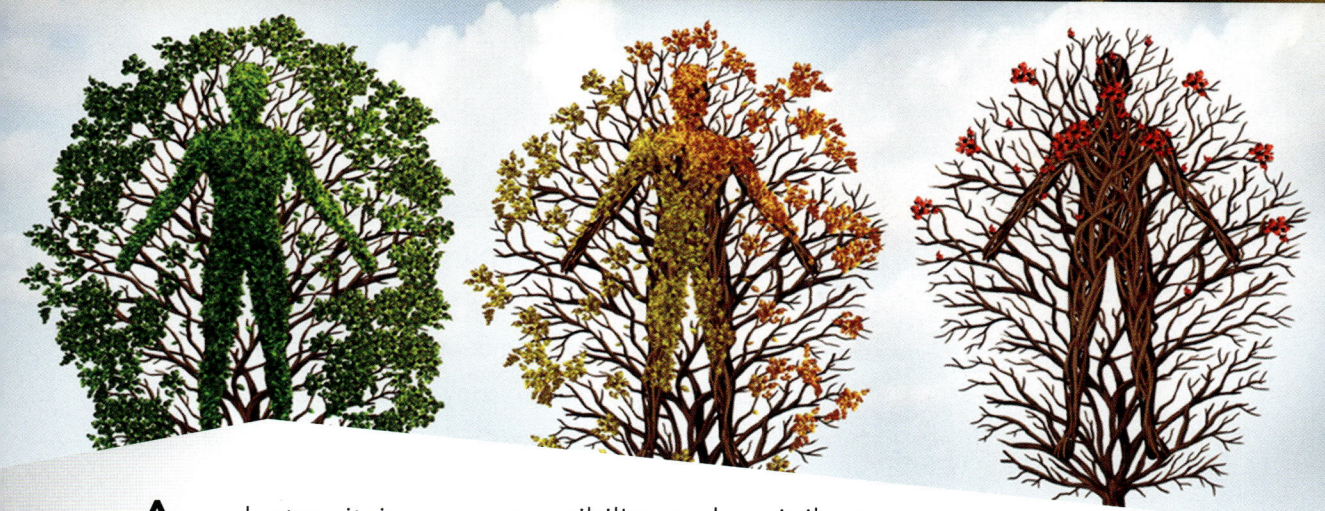

As a doctor, it is my responsibility to be vigilant, keeping my eyes sharp and my mind open to new possibilities when it comes to using natural medicine to maintain the balance of an ever-vigilant immune system & the over activity that causes self harm. Every time I travel, I can't help but explore and ask questions that could lead me to the next ingredient that could possibly help my patients. I spend hours scouring through books and articles, learning all there is to learn about chemicals and compounds, herbs and botanicals so that I can serve those who depend on me for my knowledge & experience.

It was in these pursuits that I came back to revisit Cannabis, and more specifically Cannabidiol (CBD).

Now, Cannabinoids have always been on my radar. During the time I have kept my attention on CBD, I have made several predictions that have come to pass. As I suspected, CBD has rose in popularity and has begun to stand out for its medicinal benefits. Not only is CBD non-psychoactive, it has pulled through to show the ability to influence a wide range of receptors in the brain & body that have given it the ability to alleviate many health conditions. From Stress & Depression to Seizures, Pain, Arthritis and MS, CBD has been the saving grace of hundreds of thousands of people. Although I've kept this list relatively small, it implicates the vast possibilities of CBD supplementation.

Cannabidiol is one of the primary cannabinoid molecules present in Cannabis. This molecule is so abundant, that it is second only to **THC**, the mind-altering compound.

By Focusing specifically on CBD, many people have been able to find relief and reversal of devastating health conditions that not only ruin lives, but can be proven fatal. Although many people romanticize Marijuana usage for recreational purposes, the potential of cannabidiols without mind altering THC as a treatment for symptoms and disease is remarkable. With more Scientific Trials going on every day, less people are feeding into misconceptions about CBD and are helping to create a more informed industry.

It was a common misconception that using CBD for their chronic illness, would cause them to walk around in an altered state. This is untrue! Although you may feel the positive effects of CBD, less pain and inflammation, it will come to you in the form of relief with NO HIGH! Sorry… for those of you that wanted a little somethin' extra, but Immune Gold comes with pure CBD and NO THC!!!

I cannot fault this way of thinking and completely understand the worry of obtaining a 'high' while attempting to treat your ailment. A reason why I have waited so long to work with CBD is that I wanted to be absolutely sure that a CBD extract could be made with no THC – the psychoactive cannabinoid that causes the 'high'. By patiently waiting on a process that extracts CBD while excluding and completely eliminating THC from the equation, we have been able to give those in need a true contender to consider – a CBD that can be held as the **GOLD STANDARD** for CBD Extracts without THC, marked by a chemical fingerprint proof called HPLC that guarantees purity.

As a person who travels, gives lectures, teaches and creates, I have to be present at all times and can't compromise my performance by using just any product that isn't pure CBD! I cannot trust just any CBD product in the market not being contaminated with pesticide toxins and THC.

No **THC**
No **Highs**
No **Addiction**

Although strains of the plant form with low THC and high CBD have become more popular in the last few years, they are still somewhat of a rarity. Additionally, it's hard to find cannabidiol products available commercially that have ZERO THC. Cannabis marketed for CBD use still has traces of THC that may affect the user. In **Immune Gold**, we have a solid foundation of Pure CBD, CBDa, CBG, CBGa, CBNa and CBGv, without THC that work tirelessly to activate Receptors that trigger their positive health benefits.

In **Immune Gold**, I have specifically focused on anti-inflammatory conditions by incorporating powerful Terpenes & Terpenoids. These ingredients are usually found in higher plants, mosses, algae and lichens and have been used for centuries as antibacterial, anti-inflammatory, antitumoral and anti-viral agents. This is because the ability for Terpense & Terpenoids to modulate critical cell signaling pathways involved in our body's inflammatory response. This means the Nuclear Transcription Factor kappaB (NF-kappaB) activation, specifically. NF-kappaB's role is to regulate inflammatory & immune responses, making any substance that is able to inhibit NF-kappaB an excellent anti-inflammatory agent.

5 Essential Terpene found in pure CBD of Immune Gold:

1. Beta-Mycerine: Relaxes Muscles, Eases Pain & Inflammation
2. Limonene – Immune defense. Fights Tumors, Stimulates Immune System & Fights Bacterial Infections, Relieves Depression & Anxiety, Shown to treat Gastric Reflux and Ulcers.
3. Alpha-pinene – Bronchial asthma. Found in pine trees. Helps dilate the bronchial tubes, reduce inflammation, kill bacteria, and increase cognitive function.
4. Beta Caryophyllene – Sadness and Happiness. Binds to the CB2 receptor, found mostly in the immune system. Eases inflammation, nerve pain, ulcers, and depression.
5. Linalool – Especially helpful mental effects, helping with psychosis, reducing anxiety and stress, and making SSRI antidepressants more effective. It also reduces epileptic convulsions.

By taking a few drops of **Immune Gold** sublingually, you will immediately begin to help your Immune System, protect against inflammation, stress, and improve mental wellbeing using the power of CBD, Terpenes, and Terpenoids.

Dr. Tai's Pearl

You folks probably already know that most of the products I have created were, in some way, originally meant for my own private use or for my family! That's right, each product was made with myself, or someone very close to me in mind so that they may live a long, happy and healthy life.

When I started this company many years ago it was because I could NOT find a good Daily Multivitamin. Imagine me, my counters and coffee tables littered with empty vitamin bottles because I had tried just about EVERY. SINGLE. BRAND of daily multivitamin. I spent my days tripping over those bottles because I didn't even have the energy to step over them! I stopped putting my faith in companies to uphold my seemingly impossible standard (High-Quality, Natural Ingredients that you could FEEL helping your body) and began a new project – Creating a Supplement of my Own.

I created my very first supplement, Daily Energy, using the latest in Western (American/European) technology but then I also created the Daily Wellness which was patterned after the smartest & wisest Eastern (Asian/Oriental) Methodologies of Wellness & Health. These were my first "TWINS" born to me and my company.

(Just don't tell my daughters.)

Over a HUNDRED products, past and present, shared the same origin story; born from the need of my own health & family.

Therefore, when I wanted to create a CBD formula, I was fearful of contamination as most pesticide & insecticides are "Organic Phenol Rings" based and would be highly concentrated in the oil section of the plants. As CBD is only the oil portion of Cannabis, I was terrified of possibly taking concentrated "TOXIC" chemicals inadvertently or purposely by unscrupulous salesmen selling either FAKE, crudely made, or severely contaminated CBD oil.

I searched high & low and could not find a reliable source for many years, meanwhile the market has been flooded with products claiming CBD active ingredients with NO patient improvement. When I FINALLY found a source, I was a complete hard-nose and demanded the "HPLC", the chemical fingerprint verification of all CBD's that proves there is No toxicity or Chemical Contamination, and Immune Gold was finally BORN!! With Great reviews and fabulous results, might I add (I URGE you to review the Clinical Case!). The Proof & verification is key to my success.

Directions:
SHAKE WELL!
Take 1 dropper sublingually PM. Use daily.

May add AM dosage if needed.
You may also rub a few drops on painful joints or skin problems. For further increased dosage consult your health care practitioner.

Ingredients:
Proprietary Formulation: Pure CBD, CBDa, CBG, CBGa, CBNa, CBGv, Terpines and Terpenoids, Spearamint Essential Oil, Cold Pressed Sunflower Oil

Clinical Cases:

Dr. B.C. is a Nationally known figure, bigger than life, he is probably the only person I know that travels & speaks even more than I. This means he's at least at DOUBLE the risk for all those nasty infections... I mean I WOULD feel bad for him, but a little birdie told me that he has a large private jet at his disposal. Kind of makes it hard to feel sorry for the guy.

Dr. B suffers severely from Low Immunity, Lack of Sleep, and Severe Arthritis & Skin Problems. He never had a problem with finding new supplements to try as doctors and naturopaths were always begging to treat him. Dr. B went through a number of famous doctors, protocols and BIG supplement houses that threw their all at him, begging for his endorsement... but they just didn't work. ALL to no avail, he continued to suffer consistently without ANY significant improvements.

After coming to one of my lectures, Dr. B spoke with me about his horrible health nightmares. Seriously! The things this guy had experienced and feared had me sleeping with one eye open!! For a moment, I didn't even realize he was asking for help! He jetted all the way out here just to have ME make a protocol?? Then and there we began a formal consultation and then I got to work. As you may have guessed, I recommended a natural protocol including the **Immune Gold** as both oral application at bedtime as well as local application to the itchy skin problems (with **Ultra Skin Gel**) and joint arthritis.

Dr. B is today symptom free with great improvement in his mobility, range of motion, and comfort. Dr. B told me that it was the ONLY protocol that helped him resolve all the symptoms. I'm delighted to report that he is super happy with the results and swears by **Immune Gold**! The Miracle supplement that saved him from grief, pain and despair.

Side Effects: None

Contraindications: Do not take if you are allergic to any of the ingredients.

These Statements have not been reviewed by the FDA.
This product is not intended to diagnose, treat, cure, or prevent any disease.

References

1. Blessing EM, Steenkamp MM, Manzanares J, Marmar CR. Cannabidiol as a Potential Treatment for Anxiety Disorders. Neurotherapeutics. 2015;12(4):825-36.

2. Mechoulam R, Parker LA. The Endocannabinoid System and the Brain. Annu Rev Psychology. 2013;64:21-47.

3. Morgan CJ, Schafer G, Freeman TP, Curran HV. Impact of cannabidiol on the acute memory and psychotomimetic effects of smoked cannabis: naturalistic study: naturalistic study. Br J Psychiatry. 2010;197(4):285-90.

4. Parsons LH, Hurd YL. Endocannabinoid signalling in reward and addiction. Nat Rev Neurosci. 2015;16(10):579-95.

5. Zlebnik NE, Cheer JF. Beyond the CB1 Receptor: Is Cannabidiol the Answer for Disorders of Motivation?. Annu Rev Neurosci. 2016;39:1-17.

6. Inflamm Allergy Drug Targets. 2009 Mar;8(1):28-39. Molecular basis of the anti-inflammatory effects of terpenoids.

IONIC MICRO MINERALS

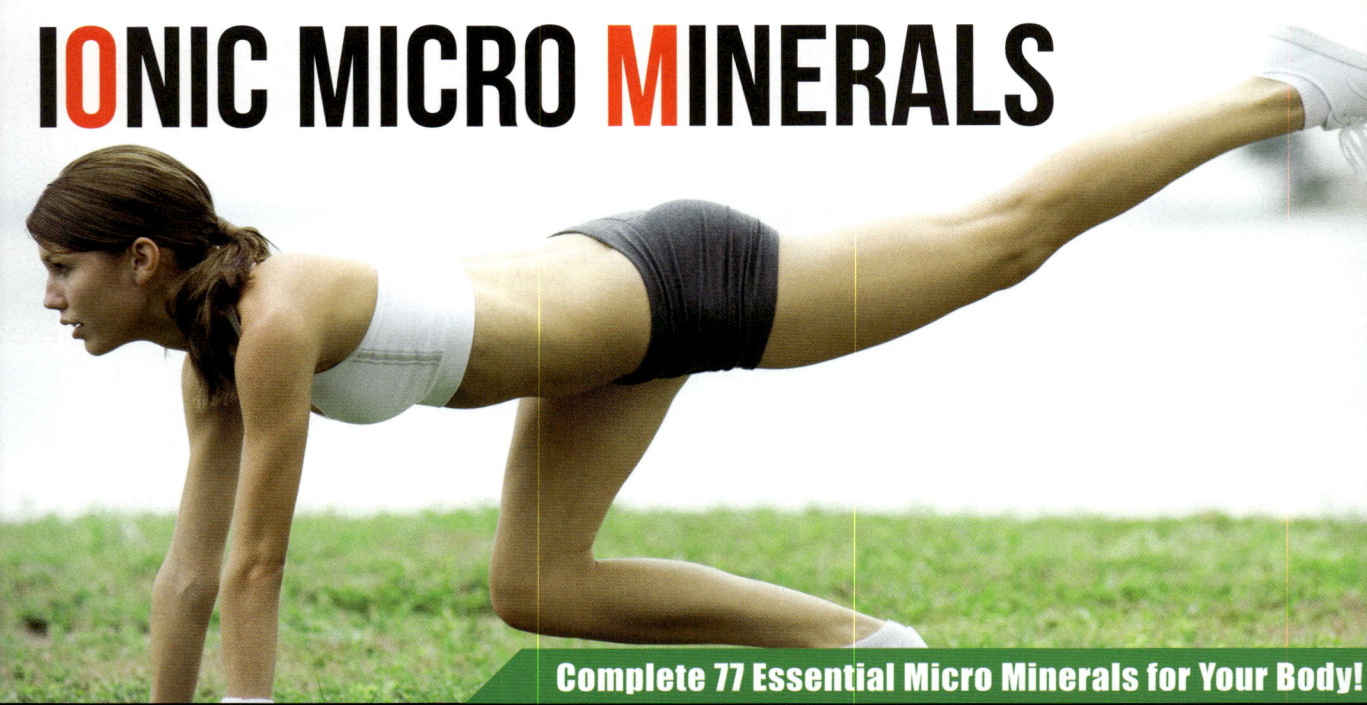

Complete 77 Essential Micro Minerals for Your Body!

Our Body's Essential Nutrients
By eating healthy and consuming daily multi-vitamins, our body automatically ingests all the micro minerals available. One of the best ways to get these minerals is by replacing low nutrient processed food with high nutrient foods. Unfortunately, most people do not take in enough of these tiny trace minerals. Back in 1936, US Senate #264 74th Congress reported: Our soils are depleted of minerals, crops grown are with deficient minerals, people who eat them get mineral deficient diseases and the only cure is mineral supplements. The US Surgeon General reports that 68% of all disease is related to one's diet!

Americas Unessential Diet
Most of Americans eat a large amount of sodium, exceeding far beyond ones daily recommended intake. Only 5% of sodium comes naturally in food. A single example of America's negligence in dieting is that most consume twice as much sodium as potassium, when an ideal diet should consist of 5 times more potassium than sodium. **A Ten-State Nutrition Survey, HANES I and HANES II** states that Americans consume a diet that is inadequate in nutritional value. **Only 20% of individuals consume nutrients at Recommended Daily Allowance (RDA)** levels. According to the **National Research Council Diet** in the National Academy Press, Washington D.C in 1989, **50% of the U.S. population shows marginal deficiency,** over two decades later, the statistics are sure to be much worse.

Dangers of Disregarded Diets
An unbalanced diet, including a low potassium, high sodium one, has been demonstrated to play a role in the development of cardiovascular disease and cancer. Whereas a diet more balanced with the proper amount of minerals and nutrients has been shown to protect against those very same diseases.

A Resolution to giving Our Body's Balance
Ionic Micro Minerals offers the versatility of an electrolyte replacement drink, while nourishing the body with a complete blend of essential minerals, without the added unnecessary sugar. The body is constantly working to stay in a state of balance. Ionic Micro Minerals is just what your body needs to get you headed in the right direction. Concentrated Trace Mineral Drop Complex also provides the balance that your body needs.

Potassium, sodium and chloride are all considered electrolytes. They function in the maintenance and distribution of water within the body. In addition, they serve in the role of controlling acid-base balance, heart contractility, kidney and adrenal function and vital neuromuscular activity.

The body needs energy, and to produce that energy, your body needs minerals to nourish the adrenals and thyroid, which are the chief organs that produce energy. Each person's daily needs are different and depend on factors such as health, age and sex. The following is a complete list of all **77 essential ingredients** to the human body's health contained in the Ionic Micro Minerals:

Magnesium, Chloride, Sodium, Potassium, Sulfate, Lithium, Boron, Trace mineral drop complex, Aloe, Bromide, Carbonate, Calcium, Fluoride, Silicon, Nitrogen, Selenium, Phosphorus, Iodide, Chromium, Iron, Maganese, Titanium, Rubidium, Cobalt, Copper, Antimony, Arsenic, Molybdenum, Strontium, Zinc, Nickel, Tungsten, Barium, Tin, Lanthanum, Yttrium, Silver, Uranium, Gallium, Bismuth, Zirconium, Cerium, Cesium, Gold, Beryllium, Hafnium, Samarium, Terbium, Europium, Godolinium, Dysprosium, Thorium, Holmim, Lutetium, Thulium, Erbium, Ytterbium, Neodymium, Praseodymium, Biobium, Tantaium, Thaalium, Thenium, Indium, Palladium, Platinum, Other elements found in sea water.

Directions: Shake Well. Add 2 drops in water or juice once or twice daily. Can be added to foods such as soup and salad dressings if preferred.

Ingredients:
Magnesium, Chloride, Sodium, Potassium, Sulfate, Lithium, Boron, Trace mineral drop complex, Aloe, Bromide, Carbonate, Calcium, Fluoride, Silicon, Nitrogen, Selenium, Phosphorus, Iodide, Chromium, Iron, Maganese, Titanium, Rubidium, Cobalt, Copper, Antimony, Arsenic, Molybdenum, Strontium, Zinc, Nickel, Tungsten, Barium, Tin, Lanthanum, Yttrium, Silver, Uranium, Gallium, Bismuth, Zirconium, Cerium, Cesium, Gold, Beryllium, Hafnium, Samarium, Terbium, Europium, Godolinium, Dysprosium, Thorium, Holmim, Lutetium, Thulium, Erbium, Ytterbium, Neodymium, Praseodymium, Biobium, Tantaium, Thaalium, Thenium, Indium, Palladium, Platinum, Other elements found in sea water.

These statements have not been reviewed by the FDA. This product is not intended to diagnose, treat, cure, or prevent any disease.

Dr. Tai's Pearls:

It is an irrefutable fact that humans date to our ancestors which really crawled out of the ocean. This is fairly logical given that salt water with micronutrients courses through our blood vessels with small particles of red blood cells which give it the red color. If you go to the hospital and need anything given intravenously, the will give it to you with a little bit of saline. It isn't difficult to understand the importance of the 77 microminerals to our bodies, as these are the same essential microminerals present in the ocean. Remember that every single one of the treatments of biochemical reactions that occurs every minute in our bodies, depends on microminerals as part of the ingredient or enzymatic exchange. Without it, these important biochemical reactions would not occur. Therein lays the reason why we do not feel well and are not as healthy as we should be.

Clinical Case:
42-year-old real estate developer in South America. Good looking, in good shape, apparently healthy with a lovely family – a physician wife and two daughters. Well-to-do, living in a beach town on a tropical isle. During conversation, he told me his nightmare is falling asleep every night. I asked him why. He explained that each night he has severe night cramps, starting with restless legs, jumping all over the bed and resulting in pain so severe he would have to jump up and stomp to make the cramps go away. He was at the point where he didn't even want to go to bed and asked me if it was okay to sleep standing up. I thought at that point it was ridiculous. The condition was so severe, it required some sort of intervention. I started him on some Super B12 and B-complex, a small, but concentrated Mineral Pak, and Max Nox to increase his circulation in the extremities, and, of course, the Microminerals. When I spoke with him again two weeks later, he was a totally different man. Grateful for the relief, he explained that he took all the supplements before going to bed, but the one that won his heart was the Ionic Microminerals. He described it as a fire extinguisher. Whenever he would feel the restless leg or cramps coming on, he would spray the Ionic Micromineral under his tongue, hold it under his tongue for about a minute before swallowing, and like a fire being put out, the pain would subside. With a smile on his face, he said he had never seen anything quite like it. Now he sleeps like a baby.

Side Effects:
Taking large doses of Ionic Microminerals all of a sudden, may create irritation of the bowels, resulting in loose stools. It is better to increase the dosage from 5 drops daily in increments of one drop per day, to get the body accustom to the Ionic Microminerals.

Contraindications:
Do not take product if you are allergic to any ingredients.

Lady Specialist

Keep Female Genitalia Healthy & Young!

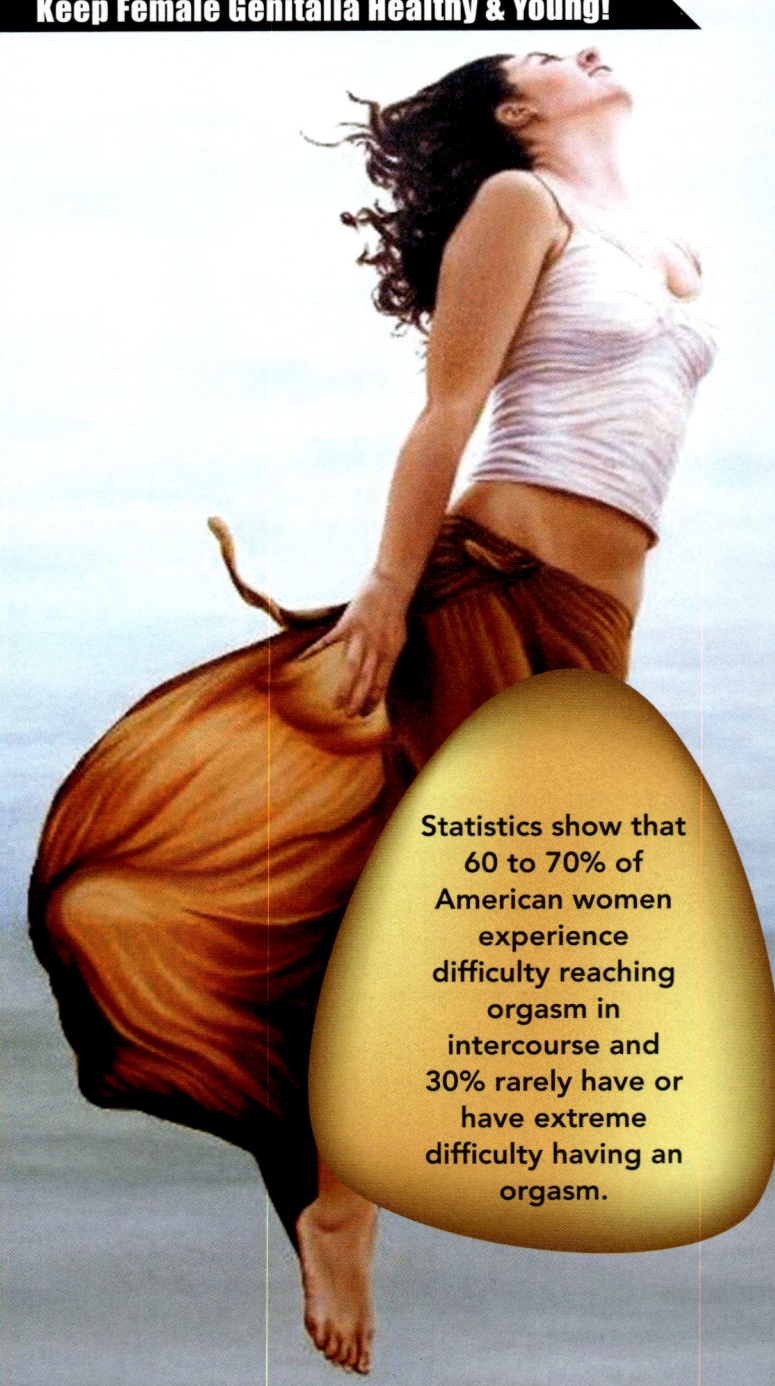

Now that their male counterparts have multiple choices of Viagra and Cialis (the infamous 36 hours), women still have to fend for themselves trying to use various techniques to overcome these difficulties which are often times useless.

Difficulty with vaginal dryness is common and affects over half of women of all ages, especially menopausal women. Symptoms of vaginal dryness include irritation, itching, burning and pain during sexual intercourse. The most common cause of vaginal dryness is declining estrogen levels. Estrogen loss not only causes vaginal dryness – but SHRINKAGE! Estrogen is a female hormone that helps keep vaginal tissue healthy by maintaining normal vaginal lubrication and tissue elasticity.

Lady Specialist is a powerful, natural, herbal combination to be used topically and may help to achieve more personal satisfaction, a much higher enhancement of sensation and a more rapid and intense orgasm. Women may achieve a new level of human sexuality by using it as a sexual enhancer and a pleasure improvement product. It may be used in conjunction with Max Nox, an oral supplement, if needed.

Lady Specialist is a water-based product, dermatologically tested, pH balanced, includes no hormones, silicones, animal byproducts or harsh chemical substances so women can expect a safe, pain-free and gentle experience.

Use outside the vaginal wall and clitoris as well as inside for greater lubrication and sensation.
Advantages of **Lady Specialist** include relief of vaginal dryness, the restoration of natural lubrication and the suppleness and contraction of vaginal tissues. It also firms, tones and tightens the vaginal wall

Statistics show that 60 to 70% of American women experience difficulty reaching orgasm in intercourse and 30% rarely have or have extreme difficulty having an orgasm.

and canal as well as increases the blood flow to the genital area for a more intense sensation.

Lady Specialist has mild antiseptic and anti-inflammatory properties to help prevent infections, stop swelling and dispel unpleasant odors.

Directions: For TOPICAL use only. Apply 1-2 pumps inside genital area and clitoris before activities. Lady Specialist can be applied as frequently as needed. For long-term results Lady Specialist should be applied daily, mornings and evenings and 5 minutes before sexual intercourse.

Ingredients:
Puresterol® standardized extract of Pueraria Mirifica, Oak Gall Extract, Witch Hazel, Collagen, L-Arginine
These statements have not been reviewed by the FDA. This product is not intended to diagnose, treat, cure, or prevent any disease.

Dr. Tai's Pearls:

Frequent usage of Lady Specialist is a woman's rejuvenation in motion. The tissues around the vaginal wall absorb the natural extract in Lady Specialist. The tissues rejuvenate and return to its former youth. Elasticity and tissue integrity is essential for a healthy vaginal wall – it keeps all the collagen and elastin in the area at peak performance. It has been said that it even helps with the prevention of urinary incontinence when used together with Max Estro E and DHEA Transdermal.

Clinical Case:
62-year-old accountant suffered quietly from vaginal shrinkage after her menopausal years. This condition is very common and occurs frequently in women after menopause when they lose the presence of estrogen. By using the Lady Specialist, she was, in the beginning, happy and relieved of the dryness and having adequate lubrication during sexual activity. As time passed by, she became elated by the fact that intercourse was no longer painful and she started to experience enhanced sensation as well as orgasm again. She said before Lady Specialist, she felt guilty that she didn't feel like having sexual intercourse with her husband, whom she loved very much, but could not enjoy due to physical limitations. Now she said all of that is in the past and she feels like a young woman all over again. Replenishment of her progesterone, estrogen and DHEA with Testosterone helped her to achieve the maximum health post-menopause with the help and guidance of salivary testing.

Side Effects: None
Contraindications:
Do Not Use if you have any laceration, infection, or inflammation in the vaginal area.
Do not take product if you are allergic to any ingredients.

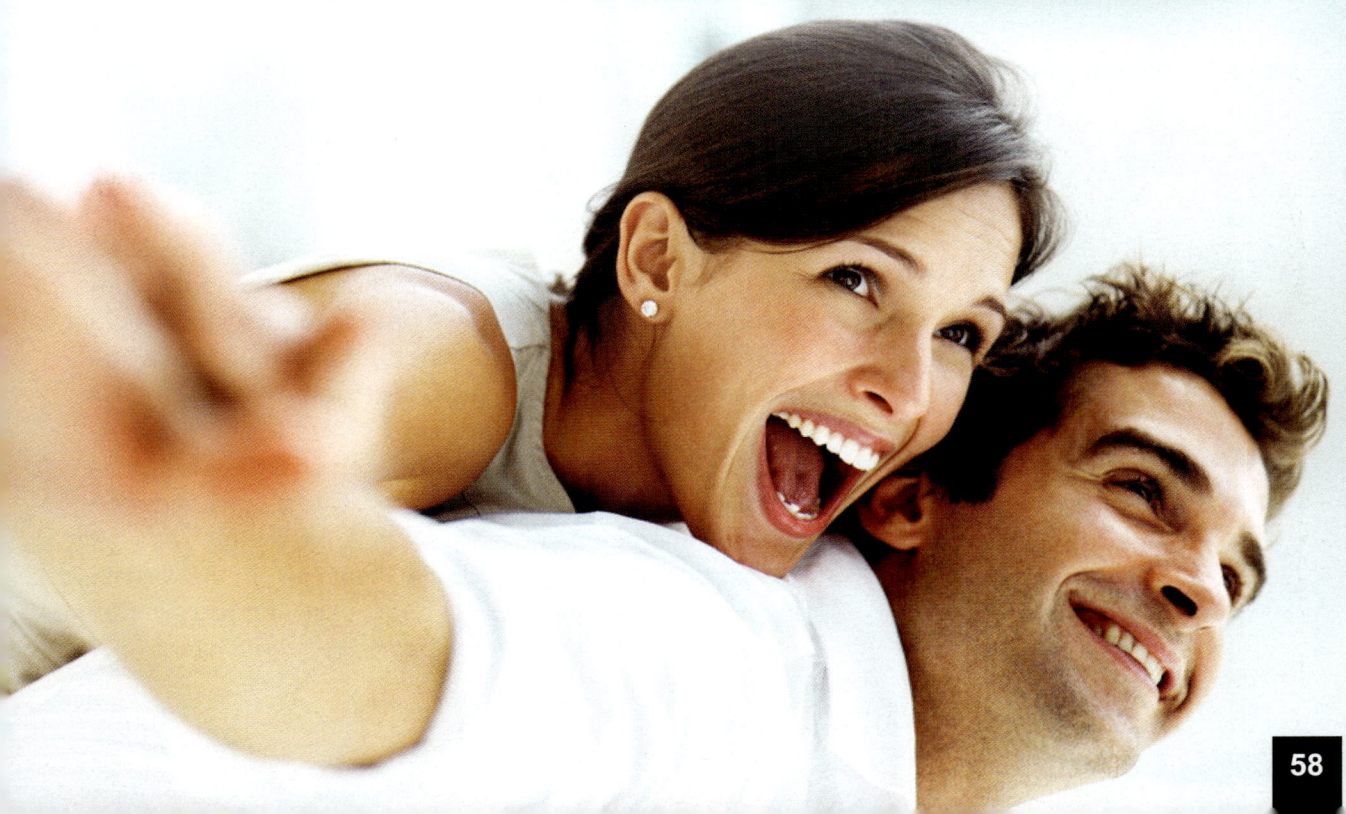

58

Liver Cleanse

Prevent GOUT and Kidney Failure!

The **liver** is considered to be the chemical processing plant of your body. Each minute, 30% of your circulating blood goes to support your liver which removes harmful toxins by filtering out & cleansing our blood and also distributes and stores essential nutrients.

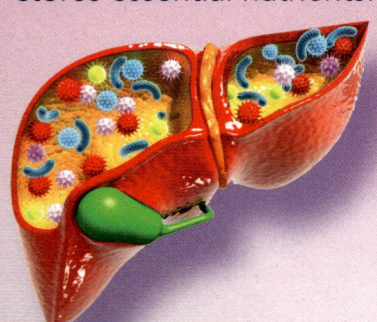

Main Functions of the Liver:
Making Bile
Building Proteins
Processing Food
Removing Toxins from the Blood

Inflammation of the liver is dangerous, interfering with important functions of the body. If a liver becomes diseased due to prolonged inflammation and dysfunction, there is no organ that can possibly take its place and do its functions. The rest of the body can't hope to receive the nutrients from food, to remove toxins from the body, or to build proteins. The absence of the liver would not only lead to poor health, but death.

The liver has an important yet thankless job. Due to its resilience, most cases of liver inflammation don't garner medical attention. The interruption in function is written off as a temporary sickness and the liver is forced to tough it out, pushing onward. You may think that this is just the natural order, but BEWARE!! Forcing your liver to work in conditions of inflammation with no additional support will make it harder and harder to bounce back later in life – leaving you devastated when you need it most!

Those who opt to help their livers are taking an important step to their overall life-long health. Unfortunately, many doctors will recommend that you begin taking prescription medications that have been shown time and time again to actually have adverse reactions from the liver. While you expressed the proper sentiment to take care of your hard-working liver, you are dragged down a path of damaging it further! We call this Drug-Induced Liver Disease.

Often drugs will injure the liver and disrupt its normal functions. The symptoms that these drugs produce are so severe that they mirror the abnormalities that can be caused by viruses and immunologic diseases that are toxic to the liver.

It is possible to have Drug-Induced Liver Disease while showing mild to NO symptoms. This is most common during the beginning stages. Once the fatigue, weakness, loss of appetite and abdominal pain set in, the disease is fully realized and you will begin experiencing symptoms that are more specific to liver failure.

Liver-Disease Specific Symptoms Include...

- Jaundice or yellowing of skin
- Easy bruising
- **Itching in the skin at night**
- Fluid accumulation in legs & abdomen
- *Mental confusion or coma*
- Kidney Failure
- Vulnerability to Bacterial Infections
- Gastrointestinal Bleeding

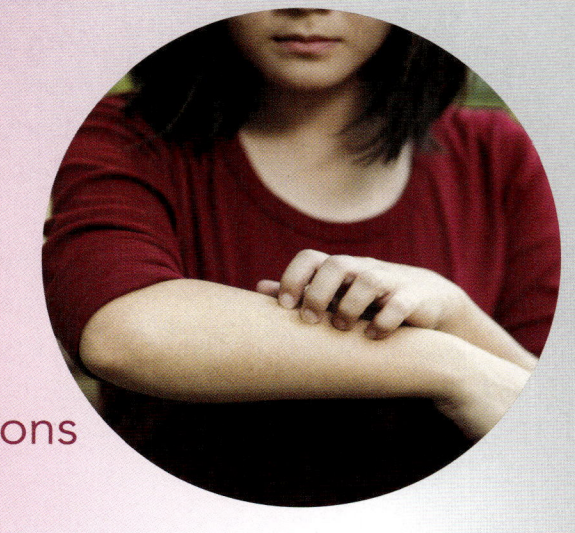

One of the most important tasks of the liver is to help purify and turn potentially harmful chemicals in the blood into harmless debris. Some drugs may harm the liver upon taking them, others can be far more ominous, only causing harm after safely passing through the liver and being transformed into other chemicals. After being converted, these chemicals may cause indirect damage, or they will attack the liver directly causing liver failure.

To avoid this dangerous condition, I always have recommended becoming more informed about your options when treating any issues within your body. The less synthetic chemicals the better – always opt to use natural if you can!!

Terrified of the hidden horrors waiting to spring out and claim my 70-year-old liver, I created Liver Cleanse to help me to maintain my liver's health. Liver Cleanse utilizes three main, powerful, and natural ingredients: **Ayuric, Graviola, and Tart Cherry Powder Extract.**

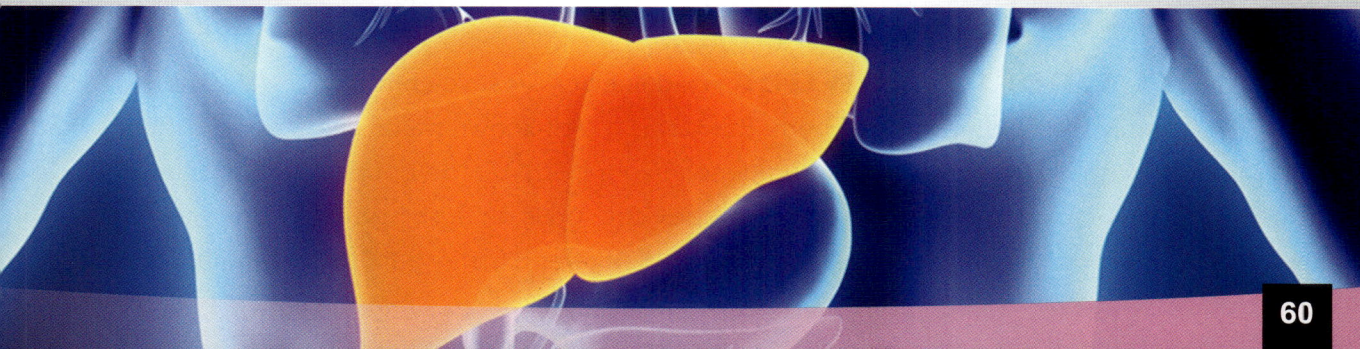

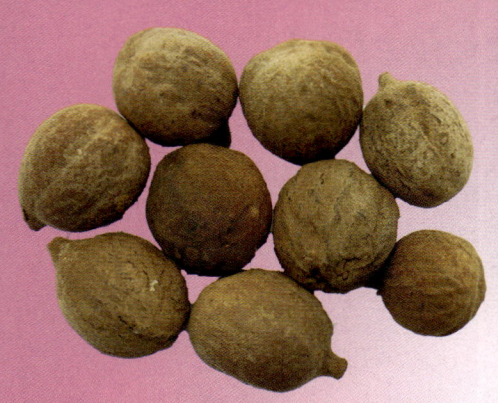

Ayuric is an ingredient that has been clinically studied for the last decade. As a water-soluble ingredient, Ayuric is able to be fully absorbed by the body to support a healthy uric acid level. Excess Uric Acid is a troubling condition that can cause irreversible damage to the Liver and Kidneys while also subjecting you to Gout, a painful type of arthritis that causes attacks of inflammation on specific joints of the feet and legs. This targeted attack on the body can cause sudden burning, stiffness, or swelling that continues to happen over and over. This constant inflammation will cause harm to all your tissues, joints and tendons.

Typically, high Uric Acid does not always equate to gout. Many people may have dangerous spikes in their Uric Acid without getting the Gout pain, but the absence of the diagnosis does not stop Uric Acid from forming hard crystals in your joints, causing debilitating pain. Not only are you experiencing these present symptoms, but increased Uric Acid levels may cause insulin resistance, oxidative stress, and metabolic syndrome, all of which progress Liver Disease.

The liver takes the blood from your digestive system and filter out toxins. While being compromised by Uric Acid, the liver cannot properly do its job!!

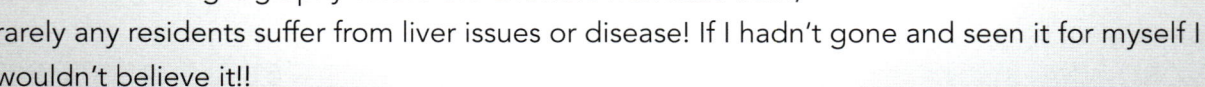

Graviola is a rather well-known ingredient that has been used time and time again for a broad spectrum of issues. The most prolific being its use against Cancers. I've included Graviola in this very special Liver Cleanse due to its history of use in the Amazon to treat Liver and stomach ailments. In the geography where the Graviola fruit hails from, rarely any residents suffer from liver issues or disease! If I hadn't gone and seen it for myself I wouldn't believe it!!

The **Tart Cherry Powder** used in Liver Cleanse comes as a welcome aid to the liver. The Malic Acid from Tart Cherry Powder is a well-known metal chelator. This means that the toxic metals, like mercury, that accumulate in your body can be bound and inactivated. By rendering these toxic metals harmless, your body can focus on flushing them to reduce toxicity! Your liver, which is left with most of the metal residue after cleansing the blood, will thank you!

Directions:
Take 1 capsule twice daily on empty stomach.

May increase to three times daily.

Ingredients:
Ayuric, Graviola, Tart Cherry Powder Extract

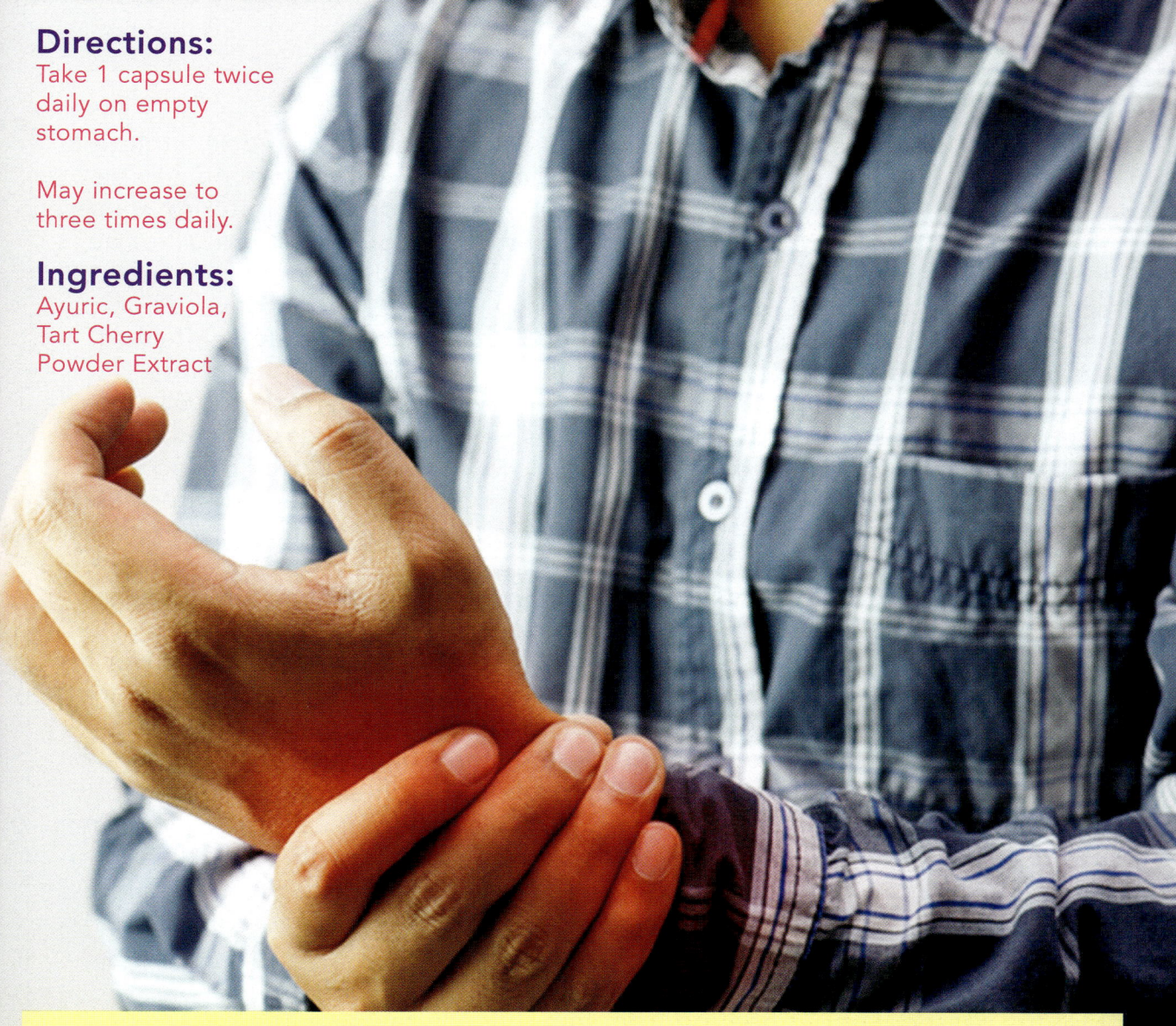

Dr. Tai's Pearl

Anyone who has suffered from Gout will tell you that the searing pain is equivalent to a broken bone. As a surgeon, I have opened and inspected many joints badly damaged by Uric Acid Crystals that have deposited in all joints of unsuspecting patients. These patients have high Uric Acid in their blood from a nonfunctioning, toxic liver. The formula of Liver Cleanse may help to clean up Uric Acid flow to help flush the Liver and Kidneys as well as protect these joints.

Clinical Cases:

One of my friends is a young and famous doctor who was a model athlete & in excellent physical shape. He came to me in tears with severe pain in his big toe joint. He was young and spry, so he had no problem ignoring it in the past, but it had grown to be so painful that he couldn't stand. After he hobbled into my office, we sat down and he confided in me that his prescription pain and gout medication didn't help at all. He had been diligently taking several pills for MONTHS and the Gout was completely unaffected. Before he had been ACTIVE – running, jumping and climbing at every moment of the day. Once, I had watched in awe as he darted around conventions, but this wasn't the same man. As we spoke, he was careful not to shift, sitting like a statue while speaking slowly. It was like the life had left him! Once vibrant and young, my friend was now so withered, so tired, and in such severe pain that he was constantly wiping away tears.

This man deserved more than constant pain and side-effects. I immediately recommended that he try Liver Cleanse to lower the Uric Acid that terrorized him and improve his diet. We worked together to identify and lower his carbohydrates and he completely wiped out sodas and fizzy drinks, sugary juices and alcohol. He was left with a diet lush in bright vegetables and delicious lean meats. Because of his severe state, he spent several weeks on the higher recommended dosage (1 capsule three times daily on an empty stomach) as the Uric Acid was cleared from his system. I cannot tell you my joy as each phone call he sounded a little more like himself. It was like waking a giant from a century long sleep. Soon, he switched to the maintenance dosage (1 capsule twice daily on an empty stomach) to continue to support his now healthy joints.

Months passed without hearing from him. I finally saw him at a conference and thanked me profusely. Since we had last spoken, he was back to hiking on trails, training in the gym and playing on the basketball court. Liver Cleanse is now a powerful staple that helped him reclaim his life.

Side Effects: None

Contraindications:
Do not take if you are allergic to any of the ingredients.

These statements have not been reviewed by the FDA. This product is not intended to diagnose, treat, cure, or prevent any disease.

References

1. Hepatology. 2010 Aug;52(2):578-89. doi: 10.1002/hep.23717.
2. Liver," Wikipedia, last modified May 3, 2015, http://en.wikipedia.org/wiki/Liver.
3. David Frawley, Ayurvedic Healing: A Comprehensive Guide (Delhi: Motilal Banarsidass Publishers, 1997), 141.
4. Jessie Szalay, "Liver: Function, Failure, and Disease," LiveScience, February 19, 2015, http://www.livescience.com/44859-liver.html.
5. Vasant Lad, Textbook of Ayurveda Volume 1: Fundamental Principles of Ayurveda (Albuquerque: The Ayurvedic Press, 2002), 96.
6. Ibid., 94-6.
7. Ibid., 59.
8. "Liver," Wikipedia, last modified May 3, 2015, http://en.wikipedia.org/wiki/Liver.
9. Lad, Textbook 1: Fundamental Principles, 116.
10. Frawley, Ayurvedic Healing, 141.
11. "Liver," Wikipedia, last modified May 3, 2015, http://en.wikipedia.org/wiki/Liver.
12. Vasant Lad, The Complete Book of Ayurvedic Home Remedies (New York: Three Rivers Press, 1998), 114.
13. Frawley, Ayurvedic Healing, 142.
14. Ibid.
15. Ibid., 144.
16. Vasant Lad, Textbook of Ayurveda Volume 3: General Principles of Management and Treatment (Albuquerque: The Ayurvedic Press, 2012), 116-118.
17. Frawley, Ayurvedic Healing, 141.
18. Ibid., 142.
19. http://www.ncbi.nlm.nih.gov/ Author: Mita Majumdar
20. Oberlies, N., Chang, C., & McLaughlin, J. (1997). Structure-activity relationships of diverse Annonaceous acetogenins against multidrug resistant human mammary adenocarcinoma (MCF-7/Adr) cells. Journal of Medical Chemistry, 17, 84-90.
21. Taylor, L. (2005). The Healing Power of Rainforest Herbs. Square One Publishers
22. http://www.cleanse-me-healthy.com/MalicAcid.html

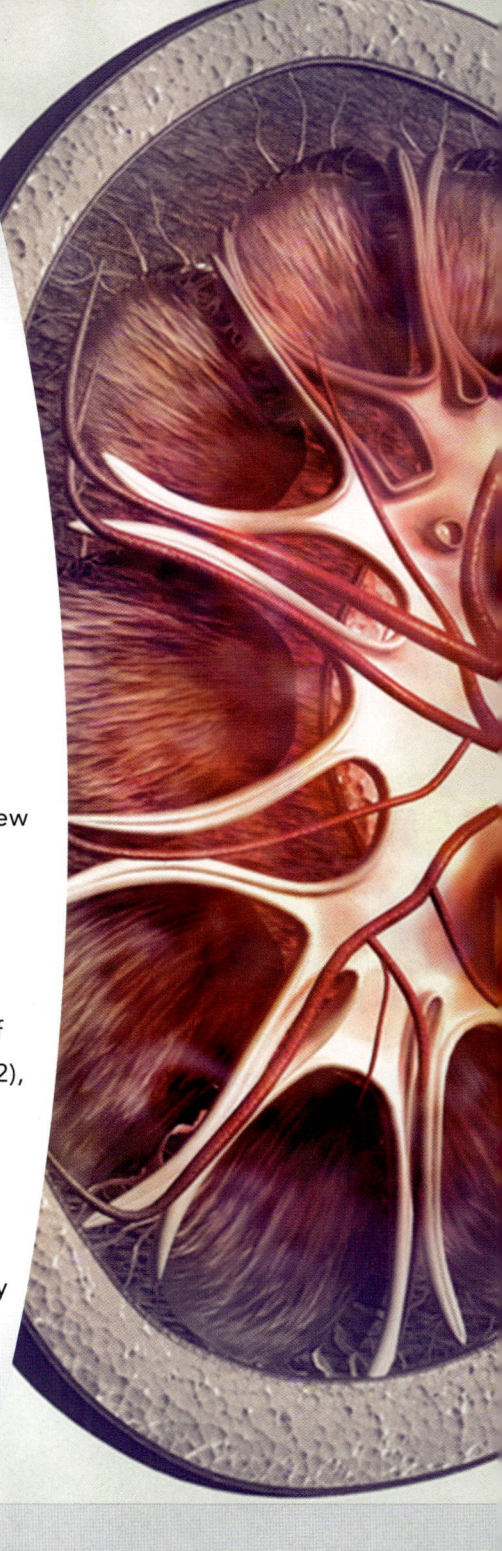

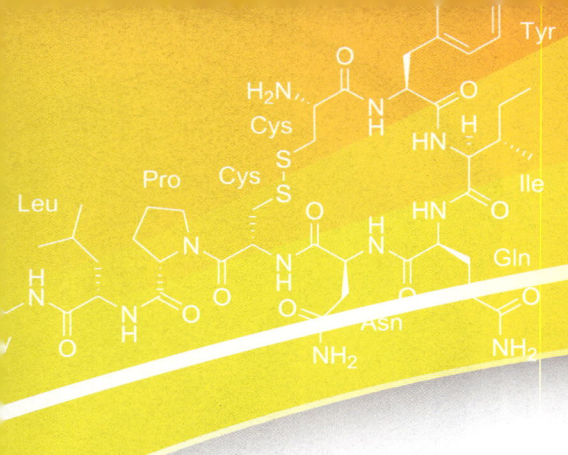

Love Factor
Support for Intimate Relationships

☑ **Do you want strong bonds of love with your family and loved ones?**
☑ **Do you want more cuddle power?**
☑ **Greater orgasms?**

Then oxytocin in Love Factor is your answer! Oxytocin is produced by the hypothalamus - the almond sized region of the brain located close to the brain stem that links the nervous system to the endocrine system via the pituitary gland. It's released either via the pituitary gland straight into the bloodstream or to other parts of the brain and the spinal cord. Modern research has shown that both men and women produce oxytocin and it is crucial for social confidence strong love bonds and sexual enjoyment.

Using Oxytocin can also help regulate sleep patterns, and have a calming effect. Research is ongoing but observation seems to cite Oxytocin's health giving benefits lying in its ability to counteract stress and the effects of the stress hormone cortisol. Nearly every disease and condition is aggravated by stress; anything that can help counteract the stress is therefore useful.

Oxytocin has a clear physical and emotional power. Not only does the hormone increase orgasm in men and women, it has the natural ability to generate meaningful bonds, calm and in turn increase personal wellbeing.

At our body's normal level of production, Oxytocin encourages a mild desire to be kissed and cuddled by your lover. In fact being touched anywhere on the body leads to a rise in Oxytocin levels. This causes a chain reaction within the body, including the release of endorphins and testosterone, which results in both biological and psychological arousal.

Oxytocin In Men & Women

Women, after menopause, will have greatly reduced levels of oxytocin which can cause major relationship problems. In women, oxytocin production in the brain is greatly affected by estrogen levels, which decline after menopause.

It is no surprise that many marriages end in divorce after mid-life. Women experience more loneliness and less life satisfaction after menopause. Before menopause, women's hormone levels increase their ability to care for others and maintain relationships and after menopause the hormones that supported these relationships decline, principally oxytocin.

In men, oxytocin is very important to help maintain empathy. Oxytocin enables men to share their emotions and be empathetic towards the emotions of others. Testosterone tends to decrease our empathetic abilities so having adequate oxytocin is very important

Interestingly, oxytocin increases male empathy while improving your stress response. For example, in a disagreement you need to understand where your partner is coming from, relay how you feel, and do this without losing your "cool". Oxytocin can help so much in this respect. It can be subtle for

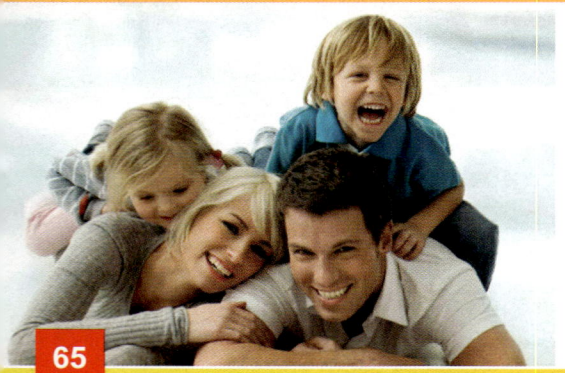

65

some men but others are likely to notice the change. Oxytocin in a sublingual form is rapidly absorbed into the blood stream. "Sublingual" means under the tongue. When formulated correctly, oxytocin levels in the brain can be augmented with a low dose and enhance social interactions. For men who have difficulties doing presentations in front of groups oxytocin can be very helpful because it allows the speaker to connect with the audience while decreasing the stress response (i.e. stage fright).

Love Factor may:

- Enhances social interactions (such as your ability to make eye contact and touch others)
   Reduces social anxiety
- Multiple orgasms in women
- Increases libido in women and helps treat impotence in men
- Generates a feeling of calmness (as one would experience after sex or being with good friends)
- Bonding – helps you connect better with others
   Reduces stress
   Lowers blood pressure in some
- Reduces cravings and addictions
- Eases depression

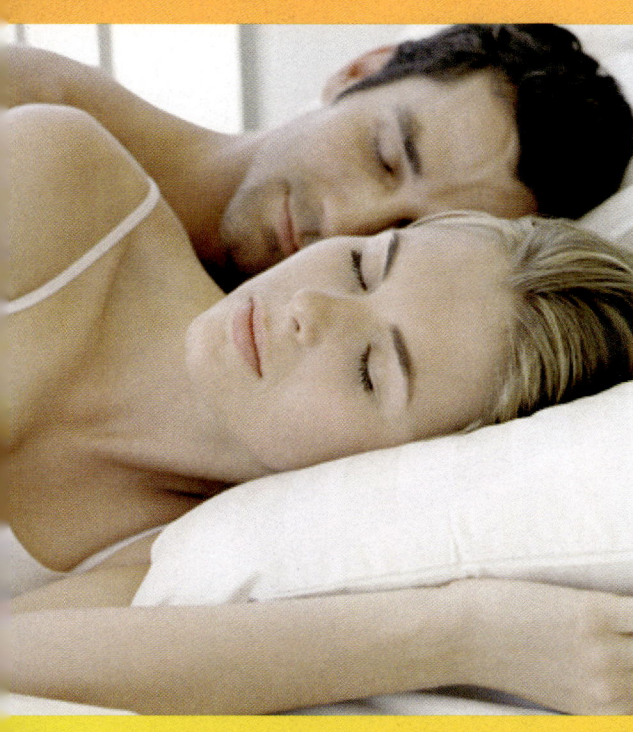

Dr. Tai's Pearl

Think what it would be like if you could live happily in the company of all your loved ones and significant partners to be a blissful dream. This can be accomplished with the help of Love Factor. Research on animals shows your partner is by your side, more loyal and with closer bonds of love. Taken before sexual activity, organisms are more enhanced. Sublingual absorption is direct to the brain, which, as you know is the largest sex organ.

Side Effects:
You will feel very close to your loved ones and family.

Contraindications:
Always take in the presence of your loved ones or significant other. It always works better when they are close when you take the supplement. Do Not take product if you are allergic to any ingredients.

Directions:
Shake well. Take 1 dropper full once daily at night by mouth sublingually.

Ingredients:
Natural Oxytocin, Homeopathic 4C Aloe Extract and Water

These statements have not been reviewed by the FDA. This product is not intended to diagnose, treat, cure, or prevent any disease.

Love Factor - Clinical Applications:
1. Mood Enhancement – Oxytocin – Social Hormone, B. Wheeler et.al, innovative Men's Health. Jan. 2013

66

MAX ADRENAL SPECIALIST

Prevention & Treatment of Adrenal Fatigue

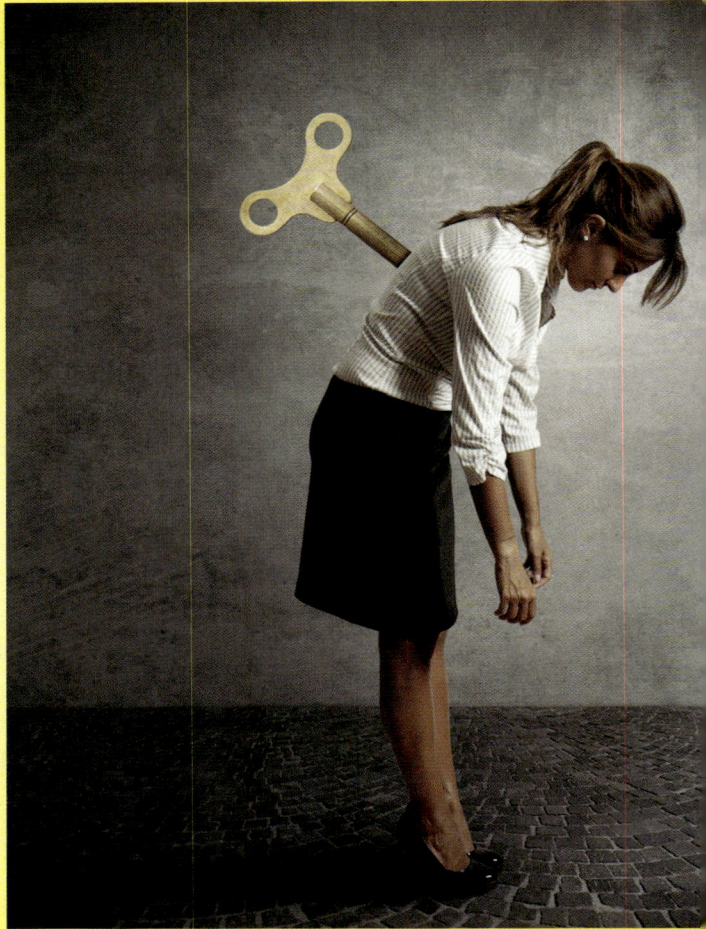

When you suffer from Adrenal Fatigue you feel your life has taken the form of the "Walking dead". You have no energy, can't sleep, you wake up exhausted, your mind is cloudy and foggy and you just feel miserable!

Most supplements don't work for this condition as evidenced by the bag full of vitamins, minerals and herbs which have failed you and thousands of dollars spend on ineffective treatment. Fear no more! Help is here! When you suffer from Severe Adrenal Fatigue or Adrenal exhaustion your Cortisol level in the morning is abnormally depressed and low. No easy treatment is available. In Adrenal Fatigue, your body is completely unable to deal with the stressful situation from your daily activity and home life.

Most of these patients have been going from doctor to doctor and have been undergoing treatment for years with no improvement. They suffer from serious problems such as extremely low energy, insomnia, digestion problems, even osteoporosis, to name just a few of the complications. Adrenal exhaustion further deteriorates the immune system to the point of causing inflammation, out of control and frequent bouts of cold, headaches and sore throat. Adrenal Fatigue is a condition which baffles both the patient as well as doctors. We are all dumbfounded by the inability of these patients to respond to any kind of treatment. They wake up tired and they go to bed tired. Mostly, they are unable to cope with their daily life, work, home and family problems.

Beyond the severe symptoms described, laboratory diagnoses of clinical Adrenal Exhaustion can be confirmed by taking a Saliva test with five samples taken throughout the day. These abnormal patterns, typical of patients suffering from low Cortisol, show the typical very low A.M. Cortisol level to be depressed and continues to be low throughout the day into the evening.

Max Adrenal Specialist incorporates powerful extractions of Glycerrhyza acid, an extract from Licorice Root. This extract has been shown to help modulate and raise cortisol levels and more importantly, Glycerrhyza acid helps to retain the cortisol

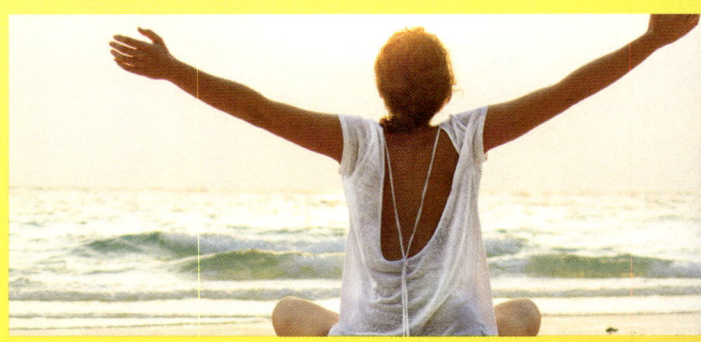

hormone in the body and its activities for greater periods of time, therefore, diminishing the loss of cortisol through excretion, leaving you an ability to keep net cortisol levels at a much higher level. Your body has the ability to tolerate stress, feels better, has more positive energy, rebuilding the tissues in the body and overcoming digestion problems, as well as circulatory abnormalities.

Max Adrenal Specialist's proprietary formula also contains centuries old Panax Ginseng, Astragulus and Eleutherococcus. These herbs are well-known, powerful and have been known to be Adaptogenic for many centuries. They are widely acclaimed throughout the world to help the adrenal gland cope with daily stress. Lastly, it contains the homeopathic Adrenalinum (3C) to help with the extraordinary job of recovering the adrenal cortex's production of its natural cortisol.

Directions:
Take 1 capsule daily as needed. See your health professional for higher dosage. Keep out of reach of children.

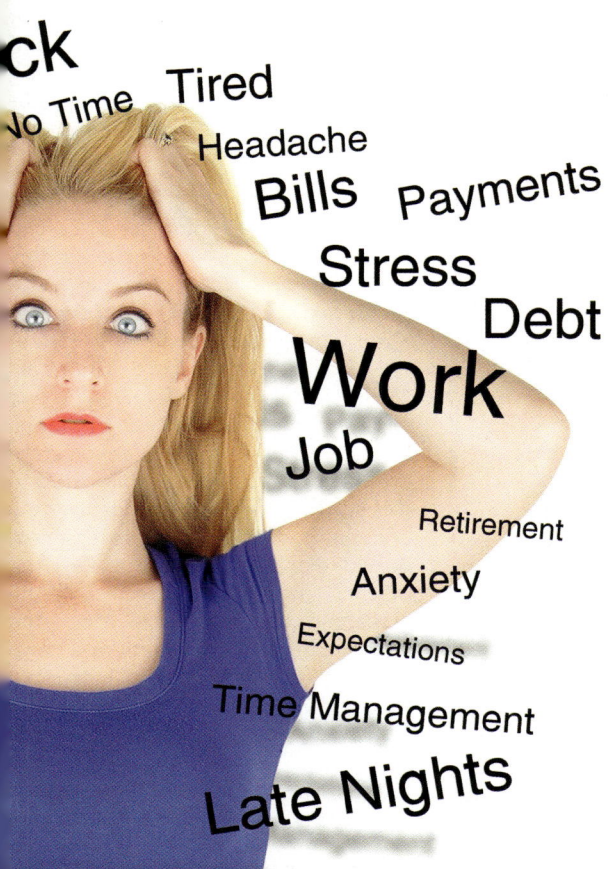

Dr. Tai's Pearl

Life has not much meaning when you have adrenal complications and fatigue. You don't seem to do anything right because you have no energy and you just want to lie down and die. It is a feeling you will never forget if you encounter it even once. It is far worse if you have to live with it for several months or years. It becomes unbearable. You see no joy and all of the anti-depressants in the world will not help you because the problem is not psychological or emotional, but physical. None of the supplements can help you if you don't address the main underlying condition of adrenal insufficiency. There is no hope in any treatment if there is not enough glucose produced from the cortisol that is made in the adrenal cortex. It is a true prerequisite health and wellness to have a properly functioning adrenal gland.

Clinical Case:
36-year-old secretary to a major executive in a Fortune 500 company. Life could not be better – great job, fortunate to work with one of the smartest men in the business world, beautiful surroundings, plush office on the 30th floor of a skyscraper. All the life and work security you could wish for. So why was she so miserable? She couldn't get up in the morning to go to work – didn't want to go to work. Throughout the day she would struggle with sleepiness and fatigue, trying to stay awake by drinking super strong Italian coffee, to the point where she was experiencing arrhythmia and jitteriness, but still tired. This is the miserable life of a woman with adrenal fatigue. Her doctor put her on a protocol using Cordyceps, Super B12 Sublingual, Ionic Microminerals, Daily Energy, Daily Wellness and Max Adrenal three times a day, morning, noon and 3 p.m. Although it is well-known that the adrenal gland recuperates extremely slowly (like watching paint dry), she was within two months, already seeing the results of her doctors protocol. She was establishing a routine of 8 – 9 hours of sleep, avoiding fast food, gluten, and dairy, and was well on her way to regaining her health and sanity.

Side Effects:
May result in water retention (rare) and could possible lead to increased blood pressure.

Contraindications:
Hypertension, kidney failure, active infection (bacterial or viral). Do not take product if you are allergic to any ingredients.

Ingredients:
Proprietary Formulation, Adrenalinum, Panax Ginseng, Astralagus, Eleutherococcus, Glycerrhyza, Panthothernin Acid, Manganese Chelate
These statements have not been reviewed by the FDA. This product is not intended to diagnose, treat, cure, or prevent any disease.

68

Max Arthro Specialist
Maintain Joint Health

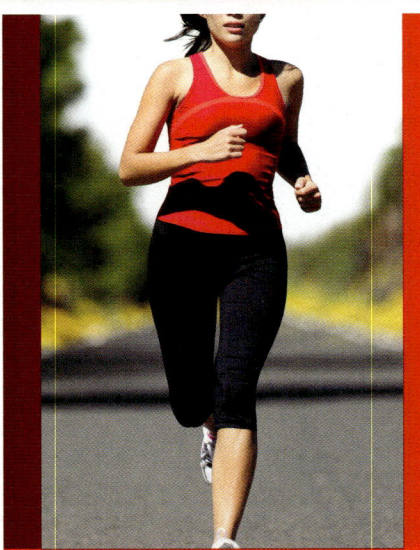

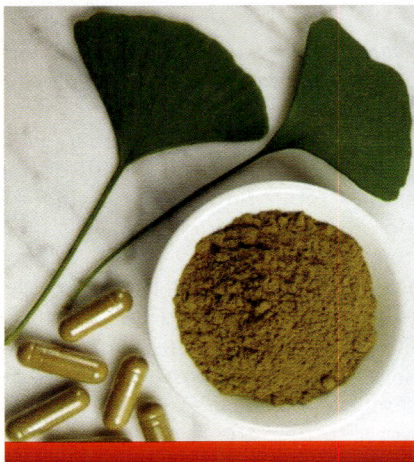

What makes Max Arthro different?

A New Formulation of purified extract of several rare and extraordinary Oriental herbs: Clematis Chinensis, Trichosanthes Kirilowii and Prunella vulgaris, ginger oil and white willow extract. These outstanding herbal extracts have been used for centuries in Asia as an anti-inflammatory for joints and arthritic diseases.

A published research paper on Clematis Chinensis, Trichosanthes Kirilowii and Prunella demonstrates the anti-arthritic effect. This was a rigid, Double Blind, controlled clinical study, evaluated for the efficacy and safety against a placebo in 96 patients with classical Osteoarthritis of the knee. This formulation demonstrated a powerful clinical efficacy, with fabulous results according to the patients and in the investigators' opinion on the positive therapeutic effect, with no significant side effects noted. In summary, this study demonstrates a new triple herbal extract with powerful anti-arthritic agents providing excellent clinical efficacy in patients with osteoarthritis and/or joint pain with arthritis.

Osteoarthritis is a degenerative joint disease that may develop into severe disability and pain. It is primarily distinguished by the progressive loss of articular cartilage and by severe reactive changes in the subchondral bone. Continuously worsening joint pain with acute flare-ups, joint enlargements and severe limitation of movement are frequent manifestations of Osteoarthritis and require immediate attention (Altman, 1991).

Over the past decade, several non steroidal anti-inflammatory drugs (NSAID) have been used to treat osteoarthritis and other kinds of arthritis. But their usefulness has always been limited because of their multiple adverse gastrointestinal and renal side effects (Murray and Brater, 1990). There were new classes of selective COX II inhibitors which have been taken off the market recently by the FDA due to severe side effects of cardiovascular diseases.

Max Arthro is a new formulation of pure extractions of herbs with multiple functions which may help with anti-inflammatory, analgesic and improved micro-circulation with protection against joint cartilage degeneration.

An analysis of six hundred (600) different oriental herbs that have been widely used in past centuries for the treatment of inflammatory diseases, such as arthritis in the Far East, resulted in researchers carefully selecting 53 herbs. They studied their anti-inflammatory, analgesic and anti-arthritic activity with blood micro-circulation enhancing activities and inhibition of cartilage degeneration enzyme.

Using different biological screening systems, they were able to identify only 3 herbs, this special combination of Clematis Chinensis, Trichosanthes Kirilowii and Prunella vulgaris (Park et al., 1995; Ahn et al., 1996; Kim et al, 1996) as most effective. In two separate medical centers in Seoul, Korea, 96 patients with classic osteoarthritis of the knee were allocated to this study. After 4 weeks of taking a combination of these three essential herbal extracts, 3 times a day, the efficacy rating reported by the research investigators, with the agreement of the patient's own assessment, showed an incredible 95.8% improvement from "fair to very good". Safety and tolerability assessment of all 96 patients showed no different than the placebo group. There were also no clinical observable changes in blood pressure, pulse rate or any significant differences in laboratory parameters, from serum biochemistry, urinalysis or hematology on all the groups. It is truly an exciting opportunity to offer a formulation of pure, natural, extraction of herbs directed exclusively to the relief of pain and inflammation with improvement of micro-circulation and cartilage.

A special ginger extract (Gingerol) has been added to this fabulous formulation. Ginger extract has been studied as an effective alternative to NSAID therapy for arthritic condition. A randomized, placebo controlled, cross-over study comparing ginger extract with Ibuprofen was performed on 75 individuals with arthritis in the hip or knee (Bliddal et al, 2000). Patients who had received ginger extract vs. Ibuprofen in the study received

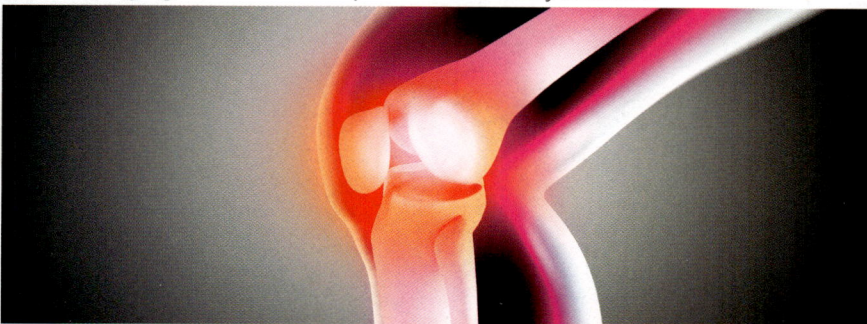

significant improvement of symptoms. (Dr. Phan, 2005, Journal of Alternative Complimentary Medicine, Division of Arthritis Surgery at John Hopkins University Medical School) The ginger extract shows that it has a positive suppression of inflammation in arthritis and is primarily attributed to the suppression of pro-inflammatory Cytokinins produced by the joints. The study found that ginger formulation may be useful in suppressing inflammation due to arthritis. Dr. Patrick B. Massey, M.D. told the Chicago Daily Herald on March 15, 2004 of the positive effects of ginger extract on knee pain in patients with osteoarthritis. This was published in the Arthritis and Rheumatism Journal, Vol 44, Nov 2001.

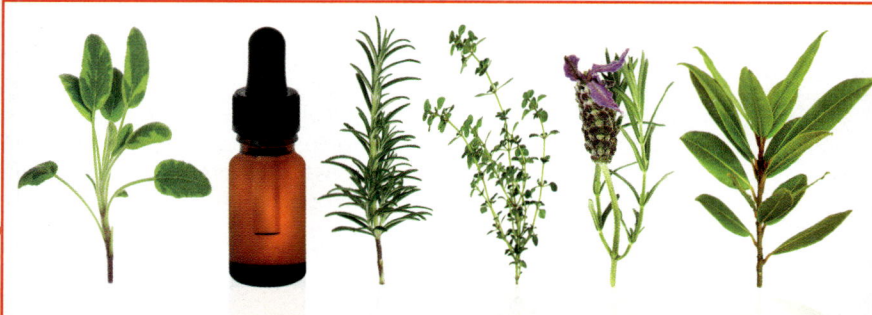

A unique, natural and clinically proven formula for arthritis with a 95.8% improvement reported by investigators and patients without negative side effects, Max Arthro may be an outstanding technological breakthrough and remarkable product.

Directions:
Take 1 capsule three times daily as needed. For additional pain control, take 2 capsules. The improvements will reach the best potential after taking for 1 or 2 months. Product must be taken with food. Keep out of reach of children.

Dr. Tai's Pearl
Most arthritis medications and supplements tend to neutralize COX-1 and interfere with its activity in the stomach. This causes major side effects and complications. The beauty of this particular formulation is that it does not have this side effect.

Clinical Case:
Ten years ago, I tore the rotator cuff on my right shoulder and there was a significant period of time during which I could not lift my arm more than 10 – 15 degrees. Most doctors who evaluated recommended surgical reconstruction of the right shoulder followed by rehabilitation. I chose to take Max Arthro together with Max Pain and begin gradual physical therapy on my own. After a few months, the shoulder went back to normal range of motion was within normal limits. Today I have absolutely no discomfort and have full activity and usage.

Side Effects:
Max Arthro is best taken with food, as it may occasionally cause irritation of the stomach lining.

Contraindications:
Untreated stomach ulcer, ibuprofen therapy. Do not take product if you are allergic to any of its ingredients.

Ingredients:
Trichosantis Kirilowii, Prunella Vulgaris, Clematis Sinensis, Ginger Extract, Dl- Phenylalanine, White Willow Extract, Piperine Extract, Gelatin Capsules, Magnesium, Stearate, Silica

These statements have not been reviewed by the FDA. This product is not intended to diagnose, treat, cure, or prevent any disease.

Max Bio Cell

Complete Herbal Protocol for Cancer Cells

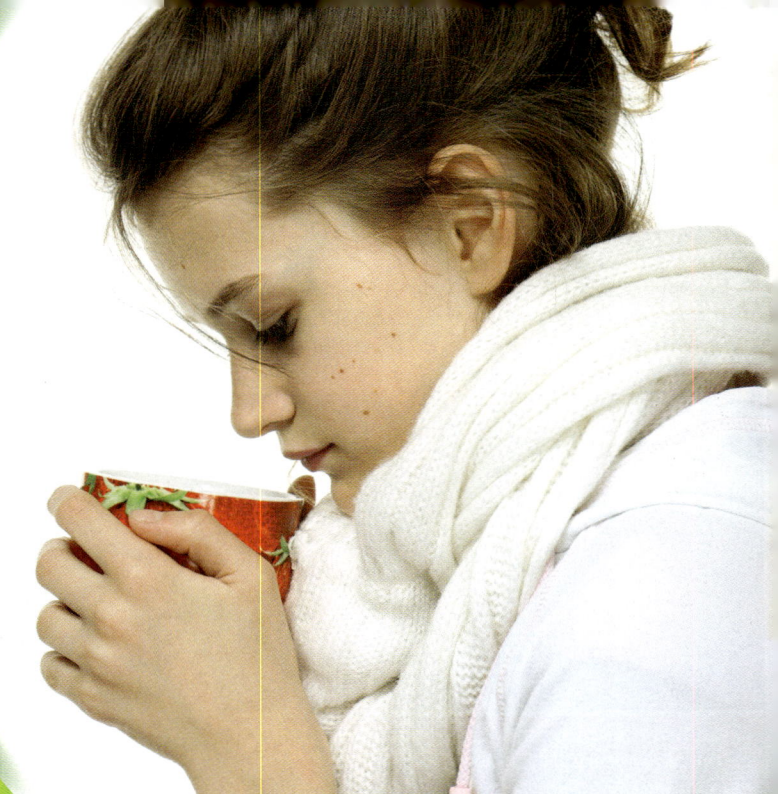

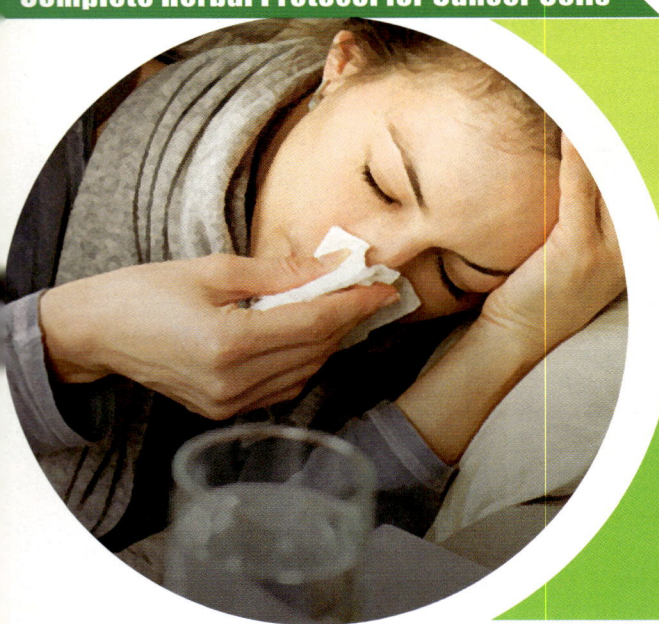

The antimicrobial properties of Poetical invitro studies show activity against bacteria, fungi and yeast, including typical fungus aspergillosis as well as Candida bacteria, such as Streptococcus, Pneumonia, Staphtococcus, H. Pylori, Tuberculosis and Dysentery. As reported by Anesini, C. et al in the Ethno Pharmacol 1993, it was strong enough to inhibit the Certimonis type of bacteria and Brucella. It shows strong activity against eleven fungus and yeast strains. In vitro studies show antiviral activity against Herpes 1 and Herpes 2, Influenza, Polio Virus and Stomach Virus as reported by Dr. Ueda, S. and Simoes, CM, et al in Phytomedicine in 1999. Many Anti-Parasitic actions were confirmed against Malaria, Schistosoma and Trypanosome.

Some of the top herbal researchers in the world have stolen the wonderful qualities of (CAT'S CLAW) Unadde Ghec One of the major herbal secrets of the Amazon rain forest is related to the species of Uncaria. The South American Indigenous People of the Amazon Rain Forest have been using cat's claw for hundreds of years.

The great history of herbal medicine in Chinese civilization stands out above all others. Singular and most powerful is Panax Ginseng. The word Panax is Greek for the root of man. Ginseng contains approximately 25 different Dammarane Saponin Glycosides called Aglycone Saponin that have been carefully isolated including capital Rf, Rb1, Rg1, Rg2, Re, etc.

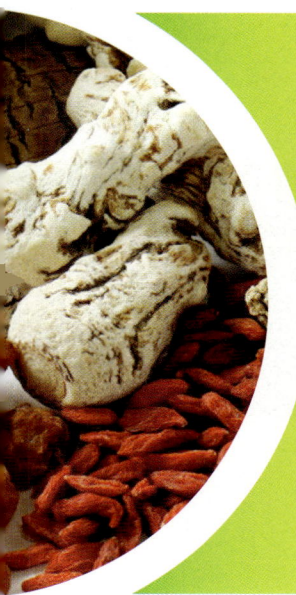

Panax Ginseng has many magnificent qualities. The anti-tumor extractions from these Saponins has been researched throughout the world with over 500 published studies showing inhibition of growth of several Cancer cell lines, as published by Matsunaga in 1989. It is confirmed with growth inhibition of Cycoma cells in tissue culture by Fugi Moto in Phyto-chemistry in 1987. In Korea, large clinical studies on the control scenario have been performed with ginseng suggesting its cancer preventive activities by Yun et al. Dr. Sharon Kruger of the department of environmental toxicology and Dr. David Williams, a professor of environmental and molecular toxicology and LPI principle investigator. They showed in their laboratory an in-vitro study that the specific Saponins were able to show great effects on the cancer cells and significant tumor cells when administered in high dosage. Within 10 days the number of cancer cells had been reduced by 98%.

The crude fraction was able to kill breast cancer cells while the other Saponins were less effective. The use of Saponins together with traditional Cancer therapy, such as Cystplatin, according to Dr. Kikuchiy, et al, from Anti-cancer Drugs in February 1991, publication showed that with the Saponins, the Cancer growth was inhibited, much more than the group that was using cystplatin alone. Dr. Matsu Naga H, from the published Cancer Chemotherapy in 1994, said that with the addition of the Panax Ginseng effect on Sarcoma Cell Line MK-1, the kill rate of the Cancer Cells was significantly higher than with Matitomycin, a typical anti-Cancer medication.

Dr. Tote T. et al, reported in the Journal of Cancer Research Clinic Oncol. 1993 that Ovarian Cancer Cells in mice had lower volume in all groups treated with the Saponins. This study group's Ovarian Cancer Cells were significantly inhibited compared to that of Cyplastin alone or in the controlled group. Research has showed that the usage of Aglycon Saponins from the Panax Ginseng has demonstrated more beneficial effects than other herbs and drugs in anticarcinogenic activity and cancer cells death by multiple fold of up to 500 times. This provides an incredible leverage and strategy in enhancing the clinical efficiency of these herbs.

Directions:
Take 1-4 capsules, 3 times daily as needed or as instructed by your physician or health practitioner. Keep out of reach of children.

Ingredients:
T-Brevifolia, Graviola Extract, Pau De Arco Ext., Una Gato Ext., Reishi/Shitaki, Piperine, P Ginseng Extract, Sapogenin

These statements have not been reviewed by the FDA. This product is not intended to diagnose, treat, cure, or prevent any disease.

Dr. Tai's Pearl

I have always wanted to create a product where most of the powerful antioxidants, such as una de gato, as well as yew tree extract, are in one formula. I had wanted to use this formula for myself because of hypertrophy of the prostate and a large tumor formation. I have suffered from this with an inability to urinate. Supplementation has been an extremely useful component of my treatment. I am, completely symptom-free and it has been confirmed by physician's examination that I no longer suffer from prostatic hypertrophy.

Side Effects:
Hexheimer reaction taken together with many cases of protocols

Contraindications:
Organ transplants. Do not take this product if you are allergic to any of its ingredients.

Max Bone Specialist
Increase Bone Strength & Mineralization 200%!!

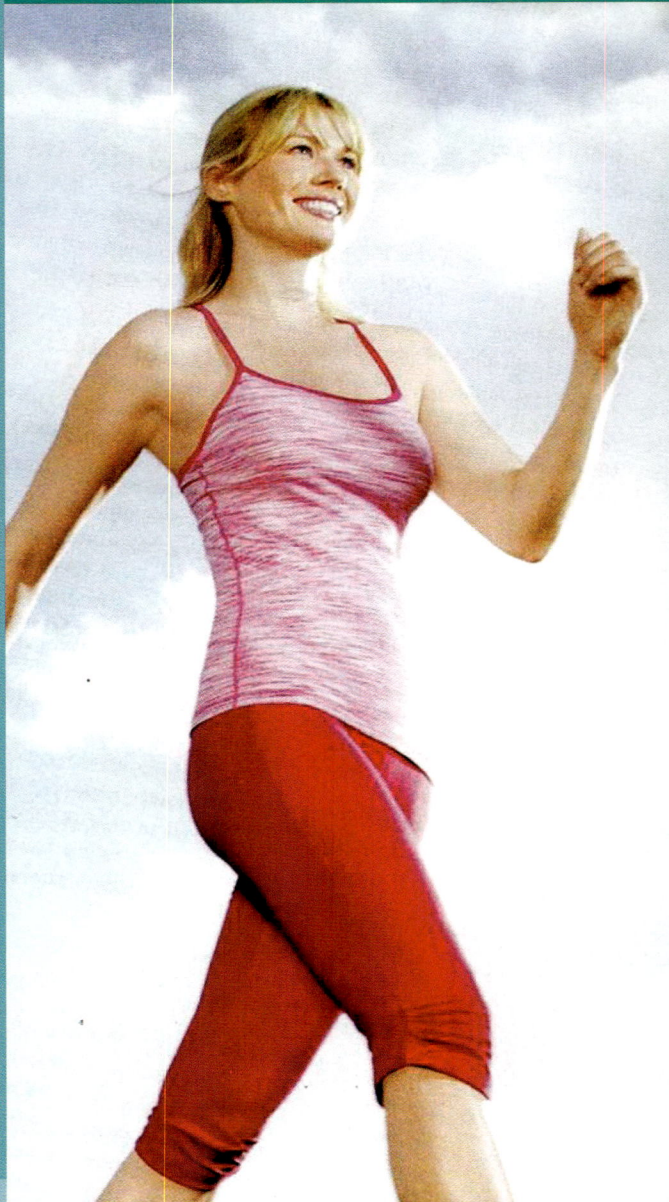

Dear Grandma and Grandpa,

Most often Osteoporosis affects both men and women over 50 (although I understand that it affects women 300 percent more than it affects men). This statistic is why I'm writing you two. I figure reading a letter from your favorite grandchild (me) will have more of an effect on both of you than if I were to just stand there and tell you.

The truth is—I love you both and I'm scared. I hear a lot of the kids in my class complain about their grandparents fracturing their hips and spines. They're in and out of the hospital constantly. According to the research conducted at the University of Southern California, Osteoporosis causes 700,000 fractures a year and these fractures have the potential to cause permanent damage or even death (knocking on wood).

And I know that you guys have osteoporosis for a variety of reasons:

1) Both of you are shrinking
2) I never see you two drink milk
3) Instead of exercising, you two sit on the couch or outside on your lawn chairs
4) Last but not least (drum-roll) I know you two are well past 50, because, well, mom told me, but please don't tell her I told you.

You both should have done something about these problems awhile ago but since you didn't, we need to work fast! I heard about Dr. Tai's Bone Specialist treatment and I really think you should give it a shot. The ingredients are all natural. It should really help you both and avoid nasty things like fractures and broken bones from happening. Anyway, here's a bottle. I used up my allowance to pay for it so you'd better use it or else I won't take my Flintstones.

With love, Pookie

Got Milk? No? Then you've got problems. 35,000,000 Americans have Osteoporosis, 1,500,000 have spontaneous fractures a year and 150,000 die from them. If that doesn't scare you—it'll probably scare someone who cares about you.

Worried about yourself or someone you love? Well, you should be! Osteoporosis is a big deal and we're glad you're thinking about it. Americans experience more than a million fractures per year!

Osteoporosis is when your bones become so porous and weak that they eventually cave in and collapse; think of a badly baked cake. We need our bones, it's our structure and it's what keeps us from standing nice and tall. It occurs mostly among women who are post-menopausal, but don't let that fool you. Men are great candidates for Osteoporosis too. As a result of demineralized bones, 2,000,000 men a year suffer from Osteoporosis.

The National Osteoporosis Foundation reported that 1 out of 8 men are diagnosed with Osteoporosis and from it other illnesses may develop (Dr. Lauren Lipson. University of Southern California—2004).

Bone Specialist is a special proprietary and unique formula that may support skeletal strength naturally so you don't have to worry about taking a pill that has more side effects than it does benefits.

But before we explain remember…

70 percent of bones are made up of protein
95 percent of that protein is Collagen

The remaining 30 percent is made up of minerals like: calcium, potassium, sodium and magnesium. Therefore, in order to make up for the bone mass you've lost you'll need to replace minerals!

Superpowers in a Super mineral

Bone Specialist's main ingredient is: Strontium, an ionic crystallized substitution for Calcium. Strontium is the Superman in Clark Kent and the Wonder Woman in Diana Prince. It is Calcium—amplified, enhanced and improved. Strontium is more effective than Calcium and this is what you'll need, especially if Osteoporosis has started to take effect on you.

Strontium works? Prove it

In 2001, BONE J. exposed a few case studies on strontium and its effects on Osteoporosis. A group of researchers gathered 353 people who suffered at least one vertebrae (back and spine) fracture due to Osteoporosis. Each study participant took strontium but some took a lesser dose than others. Those that took a daily dose of 680 mg daily had a much greater increase in vertebrae bone mineral density per year than those that did not take it on a daily basis (Osteoporosis Journal Int. 2002. Meunier, P.J., et al. The Effects of Osteoporosis Risk of Vertebral Fracture in Women That Are Post-Menopausal).

In addition, a 2004 study produced by the NEW ENGLAND J. MED. showed the subjects that consumed Strontium had a 14.4 percent increase in back-bone density and an 8.3 percent in thigh bone density. See, we told you strontium works!

Bone Specialist is formulated with Fulvic and Humate along with 80 other essential micro-nutrients, which may aid in the absorption of Strontium. The formula ensures the minerals go directly towards the bones that are in need of the most help and protects the other bones from further damage.

Directions: Take two capsules per day. Must be taken on an empty stomach

Dr. Tai's Pearl

It is always wonderful to have a formulation that address or improves a condition so easily, yet most people don't know about it. You feel privileged to have found the pearl on a vast, empty beach.

Clinical Case:

Susan, a retired CPA, 72 years of age. After her annual physical, her physician diagnosed her with osteoporosis, having run DEXA of her bone. She indicated that the prescription medications that are given for osteoporosis carry a great number of side effects that could complicate her life, but do not seem to reverse osteoporosis, but halt the progression. It doesn't get better, but it doesn't get worse. What she wasn't told was that most of these osteoporosis medications are really very dangerous and caustic and contain chemicals very much like Drain-O to clear up your bathtub sink. It doesn't help with the osteoporosis because it doesn't really help to deposit bone. Instead it mummifies the bone so that DEXA, which takes a pictures of the bones, continues to show the status quo. However, the FDA has already warned that spontaneous fracture continues to be a severe complication because the medications do not strengthen the bone. Further, dangerous side effects the physician alluded to are really things like cancer of the jaw, eating away half the face, heart attacks, and other fatal conditions. Susan instead took the Max Bone on a double-dose, including taking a saliva test which showed she had lost the Estradiol as well as DHEA and Testosterone. Supplementation with transdermal was applied at the same time and within one year she was able to return to her family physician that confirmed she no longer has osteoporosis and was now in recovery with osteopenia. Another year passed, when the physician, upon examination with DEXA, was able to tell her she no longer has osteoporosis or osteopenia, and that her bones appear to be within normal limits.

Side Effects: None

Contraindications:
Do not take with calcium. Do not take product if you are allergic to any of its ingredients.

Ingredients: Proprietary Blend: 800mg* Strontium Carbonate, Humate, Fulvate

These statements have not been reviewed by the FDA. This product is not intended to diagnose, treat, cure, or prevent any disease.

MAX
BRAIN SPECIALIST
Greater MultiTasking & Brain Power!

Do you want to have a powerful, strong mind for active and healthy living? Here lies the secret to aiding the recovery of an aging brain and reversing cognitive decline. You will become more attentive, have higher concentration ability for everyday living, and be able to apply your mind to its maximum capacity. Whether you're remembering your daughters dance recital or son's soccer practice schedule or completing the daily crossword puzzle, your mind will be sharp, clear, and quick.

As we grow older there is a loss of metabolic efficiency and lower level of the natural compounds that are part of the normal and effective brain physiology. Research reports that over 50 % of individuals approaching the age of 75 to 80 years old have some form of Dementia. Many of the natural compounds, which help with the electrical conduction, and the neural transmission of nerve cell to nerve cell are called Synapses.

Glycerophosphocholine (or GPC) is one of the beneficial ingredients of the proprietary formulation in Max Brain. GPC is a lipid which is vital for survival. It is an abundant ingredient contained in a mother's milk and provides her baby with cognitive benefits for healthy development.[1] GPC is present in almost all living things and it is an orthomolecule that is part of the body's natural biochemical function.[2] Key functions include indispensable molecular building blocks for all cells and maintaining healthy cholesterol management. GPC is an emulsifier to assist in digestion and is a messenger to other nutritional substances.[3] Studies have shown GPC boosted even a healthy mind, recovered waning cognitive function, and exhibited impressive growth-promoting effects in the brain. GPC gives significant protection to the brain's attention and memory capacity.[4,5]

Hericium Erinaceus (or lion's mane) is a Chinese edible and medicinal mushroom, progressively becoming recognized for its multitude of health promoting and anti-aging effects. In a recent study, a dose of 200 mg per kg of body weight substantially reduced plasma total cholesterol by 32.9%, low density lipoprotein cholesterol by 45.4%, triglyceride levels by 34.3% and increased plasma high density lipoprotein cholesterol by 31.1%.[6] Important physiological functions in humans include antioxidant activity, regulation of blood lipid levels and reduction of blood glucose levels.[7] Hericium Erinaceus' cognitive enhancements include, but is not limited to, nerve cell modulation, with potent inductive activity for nerve growth factor synthesis.[8]

Rhodiola Rosea is a flowering herb in the Crassulaceae family and is the only one utilized for its potential health benefits. It is the plant's roots that are most valued for their purported medicinal properties. The roots contain numerous antioxidants, tannins, flavonoids and rosavins, an active compound believed to produce antidepressant and anxiolytic (anti-anxiety) effects. Rhodiola Rosea treatment resulted in a significant improvement of mental performance, enhancing speed of visual and audio perception, increasing attention capacity and improving short-term memory.[9] Rhodiola Rosea has also been shown to have beneficial effects on creatine kinase, expressed by various tissues and cell types, after exhausting exercise.[10] Rhodiola Rosea has been traditionally used for the prevention of fatigue and the enhancement of physical and mental performance.

Benefits from Glycerophosphocholine include:
- Mental Performance
- Improved Memory
- Improved Attention
- Improved Activities of Daily Living
- Improved Mood Including Irritability and Emotional Lability
- Revitalized Mind
- Renewed Interest in Loved Ones

Additional benefits from Hericium Erinaceus include:
- Anti-tumor / Anti-cancer
- Nerve growth factor modulator
- Immuno-modulation
- Myelination augmentation
- Nerve cell modulator
- Anti-oxidant
- Anti-mutagenesis
- Cholesterol / Blood lipid lowering
- Anti-allergy / contact sensitivity
- Hypoglycemic effect (blood sugar lowering)
- Anti-atherosclerotic

Further benefits of Rhodiola Rosea which is documented for curing ailments such as:
- Fatigue
- Infection
- Alleviating physical or mental stressors
- Wide variety of illnesses and conditions
- Post stress and fatigue, restoring the body to normal healthy function
- Impotence

Directions: Take 1 capsule 2 times daily or higher dosages as needed or as directed by your doctor/health practitioner.

Ingredients: Hericium Erinaceus Extract (Lion's Mane) Rhodiola Rosea PE, Panax Ginseng PE, Glycerophosphocholine, Gelatin, Magnesium, and Cellulose These statements have not been reviewed by the FDA. This product is not intended to diagnose, treat, cure, or prevent any disease.

1. Holmes-McNary M and others. Choline and choline esters in human and rat milk and in infant formulas. Am. J. Clin. Nutrition 1996; 64: 572-6.
2. Pauling L. Orthomolecular psychiatry. Science 1968; 160: 265-73.
3. Kidd PM. Dietary Phospholipids as Anti-Aging Nutraceuticals. In, Anti-Aging Medical Therapeutics, Vol. IV, ed. Klatz RA, Goldman R. Chicago, IL: Health Quest Publications; 2000.
4. Kidd PM. PS (PHosphatidylSerine), Nature's Brain Booster for Memory, Mood, and Stress. St. George, UT, USA: Total Health Communications; 2005.
5. Canal N, Franceschi M, Alberoni M and others. Effect of L-a-glyceryl-phosphorylcholine on amnesia caused by scopolamine. Intl J. Clin. Pharmacol. Ther. Toxicology 1991; 29: 103-7.
6. Chyi, W.J., H.S. Hui, W.J. Teng, C.K. Shao and C.Y. Chen, 2005. Hypoglycemic effect of extract of Hericium erinaceus. Journal of the Science of Food and Agriculture., 85(4): 641-646.
7. Gue, S.C., S.J. Woo, C.J. Hyo, C.C. Kwan, Y.C. Heui, C.W. Tae and H.S. Hyun, 2006. Macrophage activation and nitric oxide production by water soluble component of Hericium erinaceum. International–Immunopharmacology., 6(8): 1363-1369.
8. Kawagishi H, Ando M, Sakamoto H, Yoshida S, Ojima F, Ishiguro Y, et al. Hericenones C, D and E,stimulators of nerve growth factor (NGF)–synthesis, from the mushroom Hericium erinaceum. Tetrahedron Lett 1991;32(35):4561 -4.
9. Kelly GS. Rhodiola rosea: a possible plant adaptogen, Altern Med Rev 6(3):293-302, 2001.
10. Abidov M, Grachev S, Seifulla RD, Ziegenfuss TN: Extract of Rhodiola rosea radix reduces the level of C-reactive protein and creatinine kinase in the blood, Bull Exp Biol Med 138(1):63-64, 2004.

Dr. Tai's Pearl

It is very difficult to actually have any supplement that helps with focus, attention and memory. The brain is extremely well protected and isolated by the Blood Brain Barrier. Most supplements are not able to cross this barrier. They may appear to work in a laboratory test in vitro; however individual patients actual real-life experience of taking the supplements show it does little or no good whatsoever. So it was with great pride that we were able to find the ingredients to make this supplement, which work synergistically to cross the BBB and actually work on improving focus, multi-tasking, memory, and concentration.

Clinical Case:
56-year-old physician and medical writer. Rather famous for her published books, she was a prolific writer and very accomplished. She confided in me that for the past two years she was unable to write because of either write because of either lack of motivation or having a writer's cramp. She felt very depressed over her lack of productivity. She has tried a number of different supplements to no avail. Upon taking Max Brain, together with Super B12 Sublingual, Pregnenolone transdermal, and Max Sea Extract, she was able to, within 2 weeks, start once again to go back and begin her new book. She was absolutely elated.

Side Effects:
When the dosage is too high, individuals may experience anxiety and a feeling of being hyper. In certain individuals, it may cause some hand trembling and hypertension. Lowering the dosage may help mitigate the side effects, as well as taking the supplement only every 2 – 3 days.

Contraindications:
Severe, untreated hypertension, brain tumors. Do not take product if you are allergic to any of its ingredients.

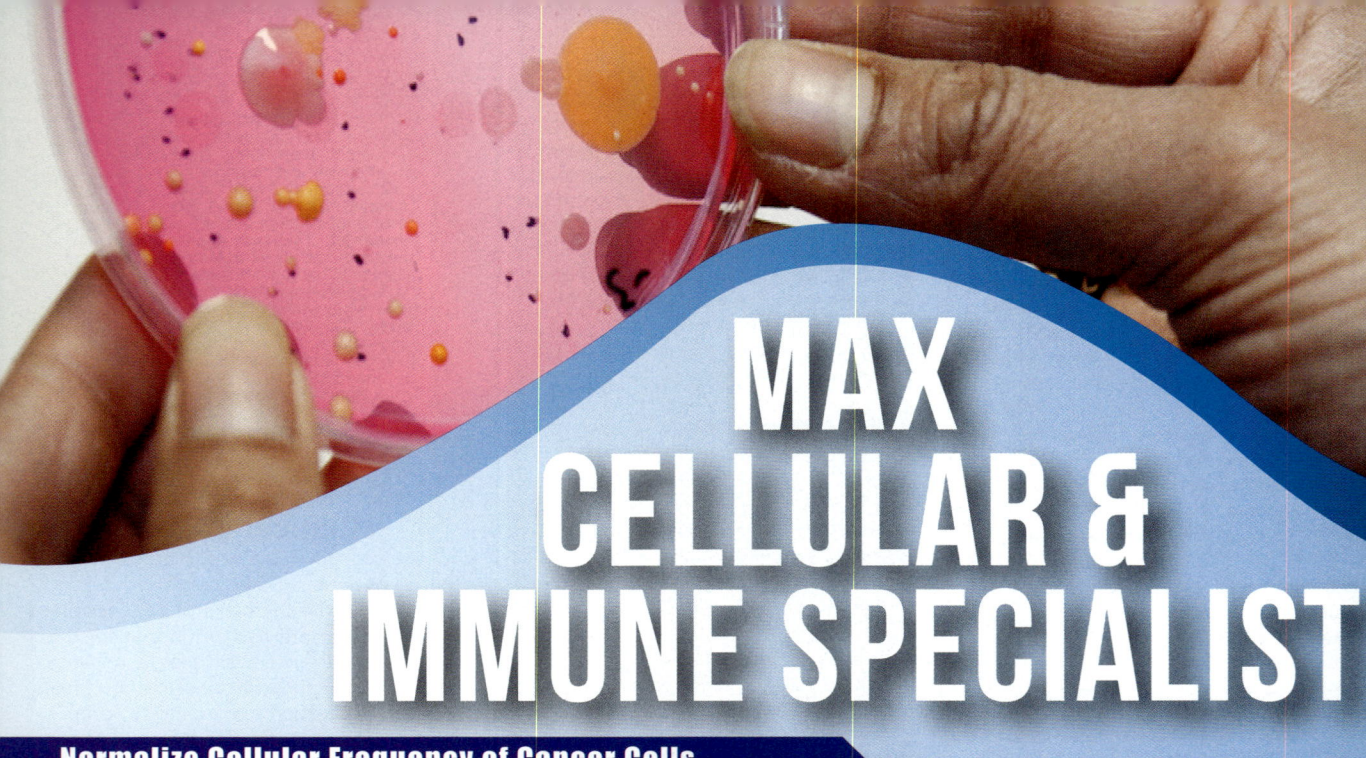

MAX CELLULAR & IMMUNE SPECIALIST

Normalize Cellular Frequency of Cancer Cells

Recently a major break thru occurred in the field of Cellular Pathology – involving Tumor growth and the cellular biochemistry of Cancer.

A group of scientist & researchers from Purdue University spent over 25 years working on the intricacies & biochemistry of what causes the rampant, uncontrolled growth of a cell leading to cysts, tumors and of course, ultimately Cancer.

The extraordinary discoveries explained why the Nobel Prize "Warburg Principles of Cause to Cancer" were correct, but actually shines a bright light on the details of Exto-Chemistry occurring on the cellular membrane of Cancer cells[1].

There is a specific Exto-Protein attached to the outer membrane of the cell only present in Cancer Cells located on chromosome Xq25-q26.2[2]. This Exto-Protein is particular only to Cancer Cells. No Exto-Protein equals NO Cancer cells, period! If a cell has the Exto-Protein then the cell definitely has Cancer activities, with the change of the Cellular Biological Oscillatory clock period length to 22 minutes. All normal proteins are in the oscillatory period length of 24 minutes[3].

Our new focus for healthy cellular physiology is to prevent and/or "knock off" this Exto-Protein pathology. Without the Exto-Protein, the cell can return to its physiologically normal growth & death cycle. Healthy cell activity involves regular Apoptosis (cell death) to create a new cell to replace the old one.

This Auto-Regeneration is healthy to our body. To achieve and maintain healthy biochemistry of the cellular membrane, we have discovered that Green Tea Extract Consumption always results in low incidence of Breast Cancer4.

It was further evaluated that very specific Polyphenols with special (-) Epigallocatechin Gallate offer very specific extracts when purified (no caffeine). This was determined in a Phase II study at the National Cancer Institute. The Research shows that the largest margins of safety and therapeutic effectiveness come with mixing Vanilloid Extracts. Therefore a Catechin-Vanilloid combination was created with applications to normalize biochemical activity of the cellular membrane knocking out the Exto-Protein. A Specific Vanillic acid of Capsicum extract was used in this Catechin-Vanilloid acid synergism[5]. We used a Proprietary Special Ratio of mixtures not known previously.

The Vanilloids attach to the Exto-Protein during the oxidative portion of the cycle, and the Catechin combines with the interchange portion of the Reducing Cycle.

The research shows that the Catechin-Vanilloid combination is up to 100 times more effective than either extract alone[6].

Both the prevention and the reversal of Exto-Protein can be achieved if we have the Vanilloid-Catechin combination in exactly the right ratio or proportions to remove the Exto-Protein from the cell membrane. Catechin must be present in the culture of Cancer cells at a level of 1nm to remove or inhibit the Exto-Protein for 72 continuous hours which is what is needed for apoptosis to be induced in Cancer Cells[7].

We know that 250 mg of Catechin is equivalent to 16 cups of tea based on pharmacokinetic studies of rodents[8]. Safety and efficacy of tea Catechins in combination with Vanilloids of Capsicum are also well documented[9].

Directions: Take 1 capsule three times daily with meals.

Ingredients: Green Tea Extract of EGCG (Decaffeinated) & Vanilloid Acid of Capsicum

These statements have not been reviewed by the FDA. This product is not intended to diagnose, treat, cure, or prevent any disease.

1. Morre & Morre 2003a.
2. Chueh et al. 20026.
3. Shinohara et al 1998.
4. Liao, et al 1995
5. Zhou et all 2004.
6. Moore & Moore 2003d.
7. Morre et al 2000a.
8. Jaule et al 2008.
9. Cooper et al 2005b

Dr. Tai's Pearl

Too much has been written about Prevention of Cancer without any Scientific Evidence to prove what these Speakers, Writers, and Promoters are talking about. Most of what I read & hear is garbage, disguised with a little Science. They never offer clarity, specificity & research backing their opinions.
I based my interest in Catechin/Vanilloid Supplementation for prevention & treatment of the Exto Protein in Cancer, based in Science. Exto Protein Science is exact & powerful. We can even correlate the type of Cancer based on the molecular Weight of the Exto Protein. This is very futuristic stuff & exciting for our patients, and yes, also for the healers & doctors themselves that want something Scientific, New, Specific, Inexpensive and Promising, I take it!

Side Effects: None

Contraindications:
Do not take product if you are allergic to any ingredients.

MAX DETOX

Improve Kidney Stones, Liver & Gall Bladder Function

The world is saturated with media advertisements about body detoxing, organ detoxification, cleansing of the body system and lymphatic cleansing. The advertisements go on and on about the benefits of detoxification!

Doctors and patients worldwide have requested a focused and powerful detoxification which provides cleansing of the liver, gall bladder, kidney flush, kidney stone and lymphatic draining. These, as most health practitioners know, are the heart and soul of the effective natural cleansing and detoxification program.

IS YOUR BODY UNDER ATTACK?

Just think of all the environmental pollutions, thousands of food additives, hundreds of thousands of agricultural pesticides, tobacco, alcohol, toxic cleaning products, garden pesticides, building material fumes, stress and pharmaceutical drugs. I can go on and on about the damages these chemicals have on our bodies.

The PubMed is absolutely replete with human and animal studies of the damaging effects of toxic chemicals on our liver, kidney, blood and lymphatic system. As your liver function becomes sluggish, metabolically it becomes ineffective. The bile flow is stagnant, producing HUGE paralyzing gall stones which will render your life with damaging signs and symptoms of headaches, anxieties, depression, mental confusion, fatigue, jaundice, decreased libido, food allergies, chemical sensitivities, PMS, senility, rapid aging, water retention, overweight and obesity.

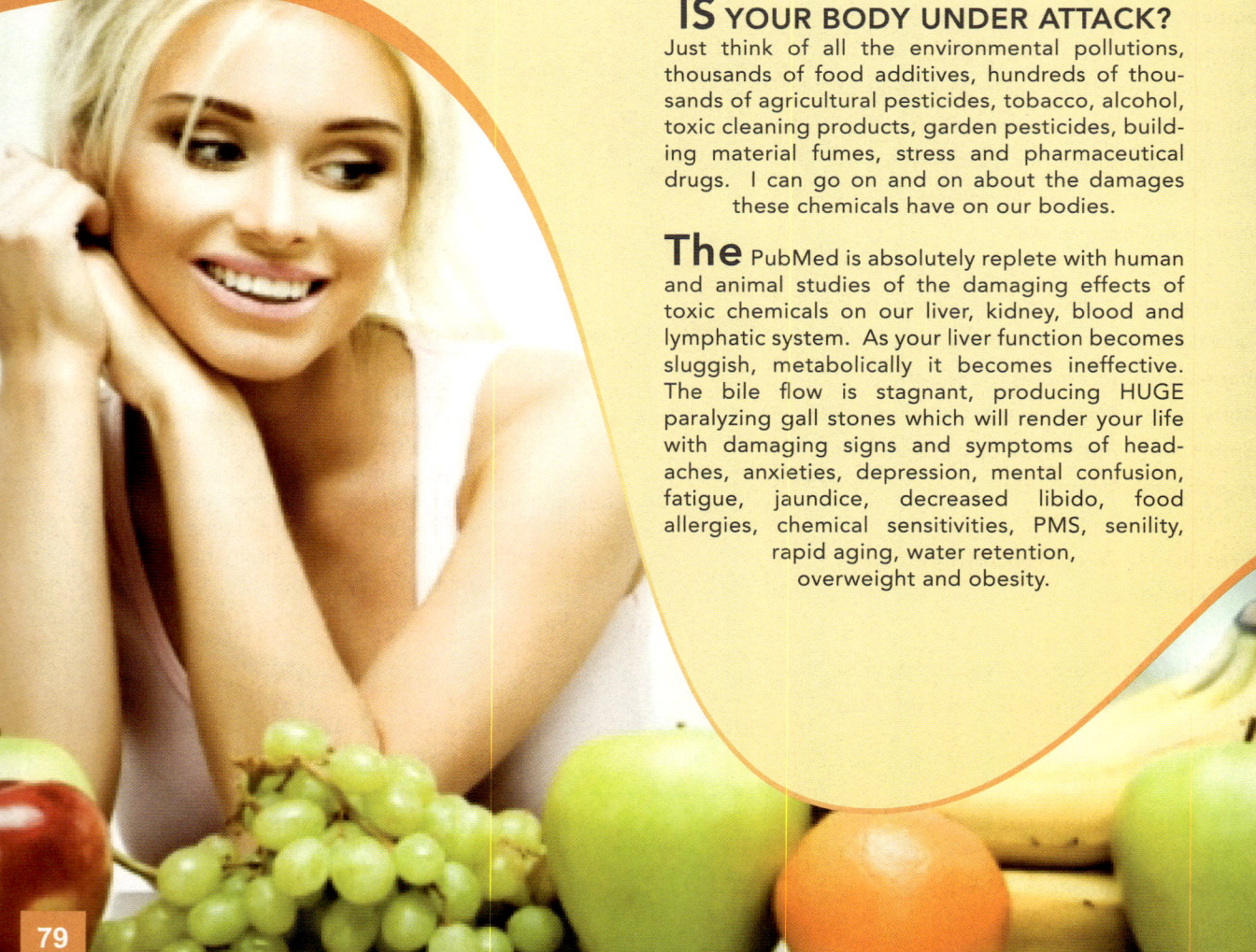

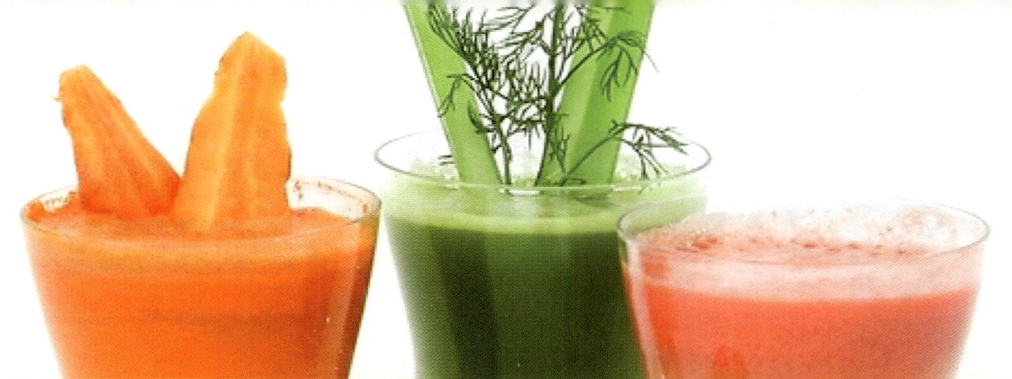

Your kidneys are the blood cleanser, blood pressure regulator, lymphatic filter and water balance controller of the whole entire body. When your kidneys are sluggish your body becomes bloated, blood and water back up, and the whole circulatory system and organs, from the heart to the brain, are under severe pressure. Crystals of calcium and other minerals start to crystallize within the filtering tubes of your kidney where the urine becomes stagnant, and urination becomes difficult and minimal. Even over concentrated urine can lead to infection, inflammation and pain, blood in the urine, low back pain, night sweats, excessive body odor and halitosis. It is said that the kidney stone is the most painful condition known to a human, equal to the intensity and pain level of childbirth and gout.

Health Secrets USA created a powerful and effective product which may Detox the liver, kidney and lymphatic by using extraordinary active ingredients from the plant Philauta Niru, Bumi Amalaky, the pure heart of the garlic called Allicin by using a proprietary formulation of Milk Thistle extract, Silica, Uva Ursi and vitamin B6.

Directions:
Take (1) capsule three times daily for maintenance and prevention. If you are suffering from kidney or gall bladder stones or severe toxicity of the liver, lymphatic or kidney, take (3) capsules three times a day with an abundance of clear water. For kidney stone removal, stay on a higher dose for a longer period, follow your health practitioner's advice and care and drink plenty of water. Must be taken on an empty stomach.

Ingredients:
Philanta Niru, Milk Thistle Extract, Silica, Uva Ursi, Vitamin B6, Magnesium Citrate

These statements have not been reviewed by the FDA. This product is not intended to diagnose, treat, cure, or prevent any disease.

Dr. Tai's Pearl

If you ever had a bout of kidney stones, then you will not need to read this next few paragraphs. It is said that for a woman, the most painful experience is childbirth and for a man it is kidney stones. Kidney stones frequently occur more among men, so after all I guess that is fair. They tell me that it is if something inside is coming apart and the pain is so severe it would be easier to die. Max DeTox is a significant relief because it works so effectively. Even if you had an ultrasound busting the kidney stones or surgery to have them removed, you will still need to know about the effectiveness of Max DeTox because neither of those procedures prevents it from happening again. Max DeTox gets to the root of the problem. It literally melts away the stones as well as preventing new stones from forming. The non-believer will quickly change their mind after a bout of kidney stones. Taking Max DeTox will seem like a tiny payment for good health.

Side Effects: None

Contraindications:
Severe renal shut-down with lack of circulation to the kidney, kidney infection, liver infection, liver tumor, kidney tumor. Do not take product if you are allergic to any of its ingredients.

MAX DIGESTION SPECIALIST | U.S. Patented Formula
Rejuvenate Your GI Tract

AMERICA'S LAST TABOO WIPED OUT

CONSTIPATION
Constipation is the slow or lack of Bowel movements of feces through the intestines.

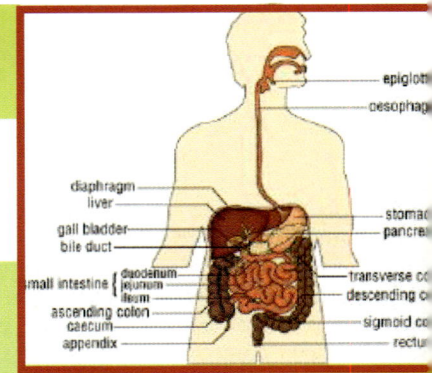

The feces often become DRY, HARD & STUCK because all the fluid is reabsorbed by the colon during this abnormal extended time. According to the American Society of Colon & Rectal Surgeons, about 80% of people suffer from Constipation at some time during their lives. The National Institute of Health published a survey showing 4-1/2 million Americans are constipated most or all the time. In the U.S. there are 2.5 million doctor visits each year from people complaining of constipation. Nearly 800 million dollars are spent each year on harsh laxatives.

Question of the Day - If you think it is important to wash your outer skin and brush your teeth then don't you think it makes equal sense to cleanse the inside of your digestive track at least once a day?
Isn't the answer obvious!!!?

You are only 30 feet away from Great Health and Abundant Energy

The digestive system from the beginning of the mouth to the end of the rectum is approximately 30 feet of flexible pipe. The entire system consists of the mouth, esophagus, stomach, small intestine, colon and rectum. Our insides are constantly smeared with gravy, mashed potatoes, chunks of meat, fish parts and ketchup, followed with ice cream, coffee or tea. Imagine all of them mixed together, what would it look like? It is first necessary that we chew the food well (basically grinding it all up together) and let the digestive juices in the stomach to mix, mash and churn to break the food into a liquid mush to expose the nutrients. These nutrients and enzymes from the Pancreas are absorbed in the upper part of the small intestines, mixing with the bile from the liver. The pulpy rotten remains are then pushed into the colon where the water is re-absorbed; the feces are compacted and disposed out of the rectum. These are the steps of a normal bowel movement which should take place from the beginning to the end (Called "Transit Time") within 15 hours and expelled out twice daily which we call <u>Regularity.</u>

THE "GUTS" OF THE MATTER

Constipation is fundamentally the slowing down process of food moving through the digestive tract and that is called "TRANSIT TIME". Back in the old days of life on the farm, Americans ate nutritional and balanced meals and then worked all day at the homestead. The typical TRANSIT TIME was 15 hours. Today, with processed food lacking enzymes and natural fibers and being heavy on sugar, the TRANSIT TIME of food through the gut is slowing down to 70 hours.

When transit time slows down, putrefied nasty material stays in your colon longer than normal, and the old feces starts to harden and stick to the walls of the colon, causing 2 million Americans to suffer. Colon diseases such as, colitis, ileitis and diverticulitis are the result along with 100,000 colostomies (surgical opening covered with a bag for collection of feces are performed each year). The average American carries an extra 5 pounds of fecal matter. A person suffering from irregularity and constipation can carry 40 pounds or more of old fecal matter. That is an awful lot of %&*@!

A Job Harder than "Mission Impossible"

When the digested food just sits there in our colon for extended periods, all the toxins, gases and poisons that are given off by the rotten fecal matter are reabsorbed with the water and re-enters our blood stream. This Self Poisoning Process is called Autointoxication. The fecal matter become dry and hard as the material becomes glued to the pockets of the colon wall, leading to a Mega-Colon. The average colon measures up to 5 inches but the left over fecal matter distend the colon up to 15 inches thick trying to push the hard stool out of a one inch hole of the rectum. These stuck and rotten fecal matter cause abnormal growths like "polyps", inflammation called Colitis, weakening and pouching of the walls called Diverticulitis (where food like corn, nuts and seeds get trapped) and lead ultimately to deadly tumors and colon cancer.

"Constipation was associated with substantially increased risk of colon cancer"

Hutchinson Cancer Research Center published in a control study of 424 cases among men and women from 30-62 years old.
Dr. Jacobs E.J. Epidemiology, July 9, 1998.

Digestion Specialist *DUAL ACTION* starts with "Washing Minerals" and follows with "Healing Vitamin Peptides" to help maintain proper gastric pH, help the stomach cells to activate the stomach enzymes from pepsinogen to enzyme pepsin, keep the stomach lining sterile and encourage the flow of bile and pancreatic enzymes. Clinical studies show decline in acid secretion of the stomach cells as we get older, preventing natural absorption of nutrients. Recent studies show 30% of all men and women past 60 have little or no acid secretion in the stomach requiring supplemental vitamin C. <u>Dr. AC Carr, published American Journal of Clinical Nutrition 1999.</u>

Dr. GS Sharp found 80% of patients with Achloalydria had soreness, burning, indigestion and excessive gas. Secretion of acid is a prerequisite to the beginning of digestion without which, you cannot absorb iron, zinc, magnesium, calcium and vitamin B complex. Dr. Sharp also reported that overgrowth of pathogenic bacteria, fungi and parasites may benefit from the supplementation of vitamin C. <u>J. America Gerontology Soc. 1967</u>

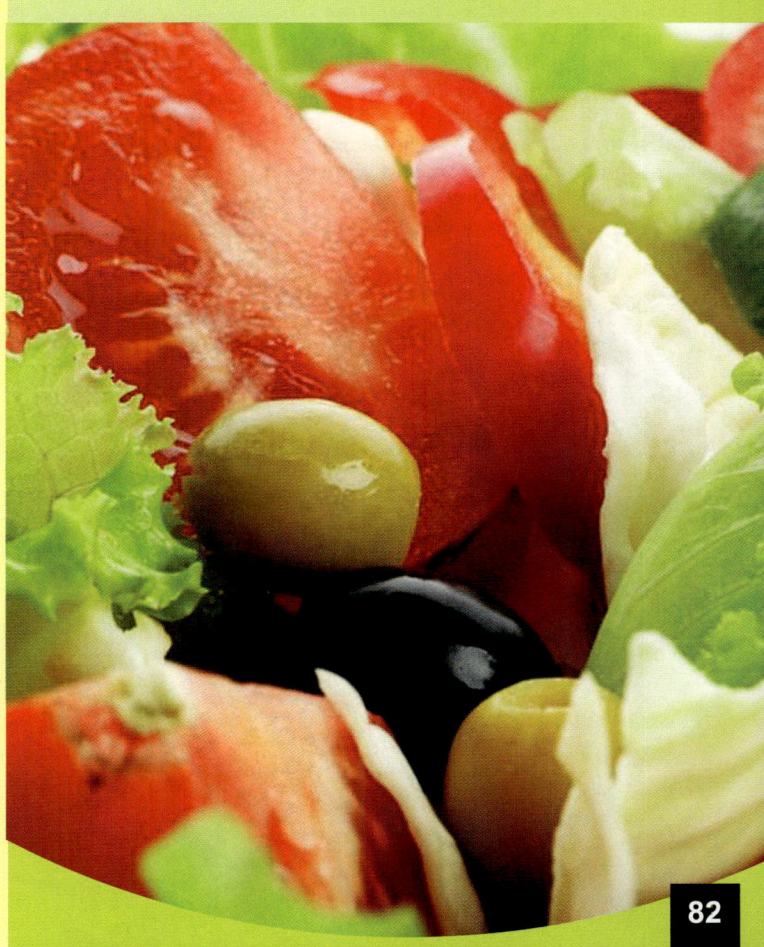

82

Researchers have found that Ascorbic acid can protect and rejuvenate aging cells from the stomach. In one study, they were feeding the cells vitamin C in growing medium and showed that it restored digestive enzyme production. But most importantly, vitamin C, an active component of "Healing Vitamin Peptides" neutralizes deadly compounds called nitrosamines a substance known to be linked to stomach cancer.

DIGESTION SPECIALIST - "Healing Vitamin Peptides"

carefully protects the intestines with a special amino acid glutamine, a principal fuel for the small intestines cell lining. Although glutamine is a major circulating amino acid for the muscles and lungs, it is the small intestines that are the primary user. Glutamine is converted in the mitochondria (cell battery) of the small intestine and colon for the energy production used in bowel movement. Researchers have shown that supplemental glutamine has incredible value in restoring and increasing the size of intestinal villi (these small fingers that actually absorbs the nutrient). The intestinal villi are damaged, cut short and blunted by the encrusted fecal matter and matted down by slimy sticky mucous.

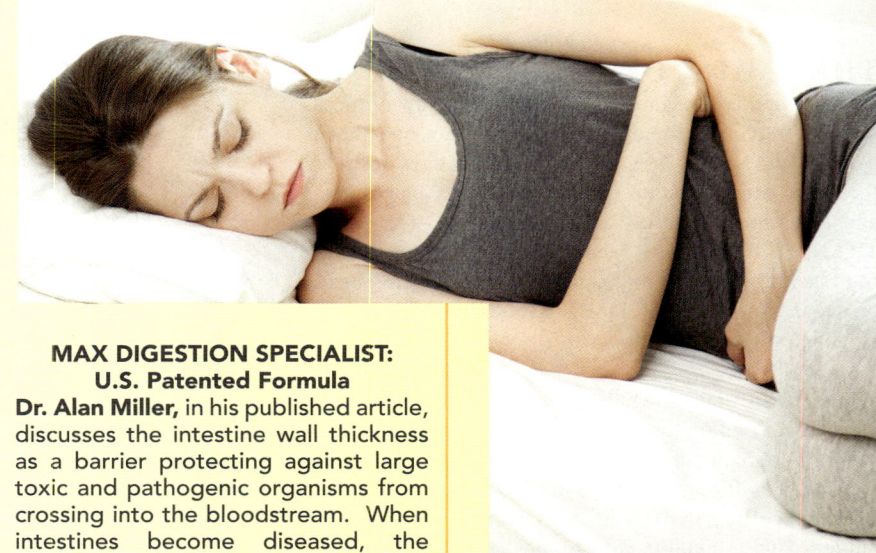

MAX DIGESTION SPECIALIST: U.S. Patented Formula

Dr. Alan Miller, in his published article, discusses the intestine wall thickness as a barrier protecting against large toxic and pathogenic organisms from crossing into the bloodstream. When intestines become diseased, the intestinal walls become thin, allowing the transport of disease, bacteria, food allergies and toxic compounds to the blood stream. Supplemental glutamine can restore the thickness of the intestinal mucosa, and increase immunoglobulin A to fight bacteria and turbo charge the immune system. It was confirmed by Dr. Klimberg V.S. that Oral Glutamine accelerates healing of the small intestine. Arch Surg 1990.

In addition, the vitamin B6 in Digestion Specialist has shown in research to protect women by reducing colon cancer by 70%. A Large epidemiologic study by **Dr. Roseil P.** shows that supplemental calcium plus vitamin D is associated with lower colon cancer in both men and women, published in Cancer 2001.

Digestion Specialist contains a unique water dissolvable Calcium whose role as one of the body's most important minerals is well known, but recent research has shown that it is also effective as an adjunct to weight loss, **Dr. Parikh S.J.** American Journal of Clinical Nutrition 2003 and confirmed by **Dr. Zemel M.B.** Journal of American College of Nutrition 2002.

What is the "Forgotten Mineral"?

Last, but not least, is Magnesium, which is the "Forgotten Mineral". Magnesium is needed to perform over 300 known biochemical reactions for metabolism and energy. Author Carolyn Dean, of Miracle of Magnesium, says that you "can't get enough Magnesium from food alone, it is nearly impossible". In fact, she announces what is not widely known that 80% of the people in United States may be "Magnesium deficient".

For most of us "Older Crowd", maintaining strong bones has been a hard fought battle and the best kept secret is that calcium alone won't do it! Magnesium is crucial to calcium absorption, so if you are taking calcium without magnesium for stronger bones, you are just kidding yourself and wasting your money.

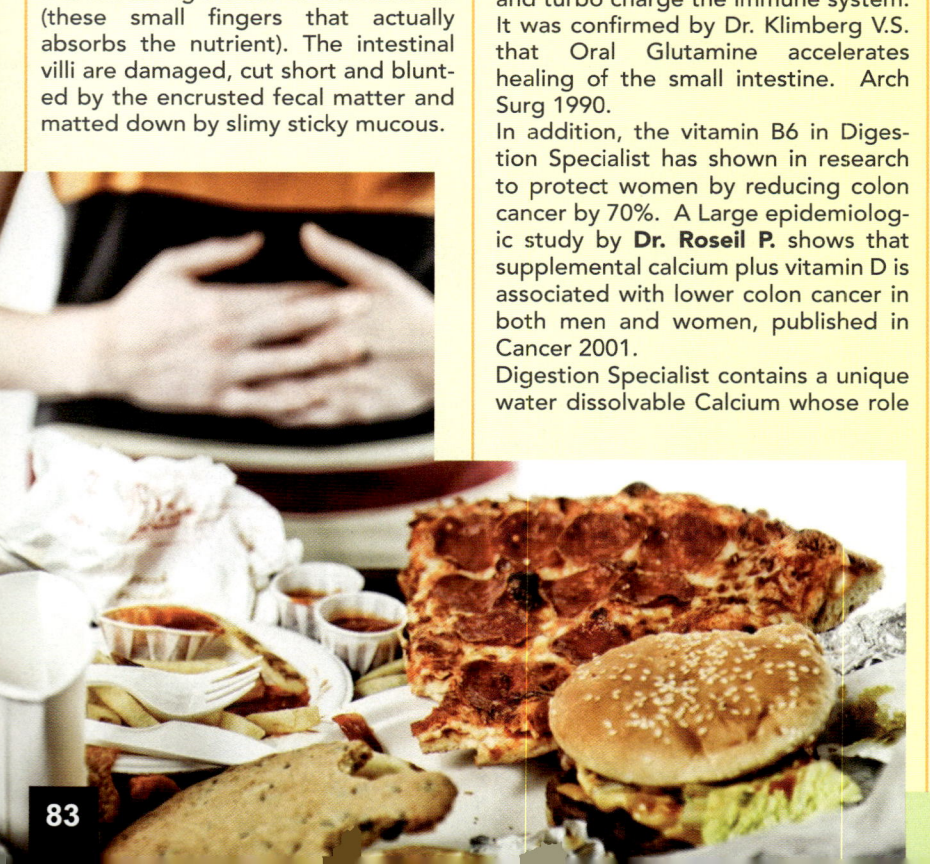

The body's ideal ratio of calcium to magnesium is a 2 to 1 ratio. And while we are on the subject of bones, may I tell you that research shows having Boron available helps calcium to stay in the bones and Boron is in Digestion Specialist.

Wait! Here comes the best part ... You won't believe your eyes!

The "Washing Minerals" & "Healing Vitamin Peptides" in Digestion
Specialist are almost completely Water Soluble. When you add a spoonful of Digestion Specialist to a glass of water, it instantaneously dissolves nearly 98% into a solution like magic. This special process makes the "Washing Minerals" even more special, containing the ingredients of Coral Calcium with all 70 micro nutrients and Vitamin D for better absorption!

DIGESTION SPECIALIST AN INNOVATIVE "DUAL ACTION" POWERFUL FORMULATION

A unique combination of "Washing Minerals" and special "Healing Vitamin Peptides" to clean and rejuvenate your intestines and colon may relieve constipation, food allergies, promote healthy repair of your digestion and even curb cravings!

U.S. Patented Formula for Satiety and Craving Control!!!

Directions:
Dissolve 1 teaspoon in 8 ounces of water. Take on an empty stomach in the morning. You may take it together with other vitamins or herbal supplements at the same time. Repeat in afternoon if needed. Add sweetener as desired.

Ingredients:
Vitamins C, D3, B6, Calcium, Fossilized Coral, Magnesium, Potassium, L-Glutamine, Boron Citrate

These statements have not been reviewed by the FDA. This product is not intended to diagnose, treat, cure, or prevent any disease.

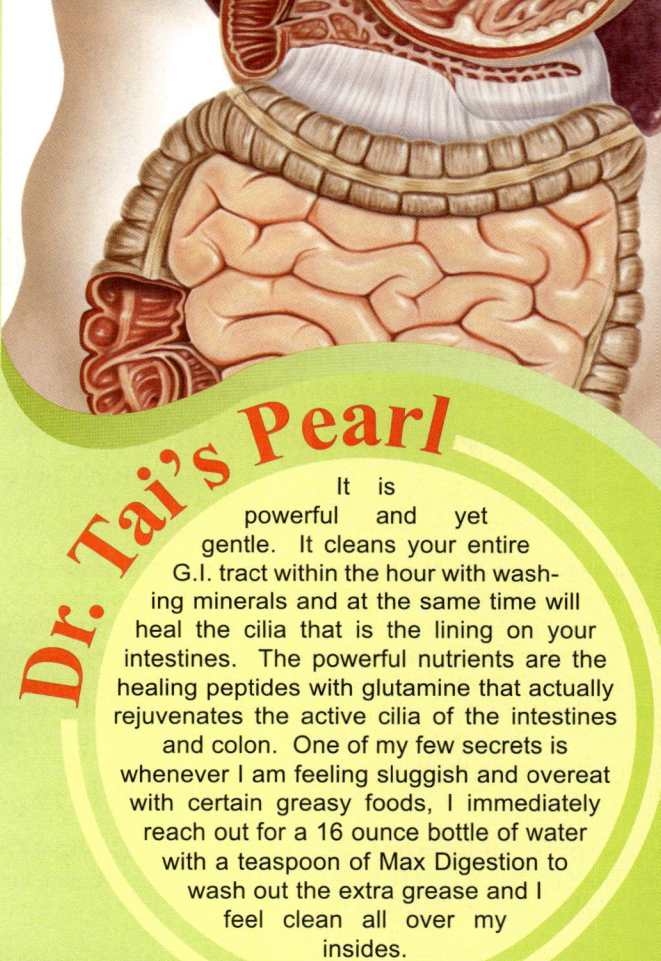

Dr. Tai's Pearl

It is powerful and yet gentle. It cleans your entire G.I. tract within the hour with washing minerals and at the same time will heal the cilia that is the lining on your intestines. The powerful nutrients are the healing peptides with glutamine that actually rejuvenates the active cilia of the intestines and colon. One of my few secrets is whenever I am feeling sluggish and overeat with certain greasy foods, I immediately reach out for a 16 ounce bottle of water with a teaspoon of Max Digestion to wash out the extra grease and I feel clean all over my insides.

Clinical Cases:
Joseph, a 67-year-old Hungarian Jew has been taking laxatives for a number of years in order to have his bowel movements. However, the bowel movements don't come except for once or twice a week. He feels sluggish and frequently has headaches. He started taking every three hours a bottle of 16 ounces of water with one teaspoon of Max Digestion. In the beginning, in order to get the bowels to move, he was taking a heaping teaspoon with every bottle of water. After one week of cleaning his system, his bowel movements became fairly regular. Every morning when taking Max Digestion, within one hour, he will have his bowel movement, as predictable as his wife's tantrums.

Side Effects:
Having bowel movements and more watery stool.
This is a welcome side effect

Contraindications:
Some people may consider kidney stones as a contraindication; however others feel that calcium ascorbate and calcium citrate are two of the nutrients that prevent kidney stones. If you have kidney stones, consider taking Max DeTox in conjunction with Max Digestion. Parathyroid abnormalities because of abnormal calcium metabolism. Do not take product if you are allergic to any of its ingredients.

MAX ENZYBIOTIC SPECIALIST

Keep a Healthy DIGESTIVE SYSTEM

When it comes to staying healthy and keeping your digestive system happy and working well, probiotics are an option used all over the world.

Heath Secrets' Max Enzybiotic is packed full of 12 species of Good Bacteria & 11 Digestive Enzymes which encouraging evidence has shown may help:

- Diarrhea especially following treatment with certain antibiotics [1-3]
- Vaginal yeast infections & urinary tract infections [4]
- Irritable bowel syndrome (IBS) [5]
- Reduce Bladder Cancer recurrence [6]
- Shorten duration of intestinal infections [7]
- Prevention of inflammation following colon surgery (pouchitis) [8]
- Prevent eczema in children [9]

Let me explain a bit about these amazing little powerhouses called probiotics.

The term probiotics comes from the Greek "for life". When ingested, these microorganisms replenish the micro flora in your intestinal tract. This results in the promotion of a number of health-enhancing functions, including enhanced digestive function. Max Enzybiotic has a remarkable formula which brings together two of the most well known probiotics- Lactobacillus and Bifidobacterium- A total of 12 Species known to work together to maintain a balance of "good bacteria" along your digestive tract. It's a probiotic powerhouse that packs 60 billion good bacteria in every capsule. Most Probiotics sold have only one, or maybe two good bacteria.

WE pack in 12 good bacteria!

The Secrets of Indigestion & Digestive problems are Overeating & Intolerance to the food you ate!
STOP…Not Another Step!! Most people take antacids…a terrible mistake which neutralizes the stomach acid essential to kick-start the ENZYMES that actually digest the food you ate. This causes even BIGGER problems.

Super Essential Enzymes
Amylase, Lactase, Cellulase, Maltase, Invertase and Bromelain, Papain, Galactosidase and Serriopeptase.

This powerful formula includes All the **Proteases (I, II, III), Carbohydrases, Lipases, Prebiotics, Probiotics** that will digest legumes, milk, soy, cereal, meat, fish and other foods.

Very Effective in wide variations of pH in your digestive tract from 3 pH to 9 pH to digest difficult Endo-Peptidase, Exo-Peptidase, Casei Nolytic and Fibri Nolytic enzymes.

Special blend of natural food grade digestive enzymes, extensive 9 probiotics from non-animal sources specially formulated for vegetarians.

Where have all the bacteria gone?

It seems that in our collective eagerness to rid ourselves of disease (and every trace of bacteria in our food supply and everything else for that matter) we may have out done ourselves. As a whole, we are less exposed to bacteria now than in the past including "good" bacteria. The problem, though antibacterial products have given us a cleaner world, is that they have also taken away the benefits of "good" bacteria. Due to strict food safety regulations, less bacteria (including the good ones) survive the manufacturing process.

That's why Max Enzybiotic should be a part of your everyday routine. It gives your GI tract and entire immune system an extra "edge"- which may allow your body to maximize the benefits of a healthy diet with 12 species of Good Bacteria & 11 Digestive Enzymes.

Dr. Tai's Pearl

Some people might turn their nose up at probiotics – **Hey! I get it!** Microorganisms aren't exactly finger food, but their benefits are so vast, you'd be CRAZY not to incorporate them into your daily routine. From Digestion to Prevention of Eczema, probiotics strengthen your body's good bacteria while maintaining a healthy and beneficial pH.

Clinical Cases:

A Dear friend of mine once suffered from **Irritable Bowel Syndrome (IBS)** so severe, that they were constantly constipated. With a gut poking out so far that he couldn't see his shoes, he always joked about being six months along. Now don't get me wrong, I was more than ready to become Uncle Doctor Tai, however this was a problem of a different sort. While my friend thought he was just packing on pounds, the tell-tale shape of the gut and absence of fat on the chest told me a different story. Although he was eating, and eating, and eating, he wasn't defecating. This gut was the result of pounds of waste backed up in his system.

Due to the complexity and severity of his problem, there was no ONE answer to help his IBS and subsequent Constipation. We got to work right away to create a solid protocol for him:

- **Max Enzybiotic** to help with the symptoms of IBS – Bloating, Pain, Diarrhea and Constipation.
- **Max Intestine** to address the constipation that had already accumulated, giving a higher dosage for those who are more resistant and prone to constipation.
- **Ultra Stomach** is added in for relief of gas & inflammation often caused by chronic infections.
- **BioFilm Testing** is an in-depth way to view the severity of intestinal issues.
- Pair your supplements with **Oral Macrophage**, which helps to clean up potential infections to achieve balance and a healthy gut.
- As always with bowel issues, we want to address **Diet**. **I recommended for him to add in more greenery that was high in fiber**, not having to sacrifice his love of red meats (although we do recommend white, lean meats most of all).

Today, he is feeling better than ever before! With his constipation corrected and his irritable bowels under control, he sports a slimmer figure that's non-bloated and not backed up!

Side Effects: None

Contraindications: Do not take if you are allergic to any of the ingredients.

Directions: Take 1 to 2 capsules with each meal. For higher doses, please consult your health care practitioner or consultant.

Ingredients: Proprietary Blend: Amylase, Protease, Lipase, Lactase, Cellulase, Maltase, Invertase, Bromelain, Serriopeptase, Papase, Alpha-Galactosidase, L-Acidophilus, L-Brevis, L-Bulgarios, L-Casei, L-Caucasius, L-Helvetian, L-Lactis, L-Plantarum, B-Fidum, B-Infatis, L-Bulgaricus, L-Reuteri, Vitamin C

Medical Journal References

1. Höcher W, Chase D, Hagenhoff G (1990). "Saccharomyces boulardii in acute adult diarrhea. Efficacy and tolerance of treatment". Münch Med Wochenschr 132: 188-92.
2. Allen SJ, Martinez EG, Gregorio GV, Dans LF. Probiotics for treating acute infectious diarrhoea. Cochrane Database Syst Rev 2010; (11): CD003048.
3. Bernaola Aponte G, Bada Mancilla CA, Carreazo NY, Rojas Galarza RA. Probiotics for treating persistent diarrhea in children. Cochrane Database Syst Rev 2013; (8): CD007401.
4. Gregor Reid, Andrew W Bruce, Nicola Fraser, Christine Heinemann, Janice Owen, Beth Henning. Oral probiotics can resolve urogenital infections. DOI: 10.1111/j.1574-695X.2001.tb01549.x
5. IBS – Maupas J, Champemont P, Delforge M (1983). "Treatment of irritable bowel syndrome with Saccharomyces boulardii: a double blind, placebo controlled study". Medicine Chirurgie Digestives 12(1): 77-9.
6. Nature Reviews Urology 5, 526-527 (October 2008) | doi:10.1038/ncpuro 1199. Does the probiotic L. casei help prevent recurrence after transurethral resection for superficial bladder cancer? Michael A O'Donnell
7. Allen SJ, Martinez EG, Gregorio GV, Dans LF. Probiotics for treating acute infectious diarrhoea. Cochrane Database Syst Rev 2010; (11): CD003048.
8. Elahi, B., Nikfar, S., Derakhshani, S. et al. Dig Dis Sci (2008) 53: 1278. https://doi.org/10.1007/s10620-007-0006-z
9. Cuello-Garcia CA, Brożek JL, Fiocchi A, Pawankar R, Yepes-Nuñez JJ, Terracciano L et al. Probiotics for the prevention of allergy: A systematic review and meta-analysis of randomized controlled trials. J Allergy Clin Immunol 2015; 136(4): 952-961.

These statements have not been reviewed by the FDA. This product is not intended to diagnose, treat, cure, or prevent any disease.

MAX FEMININE

Ultra Concentrated Phyto Extracts
More Hot flashes?
Night sweats won't stop?
Help is here!

Fighting Menopause!

Bio-Estrogen levels are very individualized and no two women are alike.

It is highly dependent on the quantities of receptor sites each person's body has, and the demand of the precise hormone level required to control menopausal symptoms.

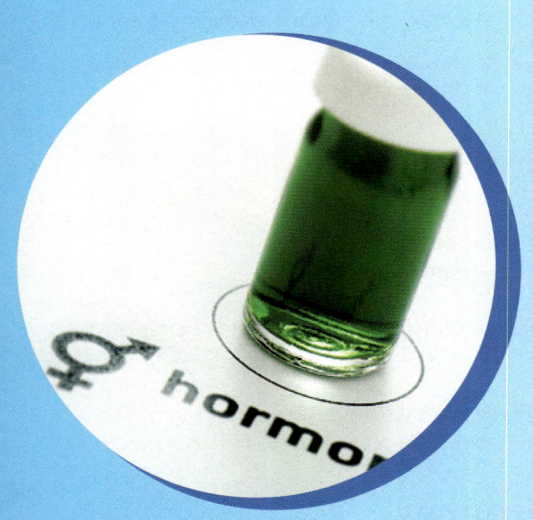

"Max Feminine" is very well balanced with the right ratio of 8:1 of Estriol (E3): Estradol(E2). The bio-hormones in "Max Feminine" are sourced from pure Genistein (E3) and Pueraria extracts (E2) to fight these protracted and resistant symptoms of menopause.

Most women believe that Estrogen is a single hormone. This, in fact, is not accurate. Essentially, we have three Estrogens. Number One is Estrone (E1). It is called a 'Bad Estrogen' because the breakdown of this Estrogen when it is in your body creates byproducts such as 4-hydroxy and 16-hydroxy.

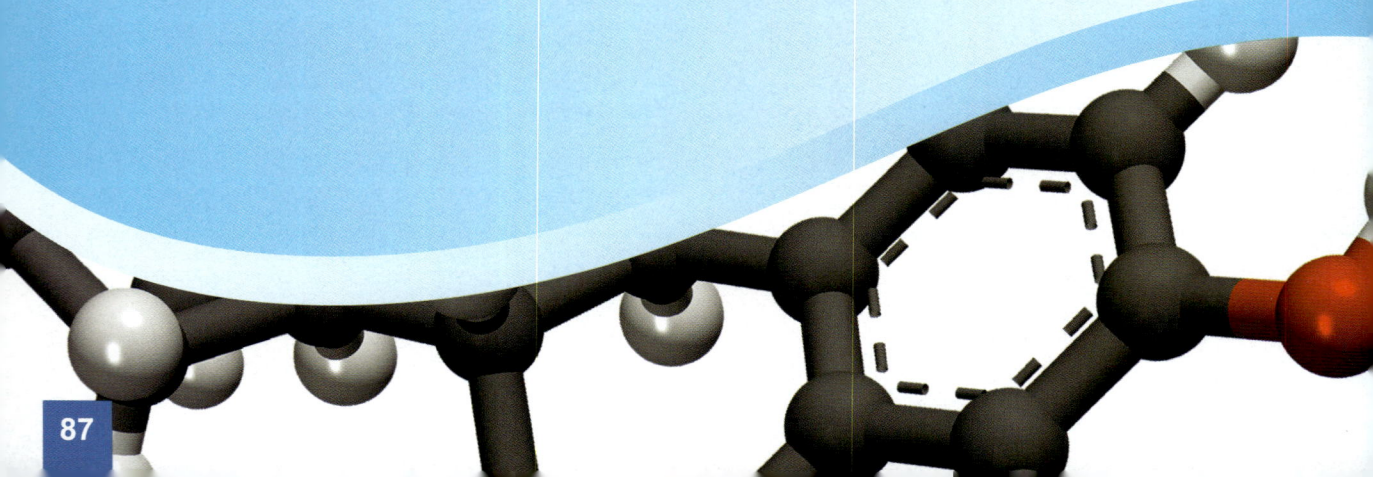

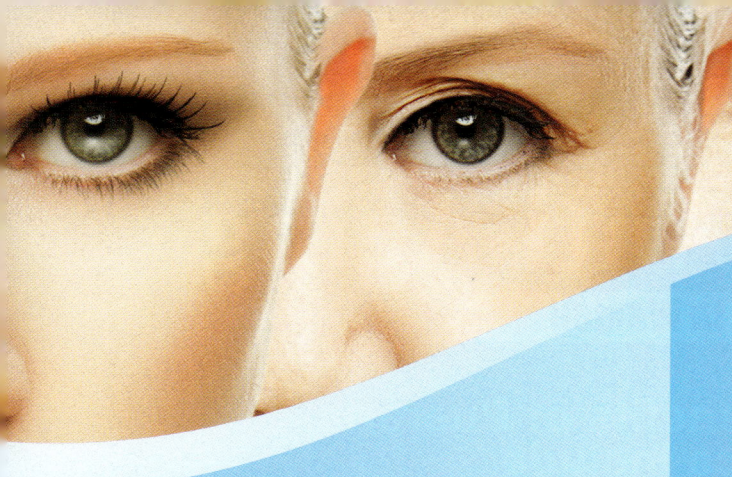

Dr. Tai's Pearl

What makes women special is the perfect balance of Estradiol (E2) and Estriol (E3), which is achievable with the help of the supplements and extracts of Ginestine and Puraria. If you'd like to have the secret to beautiful, wrinkle-free skin, then make sure you apply Max Feminine directly to your face and neck as well as your chest. It's been said that Max Feminine is a fountain to eternal youth. It will add smoothness as well as the natural beauty that every woman will appreciate. May you be beautiful forever.

These are metabolistes of Estrone that may be the significant causes for breast cysts as well as raise instances of Cancers. Number Two is Estradiol (E2). This Estrogen helps women maintain a feminine shape. It is the essential Estrogen that appears mostly during pre-menopause. This is also the Estrogen that helps women ovulate. It is an Estrogen that helps with the brain as well as provides protect on against Heart Disease. The Number Three Estrogen is called Estriol (E3). This Estrogen is considered by most to be the best Estrogen because it is so mild. It is the large amount of Estrogen produced by pregnancy. This is an Estrogen that has been shown even in severely large quantities to not cause complications. This is due to occupying the receptors without causing receptor complications. We believe that the beauty of Max Feminine is its Proper balance between Estriol (E3) and Estradiol (E2). When women have these perfect proportions they enjoy a life of great benefits, able to enjoy their femininity and still have the protection against Heart Disease with additional benefits to maintaining memory and sexuality with age.

Directions: Apply to soft parts of skin 1-3 pumps per day AM or in divided doses. Adjust dosage per your Health Professional.

Side Effects: None

Contraindications:
Don't take if you are allergic to any ingredients. FOR FEMALE USE ONLY. Keep away from children and men.

These statements have not been reviewed by the FDA. This product is not intended to diagnose, treat, cure, or prevent any disease.

Max HotFlash Specialist & Women Anti-Aging

Rejuvenation against Menopause in Women

Additional benefits of Pueraria Mirifica include:

- Softens the Skin
- Moisturizes and hydrates the skin
- Increases Blood Flow to the Skin, thereby keeping it young, supple and vibrant
- Reduces the appearance of wrinkles
- Keeps the skin elastic
- Anti-Aging
- Reduces wrinkles and freckles
- Improves Complexion
- Strengthens Bones
- Protects the Heart

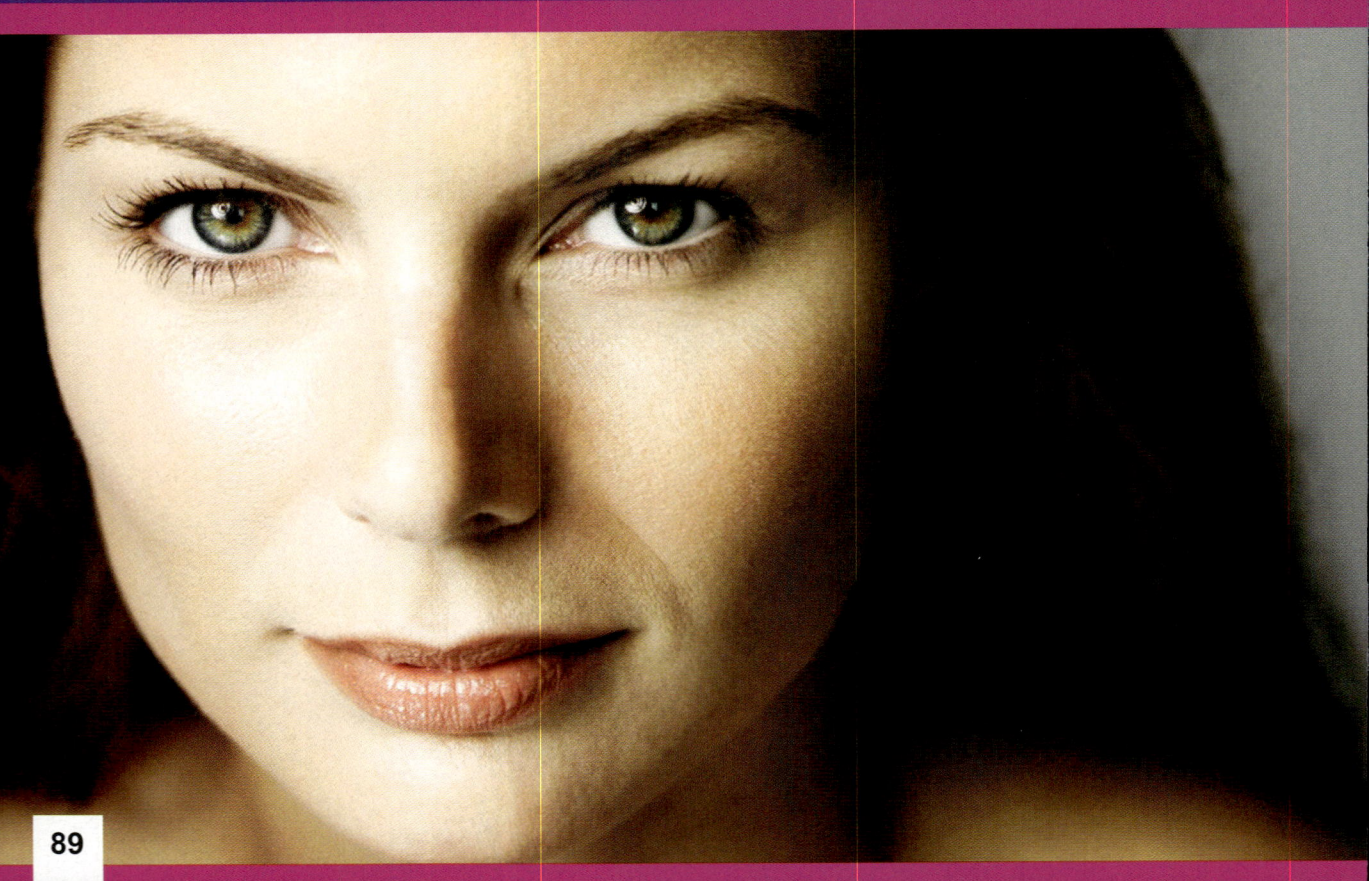

Menopause is a transition in a woman's life, during which hormonal changes occur, including decreased estrogen and progesterone production. Menstruation becomes less frequent (peri-menopause) and eventually stops completely (menopause). Symptoms of menopause include a rapid heart beat, night sweats, skin flushing, insomnia, forgetfulness, emotional instability, osteoporosis, heart disease, wrinkles, headaches, vaginal dryness and atrophy, urinary infections, and of course, the dreaded hot flash. Hot flashes may cause a woman to become irritated and extremely uncomfortable.

May alleviate the following symptoms related to Menopause:

- Heart beating too quickly or strongly
- Feelings of tension or nervousness
- Difficulty in sleeping
- Excitability
- Attacks of pain
- Difficulty concentrating
- Feeling tired or lacking in energy
- Loss of interest in most things
- Feeling unhappy or depressed
- Crying spells
- Irritability
- Feeling dizzy or faint
- Pressure or tightness in head or body
- Parts of body feel numb or tingling
- Headaches
- Muscle and joint pains
- Loss of feeling in hands or feet
- Breathing difficulties
- Hot flashes
- Sweating at night
- Loss of interest in sex

Directions:

Shake well. Take on empty stomach one (1) dropper full by sublingual at night. Hold for 30 seconds and swallow. May increase dosage to AM and PM if needed. For higher dosage consult your Health Specialist.

Pueraria Mirifica (PM) is a root extract from a plant in Thailand which provides all the benefits of estrogen without any known risks. In the area of Thailand where the plant is derived, there are almost no cases of breast or prostate cancer, people rarely suffer from osteoporosis and the difficulties associated with menopause and andropause are nonexistent. The locals eat the root in their salads and these individuals are virtually devoid of hormone related degenerative disease, including Prostate or Breast Cancer. Pueraria Mirifica is loaded with the phytoestrogen miroestrol which also improves cardiovascular function and reduces cardiovascular risks.[1]

Pueraria Mirifica phytoestrogens relieve symptoms in peri-menopausal women using the Greene Climacteric Scale covering twenty-one symptoms of menopause.[2] PM has an estrogenic effect similar to conjugated equine estrogens without the serious health risks of breast cancer, endometrial cancer, uterine cancer and ovarian cancer related to synthetic estrogen.[3] PM has proven to exhibit estrogenicity on the vaginal tissue, to alleviate vaginal dryness symptoms and dyspareunia, to improve signs of vaginal atrophy and to restore the atrophic vaginal epithelium in postmenopausal women.[4]

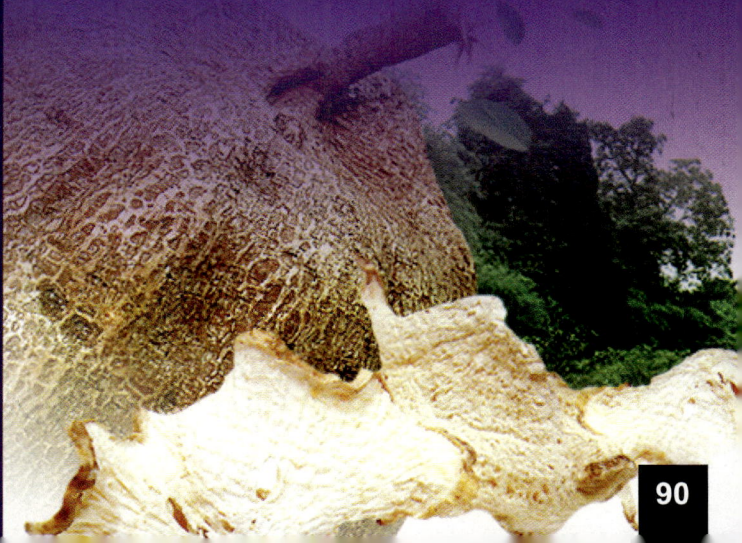

Max HotFlash Specialist & Women Anti-Aging

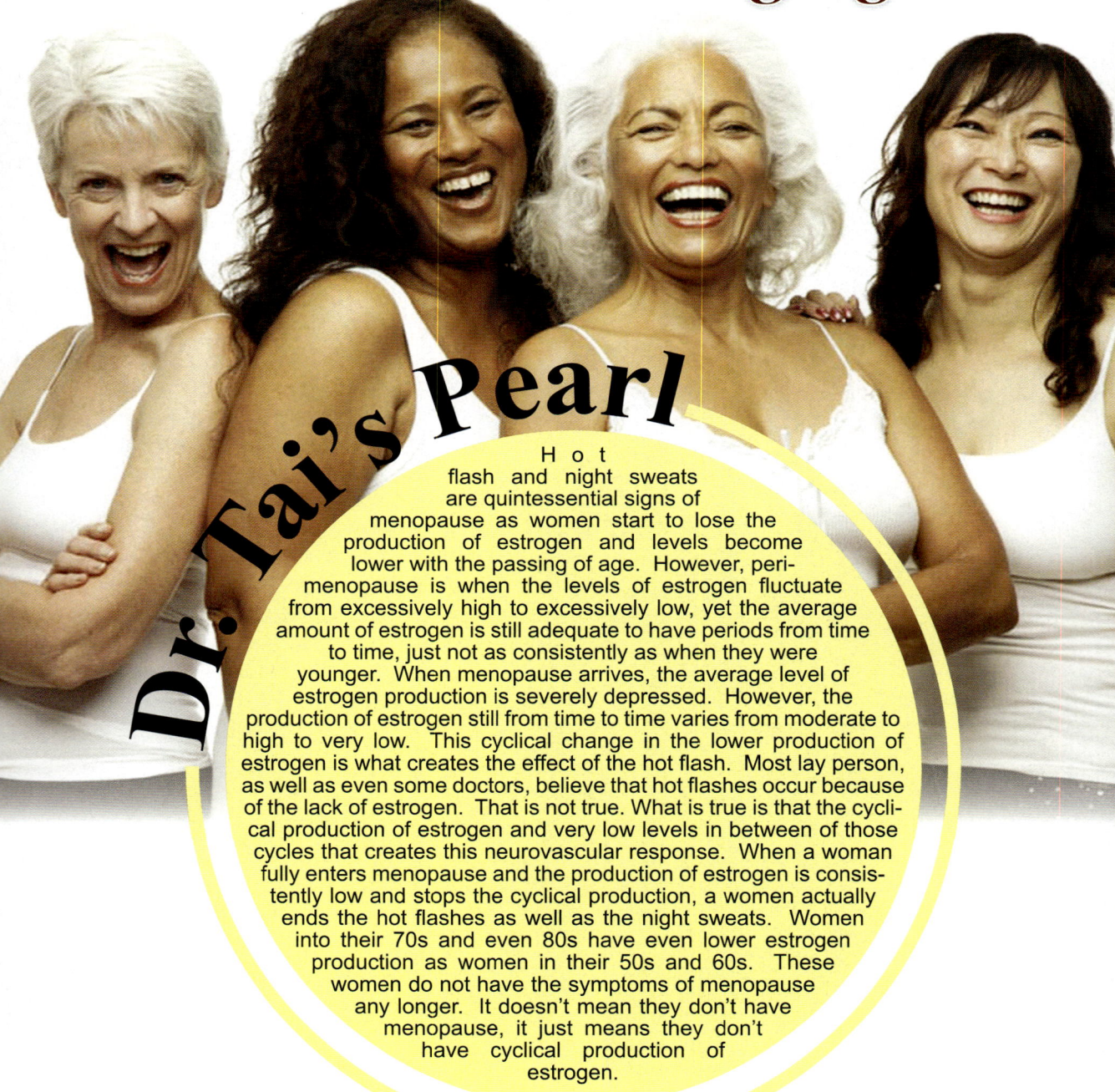

Dr. Tai's Pearl

Hot flash and night sweats are quintessential signs of menopause as women start to lose the production of estrogen and levels become lower with the passing of age. However, peri-menopause is when the levels of estrogen fluctuate from excessively high to excessively low, yet the average amount of estrogen is still adequate to have periods from time to time, just not as consistently as when they were younger. When menopause arrives, the average level of estrogen production is severely depressed. However, the production of estrogen still from time to time varies from moderate to high to very low. This cyclical change in the lower production of estrogen is what creates the effect of the hot flash. Most lay person, as well as even some doctors, believe that hot flashes occur because of the lack of estrogen. That is not true. What is true is that the cyclical production of estrogen and very low levels in between of those cycles that creates this neurovascular response. When a woman fully enters menopause and the production of estrogen is consistently low and stops the cyclical production, a women actually ends the hot flashes as well as the night sweats. Women into their 70s and even 80s have even lower estrogen production as women in their 50s and 60s. These women do not have the symptoms of menopause any longer. It doesn't mean they don't have menopause, it just means they don't have cyclical production of estrogen.

Ingredients:
Aloe Vera Extract, Pueraria Mirifica Extract, Sterol, and Distilled Water

These statements have not been reviewed by the FDA. This product is not intended to diagnose, treat, cure, or prevent any disease.
References

1. Wattanapitayakul SK, Chularojmontri L, Srichirat S. Effects of Pueraria mirifica on vascular function of ovariectomized rabbits. J Med Assoc Thai. 2005 Jun;88 Suppl 1:S21-9. PMID: 16862667

2. RefLamlertkittikul S, Chandeying V. Efficacy and safety of Pueraria mirifica (Kwao Kruea Khao) for the treatment of vasomotor symptoms in perimenopausal women: Phase II Study. J Med Assoc Thai. 2004 Jan;87(1):33-40.

3. Chandeying V, Sangthawan M. Efficacy comparison of Pueraria mirifica (PM) against conjugated equine estrogen (CEE) with/without medroxyprogesterone acetate (MPA) in the treatment of climacteric symptoms in perimenopausal women: phase III study. J Med Assoc Thai. 2007 Sep;90(9):1720-6.

4. Manonai J, Chittacharoen A, Theppisai U, Theppisai H. Effect of Pueraria mirifica on vaginal health. Menopause. 2007 Sep-Oct;14(5):919-24.

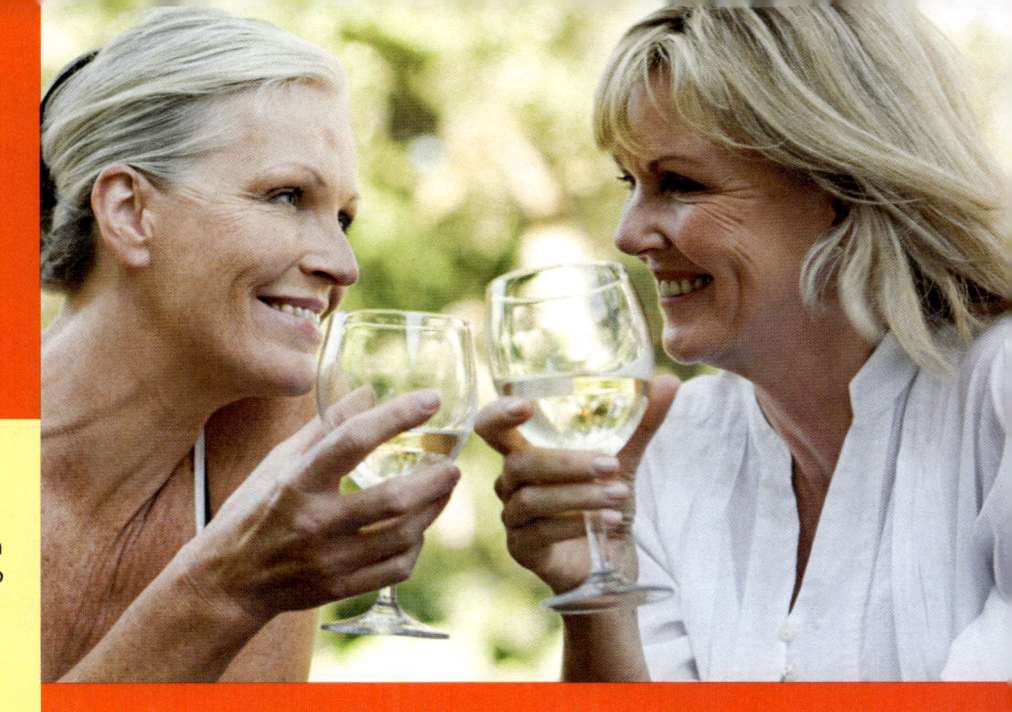

Clinical Case:

Joanne was a 54-year-old physician that had been undergoing peri-menopause for two hell-filled years before I met her. When we were finally introduced, she was the DEFINITION of female-aging, already approaching eight months without a period. The symptoms of menopause grew stronger each day and she found herself constantly in excess – too tired, too hot, and too emotional. She suffered non-stop with no sense of relief. In BOTH the United States and England, in the world of mainstream medicine she was so familiar with, the primary treatment for hot flashes and peri-menopause symptoms were anti-depressants. Although this may help to stabilize the moodiness, the main issue here was far from solved. Some women who suffer severely from Menopause may not experience ANY mood swings. What will antidepressants do for them?? I hoped to address the obvious deficiency in the market for a product that addressed the needs of ALL Peri & Menopausal women

I knew from published research that any product I made to properly help would center around Pueraria Mirifica. This root, devoid of side effects and equipped with a compound very similar to good estriol, helped to increase the presence of the receptor without stimulating it – which could increase potential tumors. Dr. Joanne chose to use the Max Hot Flash Specialist together with balancing her progesterone in order to resolve all of her menopausal symptoms. By initially using a higher dosage in order to quiet the neurovascular response & receptor activity, she stabilized and was able to further decrease the amount of product she used. Through monitoring her progress and continuously adjusting her dosage, Dr. Joanne found herself completely symptom-free! In addition, results from clinical testing came back with optimal results, too!

Another Bonus: Women who associate stress with their HOT FLASHES and Excessive sweating have reported WONDERFUL results using a supplement called "Stress & Anxiety Specialist". In just 2 days, they noticed they had NO MORE STRESS!

Smart Ladies!!

Side Effects: None

Contraindications:
Do not take product if you are allergic to any of its ingredients.

MAX INTESTINE SPECIALIST

Prevent & Treat Intestinal Inflammation

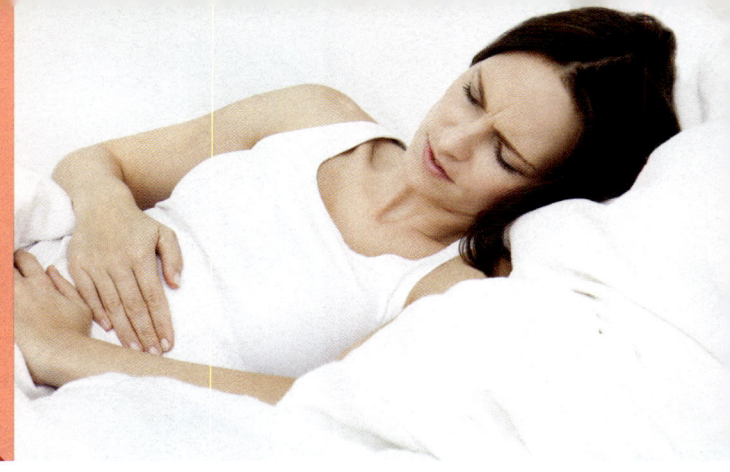

Most people suffer from constipation at some point in time, but some may complain of more frequent bouts than others. For most people constipation is a discomfort that's best not discussed as it is in some cases temporary, and for most people not being able to go to the bathroom is an awkward subject. If the problem is severe or frequent and causes you a great deal of discomfort however it is important that you discuss it with your health care provider. In most cases, dietary and lifestyle modifications alone suffice and there is no real need for medical treatment.

For chronic cases, where the problem of constipation frequently recurs or is long lasting, a more aggressive form of treatment with natural supplements may be necessary. Infants, children and adults can all suffer from constipation due to a variety of reasons.

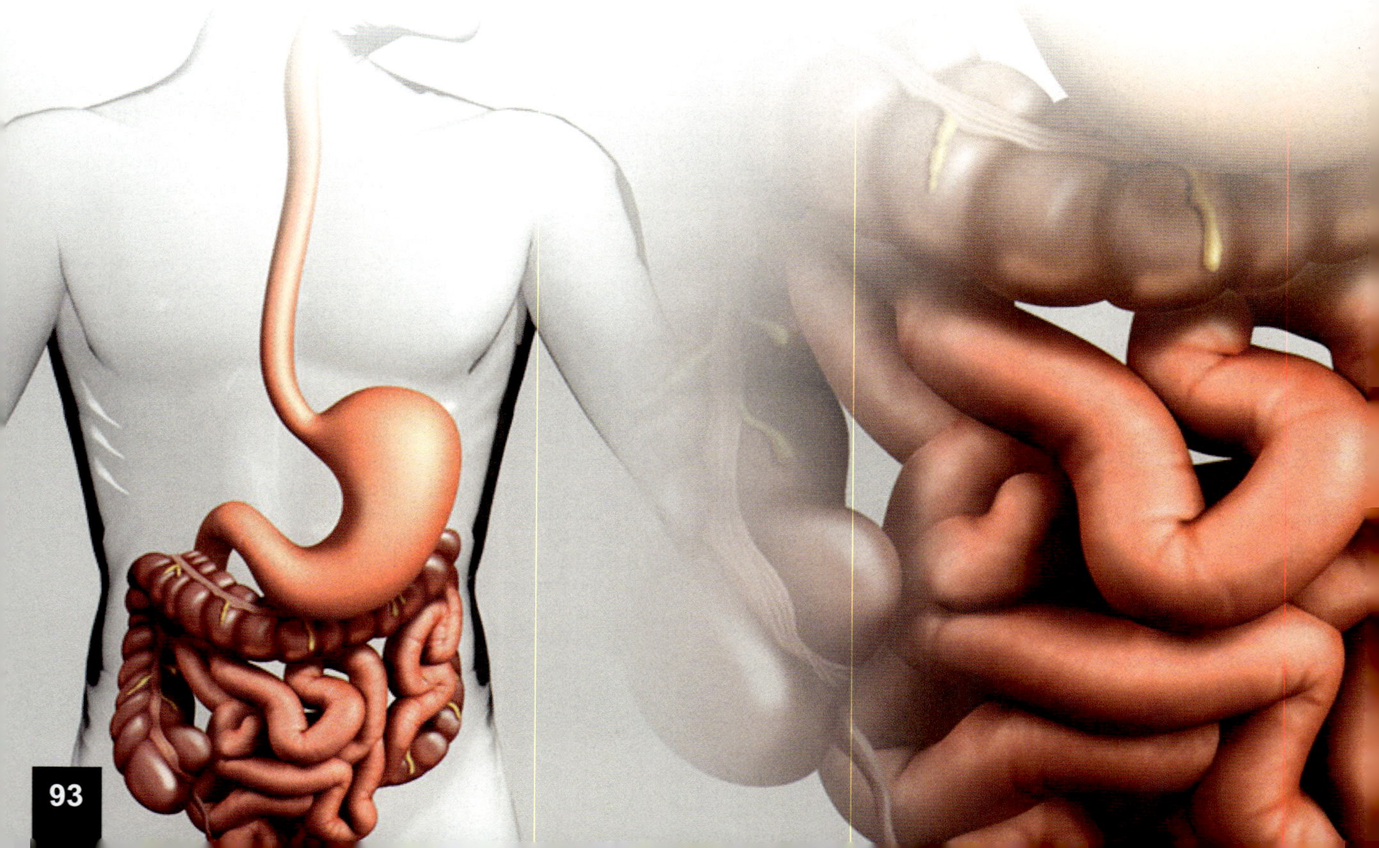

Symptoms of Constipation

Other symptoms of constipation may include:

- Irregular or less frequent bowel movements or anything less than thrice a week (severe constipation refers to only one or less bowel movements per week)
- Sudden change in regularity
- Harder stools that are more difficult to pass
- A bloated feeling in the lower abdomen
- Straining while passing stools
- Coated tongue
- Bad breath
- Depression and anxiety
- Headaches
- Insomnia
- Loss of appetite
- Dark circles under the eyes
- Mouth ulcers
- Dizziness
- Nausea
- Feeling of fullness in the abdomen
- Gas and bloating
- Varicose veins
- Heartburn
- Children who suffer from constipation may be easily fatigued and have no appetite
- Infants tend to be uneasy and fussy and suffer from gas and bloating

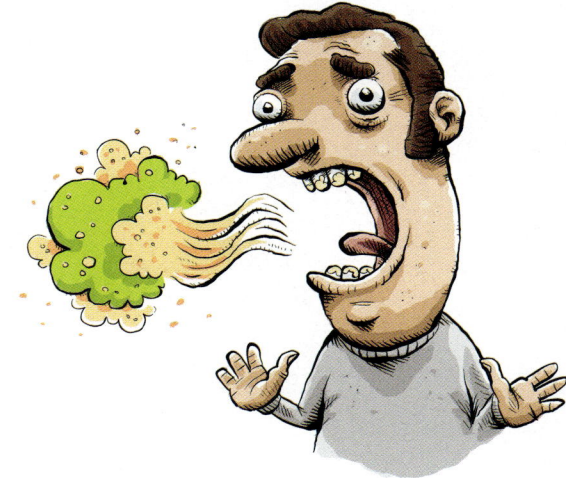

Diet for Constipation

An ideal diet to cure constipation and prevent its recurrence is one that contains high amounts of fresh fruits and vegetables, especially those with high fiber content. Dried fruits, whole grains, cereals, and vegetables are the best ways to get fiber into your diet. For the best results, you must increase your intake of water as well. Keep hydrated at all times to prevent the hardening of stools and, to encourage regularity. For some people, suddenly adding high amounts of fiber into their diet may cause gas or bloating, and even worsen the constipation. If this is the case, try introducing small amounts of fiber at a time until the digestive system gets used to it.

Suggestions for Constipation

The best way to treat constipation is to try and prevent it. To avoid constipation you must:

- Include lots of fiber in your diet
- Drink plenty of water daily but avoid too much caffeine and alcohol
- Start a regular exercise routine
- Do not delay a bowel movements if the urge occurs
- Chew food slowly and well when eating
- Do not eat on the go or at irregular times
- Avoid foods that are high in fats and refined sugar
- Avoid over processed and junk food

If you are pregnant and suffer from constipation stay away from laxatives and over-the-counter medications as these can cause premature contractions. Opt for natural remedies and dietary changes to prevent constipation instead.

Yoga can help regularize bowel movements. Certain yoga poses and asanas stimulate the digestive tract and encourage bowel movements. Deep breathing exercises and meditation also help relieve stress and anxiety that may be causing the constipation.

Directions:
Take 1 capsule 4 times daily. For higher dosage check with your health practitioner. Adjust dosage for Regular Maintenance of daily bowel movement.

Ingredients:
Psyllium Husk, Casara Sagrada, Citrus Pectin, Aloe Vera, Senna, Parsley, Horsetail, Goldenseal Root, Lactobacillus Acidophilus, Buckthorn Bark, Gentian Root

These statements have not been reviewed by the FDA. This product is not intended to diagnose, treat, cure, o prevent any disease.

Max Intestine Specialist Clinical Applications

1. Xu J, Zhou X, Chen C, Deng Q, Huang Q Yang J, Yang N, Huang F. Laxative effects o partially defatted flaxseed meal on norma and experi mental constipated mice. BMC Complement Altern Med. 2012 Ma 9;12:14. doi:10.1186/1472-6882-12-14 PubMed PMID: 22400899; PubMed Centra PMCID: PMC3353840.

2. Marlett JA, Li BU, Patrow CJ, Bass F Comparative laxation of psyllium with and without senna in an ambu lator constipated population. Am Gastroenterol. 1987 Apr;82(4):333-7 PubMed PMID: 3565338

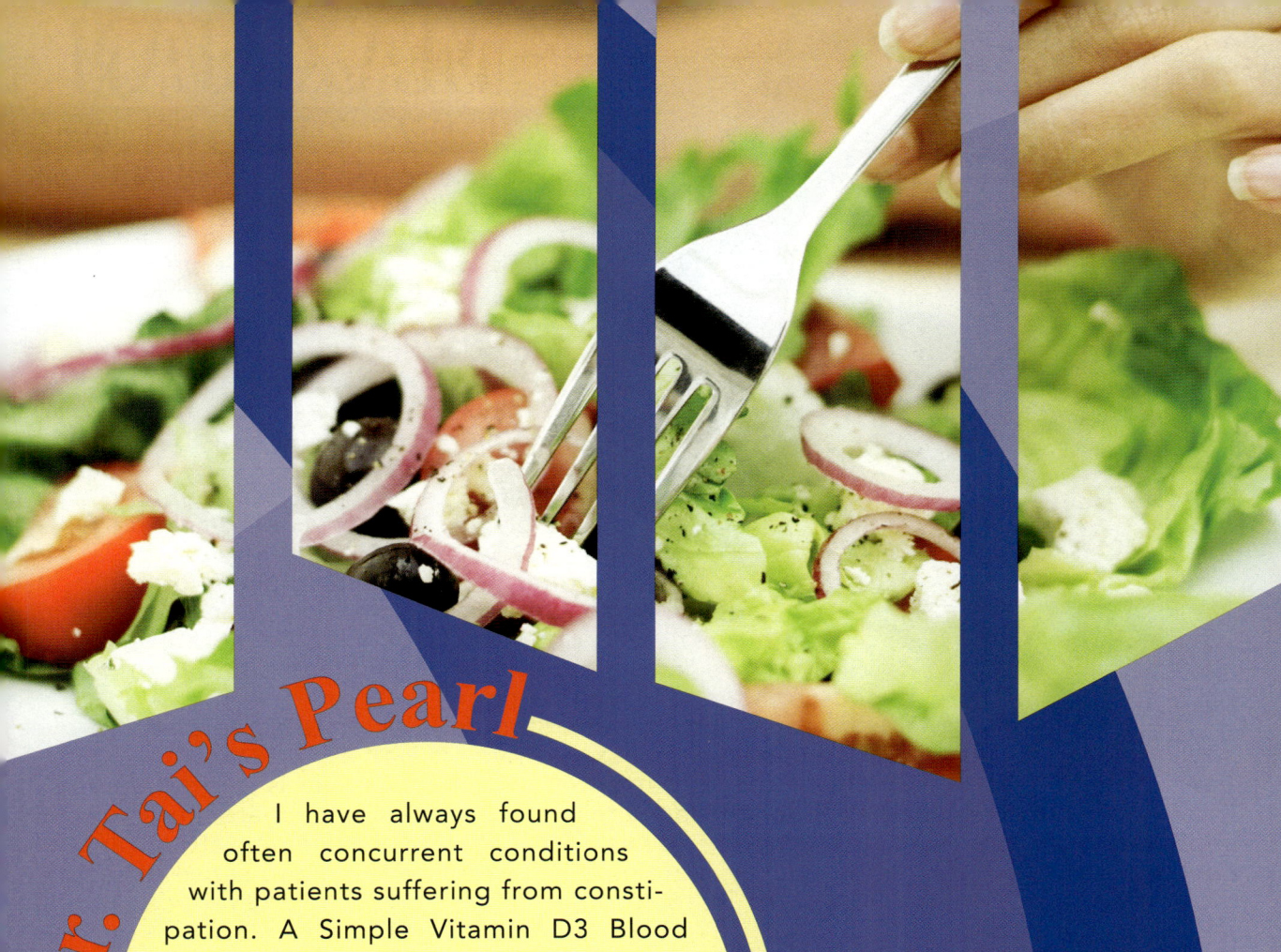

Dr. Tai's Pearl

I have always found often concurrent conditions with patients suffering from constipation. A Simple Vitamin D3 Blood Spot Test can help as well as Thyroid Profile Testing to rule out Hypothyroid condition of lack of energy to create Gastric Motility. All of these tests can be run with one single blood collection drawn from a finger in a simple test. Don't forget to test for Food/Chemical Sensitivity which can create constipation. You may call for additional information.

Side Effects: None

Contraindications: Do not take product if you are allergic to any of its ingredients.

This will get to the REAL cause & the root of the problem of constipation.

MAX MAN
Elevate your Intrinsic Testosterone!

Testosterone level peaks in both men and women in their early twenties. Afterwards, testosterone levels quickly, and drastically, decline with age. By the time we are 50 years old, we have lost over 50 % of our Testosterone, leaving us with flabby muscles, increased fat in the middle, loss of bone mass, non-existent sex life, diminished mental logic & memory, less confidence and less protection from heart diseases.

Much less discussed but far more important is the psychological and emotional effects from the loss of Testosterone. The diminishing level of Testosterone may leave us depressed, less enthusiastic and optimistic about life or more likely to cry easily. There is no greater harm to a human being than the loss of self-confidence through aging.

Major research shows that optimum level of Testosterone improves the essence of sexuality, sexual drive, as well as enhancement of sexual performance. Testosterone is a great source of energy, self-confidence and vitality; our thinking is clearer and memory improved with optimum Testosterone levels. Testosterone supplementation can help develop more strength, vigor, energy, stamina, better muscle tone, and sense of security. Most importantly, optimum levels of Testosterone will firm body tone and reduce fat in the middle of the body.

However, be careful of over doing it! Aggressiveness and bossiness are typical signs of too much Testosterone, as well as unwanted hair growth and acne. These negative symptoms are easily controlled by reducing Testosterone Supplementation when you see these signs, and your body will adjust accordingly.

MAX WOMAN

I know everyone thinks Testosterone is a "man's thing". Testosterone is not just for men, Woman need testosterone as well.

"Do I need Testosterone?"

Women are always surprised to know not only that they have Testosterone, but they also need Testosterone as they age to keep them looking and feeling younger. Use AndroWoman to benefit your health. Learn to take higher doses when appropriate for greater confidence, aggressiveness and sexuality.

Max Man and Max Woman are formulated with a natural super blend of herbal extracts and Hydroxyprogesterone Caproate in which your own body quickly and efficiently converts and metabolizes into Testosterone.

Max Man & Max Woman may:

- **Increase Energy**
- **Protect from Heart Disease**
- **Improve Mood & Memory**
- **Improve Self Esteem**
- **Build Lean Muscle**
- **Decrease Body Fat**
- **Improve Sexual Performance**
- **Increase Auto-Immunity**
- **Enhance Sex drive**
- **Lower Cholesterol**

Dr. Tai's Pearl
Not for use in athletes — May interfere with testing or doping.
Check with proper authorities for final approval before using this supplement for national and international competition.

Side Effects: None
Contraindications: Check with your health practitioner if you have prostate cancer prior to usage. Do not take if you are allergic to any of the ingredients.

Directions: Apply 2-5 pumps to hips or thighs for 5 days off for 2 days. Repeat cycle. Adjust dosage per your Health Professional.

Ingredients: Fulvic Ext., Essential Phospholipids, Evening Primrose Oil, Shea Butter, Glycerin, Aloe Vera, Hydroprogesterone, Eurycoma, Tribulus, Cnidium, Evodia, Cistanche, Lavender Oil, Almond Oil, Hemp Oil, Alpha Lipodic Acid, Vitamin E, Vitamin A, Allantoin, Na Pca

These statements have not been reviewed by the FDA. This product is not intended to diagnose, treat, cure, or prevent any disease.

Max Man & Max Woman - Clinical Applications:

1. Reduced Libido, Haffar et.al, J. Clin, Endoc. 1997
2. Alzheimer's, Hogervost E., et al. Int. J. Ger. Psy. 2002 Oct
3. Parkinson's disease, Okun. M.S. et al. Arch Neur. 2002 Nov.
4. Memory, Moffat S.D. et al, J. Clin. Endoc 2002 Nov.
5. Depression, Pope HG.et al., Am. J. Psych. 2003 Jan
6. Angina Pectors, English K.M. Circulation 2000 Oct.
7. Cardiac Eschemia, Rosano GM., et al., J. Clin. Endoc. 2002
8. Andropause, Jenever J.S. Ewooc & Met. Clin, North AM. 1994; Ravaglia G. et al., Boll. Soc. Itat. Biol. Exp 1995; Morley J. Metabolism 1997 April
9. Cardio Vascular Disease, Barrett0Connor E.C., Diabe tes & Metab. 1995
10. Muscle Strength, Bhasin S et al., N. E. J. Med. 1996

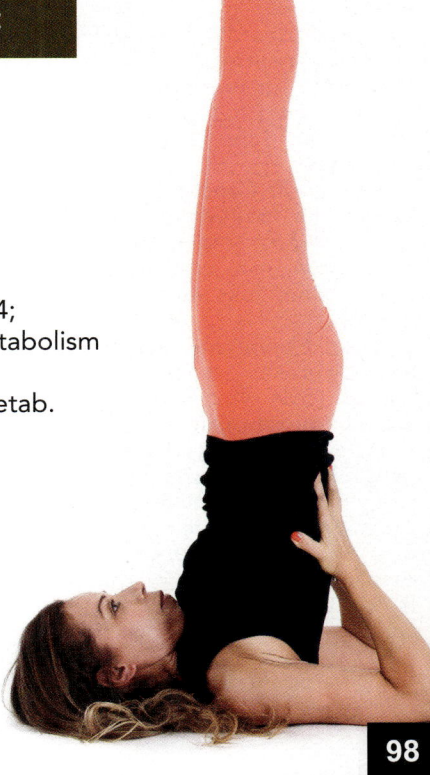

MAX MENOPAUSE SPECIALIST

Herbal Healing for Symptoms of Menopause

Natural "Miracle Healing" for Menopausal Problems

Bio-equivalent Phyto-Estrogen is a natural plant that is chemically and structurally similar but a weaker version full of good Estriol.

1. Isoflavones – Concentrated active ingredient of soy.

Published Research on Isoflavones

Dr. McKenna 2001 – Using Isoflavones concentrate, he found Positive treatment for menopause and symptoms of PMS. It was shown to be safe, with low toxicity and good tolerance.

Dr. Xu 2000 Cancer Epidemiology – shows the Isoflavones decrease the risk of breast cancer and increased protection from bone loss by reducing calcium loss in research animal models.

2. Red Clover has active Genistein and Daidzen. It also provides 18 amino acids which are important in protein metabolism. Research shows it is good for heart disease, decreases cholesterol and decreases cancer risk in the colon and breasts by blocking estrogenic cells.

3. Black Cohosh is very well researched with lots of clinical study. It is approved by the European German Commission E (European FDA) and US: Pharmacopeia 1928.

Published Research on Black Cohosh

Dr. Lieberman 1998 - Black Cohosh is shown to be effective against Menopause

Dr. Lehmann 1988 - 80% of women using Black Cohosh had improvement of their symptoms of Menopause and PMS.

Dr. Ducker 1991 - Proved that Black Cohosh stabilizes the luteinizing hormone and improved the symptoms of menopause

Phyto-Progesterone: The forgotten hormone is made by the ovary after ovulation. Among other sources, a Natural health practitioner calls the symptoms estrogen dominance because the progesterone drops even more severely than estrogen and the theory is that progesterone is the replacement hormone of choice.

1. Chaste tree - VITEX AGNUS - This bush comes from the Mediterranean. It restores and balances reproductive hormones. It works primarily on the pituitary to send messages to the ovary to increase progesterone.

Published Research on Chaste tree

Dr. Veal 1998 – Oral Chaste tree study shows hormonal imbalances were restored in menopause patients.

Dr. Halaskun 1998 – Clinical relief of menstrual and breast pain when patients take Chaste tree treatment.

Dr. Amann 1979 – Used Chaste tree for relief of menstrual water retention. A large clinical study of 1,500 patients on Chaste tree for 5 months, showed 35% of patients had total menopausal relief with no symptoms at all and 90% of all patients had improvement of symptoms from menopause.

Balancing organs means strengthening the kidney, adrenal, ovaries and blood which carry the hormones and all fluids. The first ingredient:

1. DONG QUAI - Angelica Sinensis - comes from the carrot family known in Asia as the female tonic, smooth muscle relaxant, helps convert all androsterones to estrogen, progesterone and testosterone in the liver.

99

Published Research on Dong Quai

Dr. Osaka 1990 – Dong Quai research shows clinical smooth muscle relaxation which improves blood flow by opening blood vessels for better hormone distribution. Ovaries and uterine pain is also relieved. Vasomotor Relaxation also relieves sweating, heat to cold chills and also has positive changes on the skin and blood vessels.

Dr. He et al 1986 - Research showed that patients taking Dong Quai were able to regulate menstrual abnormality and obtained relief of symptoms of PMS.

PANAX GINSENG - A root prized for centuries, the most used herb in the world. Benefits are tonify, vigor, health, longevity, anti-fatigue, increase libido, strengthen immunity and retard the aging process.

Directions: Take 1 capsule twice daily or more as needed and recommended by your physician or health practitioner. Do not take if bleeding occurs or while bleeding. Keep out of reach of children.

Ingredients:
Isoflavone, Black Cohosh Ext., Chastetree Berry Ext., Dong Quai Ext., Pueraria, Rhodiola Rosea, Red Clover Ext., Piperine Ext

These statements have not been reviewed by the FDA. This product is not intended to diagnose, treat, cure, or prevent any disease.

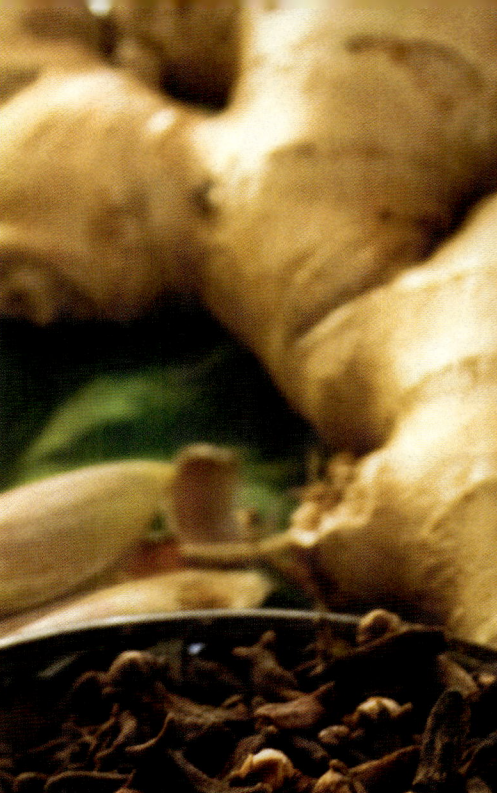

Dr. Tai's Pearl

Max Menopause Specialist is key to having an alternative of controlling the symptoms of menopause without any of the effects of estrogen. Most people erroneously think that soy isoflavones have estrogen. This is absolutely completely false. The isoflavones that work on the receptors and calms them are called genistein and daidzein. They are not hormones and do not have hormone effects. They do, however, have the affinity to the receptors of the hormone which when attached gives the calming effect of symptoms of menopause. Asian women have been using these herbs for thousands of years and we know that the Asian women have the lowest incidence of breast cancer among the population of the world.

Side Effects: None

Contraindications:
Do not take during the menstrual (bleeding) period; can re-take supplementation upon cessation of bleeding. Do not take product if you are allergic to any of its ingredients.

Clinical Cases:
Emanuella, 60-year-old Portuguese woman. Since struggling with menopausal symptoms since the age of 56, she attempted anti-depressants, but had to stop using them because of the side effects it created for her. What disturbed her greatly was the night sweats. They would wake her up in the middle of the night in a severe panic, completely dreanched in sweat. She described her husband as a saint because he never complained about her symptom episodes and was completely baffled by the horrific occurrences. She felt extraordinary dryness of her eyes and skin, her C-cup breasts were drooping severely and intercourse was extremely painful. She decided to try the Max Menopause capsules, taking double doses in the first few weeks to re-establish her receptor activity. She started to immediately notice the dryness resolving itself. She also used topical Pueraria on her vaginal opening and quickly noticed the intercourse became a more pleasurable experience without severe pain and dryness. When I last spoke with her, she was very happy with her progress and very grateful for natural supplements without any side effects.

MAX MITOCHONDRIA

Power Proper Function in Cells

Every single activity your body does to stay alive requires *ENERGY*.
Mitochondria are the only original source of energy in your body!
Without it? You'd DIE!

As a physician in the past 45 years, I am seeing an extraordinary group of New Age diseases never understood before, but now, for the first time, an excellent understanding for underlying pathogenesis, treatment with excellent results and prevention.

A simple, concise, all natural treatment plan helps physicians and health professionals control pathology, regrowth of Mitochondria in quantities and qualities for restoring normal, even excellent activities never seen possible before.

What Are Mitochondria?

This magical sub-cellular unit is the "Battery" and the "Power House" that provides for more than 90% of human energy and found in every cell of the body. It is what makes life a divine electrical power for All Human Functions, from your Brain, Muscle, Heart, Liver (Hood, 2006) to energizing all essential biochemical changes in our body and from Cell Replication, Cell Messaging, Aging & Cell Death (Schardt 2008), without which LIFE CANNOT EXIST! OR IT'S JUST PLAIN MISERABLE!!!

This miracle tiny organelle is so important that it has its own DNA!

It is this Food-Burning furnace in our body's cell (Schardt 2008) that Burns Fat (Triglycerides) controlling our weight, obesity and total nutrition. A MUST Science for the fitness and weight loss doctors and coaches.

From muscle growing and enlarging to endurance training, the mitochondrial is key to using and burning fat and less dependent of glucose. (Hood 2006) This is the essential knowledge for fat in Metabolic X Syndrome, Diabetes, Obesity and lowering cholesterol.

This Essential Breakthrough knowledge used by the young and old patients alike, is enhancing the quality of life of the exercising athlete and individual (Melov 2007).

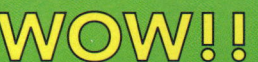

Remember that our brain and nerve cells require tremendous energy to communicate with the billions of Neurons and Mitochondria to power on thoughts, maintain a sharp mind, wipe out Brain Fog and restore excellent hearing, memory and concentration for older patients and young students alike. **Max Mitochondria** is the simplest, most powerful answer to slow aging, extend life with excellent health and to reverse your signs of aging.

R-Alpha Lipoic Acid (only Human Form) is of course unique in Antioxidants because it is Natural, Broad Spectrum, and unique in luring other antioxidants to regenerate the power to work. No other antioxidant is both water and fat-soluble, working to regenerate cell membranes in the Muscles, Liver, Kidneys, Skin and the Brain!

WOW!!
I call it A Super Antioxidant!

- Lower body levels of toxic metals, especially mercury
- Protecting LDL cholesterol (bad cholesterol) from oxidation by copper
- Brain and nerve cell health by stimulating Nerve Growth Factor (NGF)
- Improve memory in aged animals, reversing brain cell receptor defects
- Protect brain cells damaged by toxins and chemicals
- Recycle CoQ10 back to active antioxidant form
- Normalize elevated lipid peroxide, reducing risk of oxidation damage, cardiovascular disease and Cancer
- Restore antioxidant in old animals to normal, young animal levels

Acetyl L-Carnitine in Max Mitochondria gives power to cells, especially those that help in all functions of the Human body and also Heart Function and Brain Power. Acetyl L-Carnitine can Re-Energize Mitochondria without the damages often seen with higher Free Radical production associated with Mitochondrial Function

- Significantly improve Mitochondrial function to lower oxidative stress and free radical generation
- Restore age-related dysfunction and key mitochondrial enzymes used in energy production
- Improving mitochondria function and energy production
- Improved memory in old rats

The only formula in the world that consists of Cordyceps Sinensis, which is fermented in special low temperatures and in low pressure, just as found in Nature at the high 20,000 feet mountains of Tibet, where it was first discovered thousands of years ago by Buddhist Monks. It includes the previously unavailable Cordyceps Militaris and Cordycepis Oophioglosoides which provides unique WBC training and T-cells production up to 800% to protect the Mitochondria from damage and fight off the millions of Fungus, Yeast, Viruses and Bacteria.

If you are looking for relief, prevention of Disease, and symptom relief of Adrenal Fatigue, Chronic Fibromyalgia, Hypothyroid, Hashimoto Thyroids, Energy drain and Malaise, lack of Immunity, G.I tract dysfunction, endocrine malfunction and deficiency, Advanced Aging, Arthritis and Pain, Overwhelming Inflammation, Atherosclerosis, Heart Disease, Dementia, Lung and breathing symptoms, Recurrent Stress, and unrelenting Depression with frequent colds and infection, Max Mitochondria is the powerful answer. It is a highly effective first step of a return to awesome Health.

Directions:
Take 1 capsule AM & Bedtime with a large glass of Water on an Empty Stomach
Do not eat for 1 Hour After Taking.

Ingredients:
Zinc, Manganese, Selenium, Proprietary Formulation: Acetyl L-Carnatine, ALA, CoQ10, C. Sinensis, C. Militaris, C. Ophioglossoides, D. Ambrosioides, Una de Gato, Thyroidinum, N-Acetyl-Cysteine

These statements have not been reviewed by the FDA. This product is not intended to diagnose, treat, cure, or prevent any disease.

Dr. Tai's Pearl

I, too, once took my mitochondria for granted. I spent all my time chasing symptoms, and for the most part finding relief, but without addressing the one, HUGE underlying cause. When I started to pay special attention to my mitochondria, that's when everything changed for the better!

I'll let you in on a secret - Learning to charge up my mitochondria was ultimately the key to my 60lb weight loss. When my dormant mitochondria WOKE UP and got to work, they created more and more energy for my cells and my body – using all the glucose, amino acids and FAT they could get their hands on. My body turned into a calorie-burning furnace and before I knew it I had to wrap my old belts around me twice! Looking and feeling great wasn't even the biggest bonus – my awakened mitochondria, which were now growing younger, began to energize my brain and help protect me from major neurodegenerative diseases. Although no one is unsusceptible from developing Alzheimer's or Dementia, to reach a whopping 70 years old and still being able to come to my office every day, consult with members and patients, and write to you like this... well, it feels **FANTASTIC!**

Side Effects: None

Contraindications: Do not take if you are allergic to any of the ingredients.

Clinical Cases:

Dr. George is a 62-year-old doctor who struggled with being overweight along with low libido, severe fatigue and frequent bouts of colds, flu and even shingles. With all these problems, he told me that he was planning to retire soon because, in his words, "I just don't have it anymore."

Of course, his laboratory blood work up looked normal with nothing salient to justify his crippling symptoms. His own doctor threw up his hands, saying "GEORGE! You are just GETTING OLD!"

I worked with Dr. George and focused my attention on the thyroid & mitochondrial activity. As part of the treatment, the nutritional diet was simple vegetables, salads and protein. Dr. George committed fully to removing all sugars, fruits and carbohydrates from his diet.

He supplemented with Cellular Energy, Ultra Charge and Max Mitochondria. Of course, Super B12, Max Sea and Vitamin D3-K2 helped to increase & strengthen immunity.

I am happy to report after 6 months, that Dr. George has lost 32lbs, no longer suffers from colds or the flu and his stamina and vigor has returned!!

REFERENCES

1. Melov, S., Tamopolsky, M., Beckman, E., Felkey, K., and Hubbard, A. Resistance training reverses aging in human skeletal muscle. PLoS ONE (5), 2007.
2. Sagan, L. (1967). On the origin of mitosing cells. Journal of Theoretical Biology, 14(3), 225-274.
3. Lino A, Boccia MM, Rusconi AC, Bellomonte L, Cocuroccia B. "Psycho-functional changes in attention and learning under the action of L-acetylcarnitine in 17 young subjects. A pilot study of its use in mental deterioration." Clin Ter. 1992 Jun;140(6):569-73
4. Schardt. D. (2008). Manipulating Mitochondria. Nutrition Action Healthletter, 35(10), 8-10.
5. Sano M, Bell K, Cote L, Dooneief G, Lawton A, Legler L, Marder K, Naini A, Stern Y, Mayeux R. "Double-blind parallel design pilot study of acetyl levocarnitine in patients with Alzheimer's disease." Arch Neurol. 1992 Nov;49(11):1137-41
6. Bowman BA. "Acetyl-carnitine and Alzheimer's disease." Nutr Rev. 1992 May;50(5):142-4.
7. Postiglione A, Soricelli A, Cicerano U, Mansi L, De Chiara S, Gallotta G, Schettini G, Salvatore M. "Effect of acute administration of L-acetyl carnitine on cerebral blood flow in patients with chronic cerebral infarct." Pharmacol Res. 1991 Apr;23(3):241-6.
8. Rosadini G, Marenco S, Nobili F, Novellone G, Rodriguez G. "Acute effects of acetyl-L-carnitine on regional cerebral blood flow in patients with brain ischaemia." Int J Clin Pharmacol Res.1990;10(1-2):123-8.
9. Bella R, Biondi R, Raffaele R, Pennisi G. "Effect of acetyl-L-carnitine on geriatric patients suffering from dysthymic disorders." Int J Clin Pharmacol Res. 1990;10(6):355-60.
10. Gregus Z, Stein AF, Varga F, Klaassen CD. "Effect of lipoic acid on biliary excretion of glutathione and metals." Toxicol Appl Pharmacol 1992 May;114(1):88-96

11. Lodge JK, Traber MG, Packer L. "Thiol chelation of Cu2+ by dihydrolipoic acid prevents human low density lipoprotein peroxidation." Free Radic Biol Med 1998 Aug;25(3):287-97

12. Murase K, Hattori A, Kohno M, Hayashi K. "Stimulation of nerve growth factor synthesis/secretion in mouse astroglial cells by coenzymes." Biochem Mol Biol Int 1993 Jul;30(4):615-21

13. Stoll S, Hartmann H, Cohen SA, Muller WE. "The potent free radical scavenger alpha-lipoic acid improves memory in aged mice: putative relationship to NMDA receptor deficits."Pharmacol Biochem Behav 1993 Dec;46(4):799-805

14. Stoll S, Rostock A, Bartsch R, Korn E, Meichelbock A, Muller WE. "The potent free radical scavenger alpha-lipoic acid improves cognition in rodents." Acad Sci 1994 Jun 30;717:122-8

15. Muller U, Krieglstein J. "Prolonged pretreatment with alpha-lipoic acid protects cultured neurons against hypoxic, glutamate, or iron-induced injury." J Cereb Blood Flow Metab 1995 Jul;15(4):624-30

16. Nohl H, Gille L. "Evaluation of the antioxidant capacity of ubiquinol and dihydrolipoic acid." Z Naturforsch [C] 1998 Mar-Apr;53(3-4):250-3

17. Arivazhagan P, Juliet P, Panneerselvam C. "Effect of dl-alpha-lipoic acid on the status of lipid peroxidation and antioxidants in aged rats." Pharmacol Res 2000 Mar;41(3):299-303

18. Hagen TM, Liu J, Lykkesfeldt J, Ames BN, et al. Feeding acetyl-L-carnitine and lipoic acid to old rats significantly improves metabolic function while decreasing oxidative stress. Proc Natl Acad Sci USA. 2002 Feb 19;99(4):1870-5.

19. Liu J, Killilea DW, Ames BN. Age-associated mitochondrial oxidative decay: improvement of carnitine acetyltransferase substrate-binding affinity and activity in brain by feeding old rats acetyl-L- carnitine and/or R-alpha -lipoic acid. Proc Natl Acad Sci USA. 2002 Feb 19;99(4):1876-81.

20. Liu J, Head E, Gharib AM, Ames BN, et al. Memory loss in old rats is associated with brain mitochondrial decay and RNA/DNA oxidation: partial reversal by feeding acetyl-L-carnitine and/or R-alpha -lipoic acid. Proc Natl Acad Sci USA. 2002 Feb 19;99(4):2356-61.

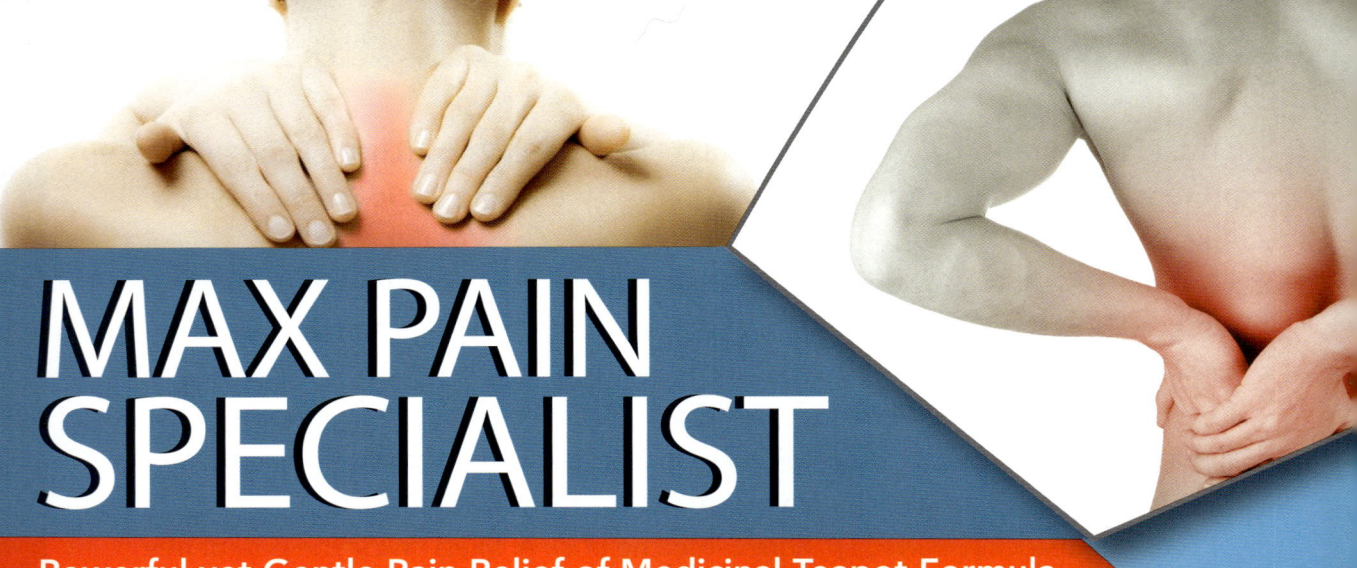

MAX PAIN SPECIALIST

Powerful yet Gentle Pain Relief of Medicinal Teapot Formula

Corydalis, Poeonia, Dong Quai, Notoginseng, Shefflera, Angelica, Licorice

This Astonishing PRINCE OF PAIN RELIEF, a concentrate of Traditional Chinese Medicine Extracts, was discovered after monumental laboratory work. Using 4,605 extracts of natural plants, they patiently evaluated each of the extracts against the "Gold Standard" Morphine for pain relief and anti-Inflammatory activities and then the best analgesic extract was chosen those reaching 60% analgesic of morphine and processed using the "Medicinal Teapot" technology. Now you have the Prince of Pain Relief with all the benefits of morphine without the negative side effects.

THE SCIENCE BEHIND MAX PAIN SPECIALIST!

The Amazing miracle formula to relieve all kinds of pain from all over your body: Glucosamine Sulfate –This is the most fundamental and natural component of our joint cartilage, tendons, bone, ligament, nails, hair, etc. There are multiple clinical studies and published reports proving its value in reducing symptoms and rebuilding the damaged cartilage of your joints. Our own body's cartilage cells use it for the repair of joints as well as inhibiting enzymes that destroy cartilage. Capable of increasing flexibility and resistance to corrosion to counteract joint stress, Dr. Phoon reported its unique ability to repair cartilage and damaged joints. By blocking the destructive mechanism of cartilage degeneration, glucosamine can halt and even reverse the disease process and relieves symptoms.

However, be aware that there are several forms of glucosamine. All clinical studies have used only one kind. Do not buy the wrong one just because it is cheaper, as it does not work. Helme, et al, conducted a clinical study of 68 patients with knee joint arthritis. Loading pain improved by 80%.

MSM (Methyl Sulfonyl Methane) – This is critical sulfur required for proper repair of injured cartilage, ligaments and tendons. Although naturally present in foods like vegetables, fruits, fish and meats, it is not available at sufficient quantities for our joint needs (Qie et al, 1998). Reports show that a strategic use of MSM increases the therapeutic efficiency of glucosamine because of the sulfur presence. This combination really works. Dr. Lawrence UCLA Medical School found 80% of arthritis patients improved their pain symptoms.

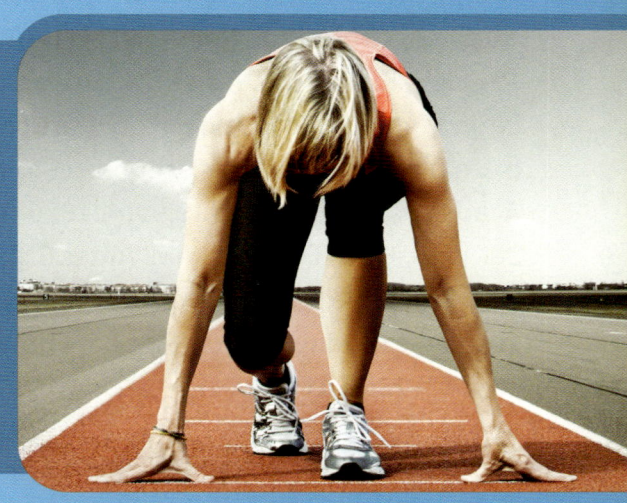

Ginger –

Often overlooked and forgotten. This is one of the oldest anti-inflammatory and pain relievers known to mankind. A special concentrated extract of gingerol (the active ingredient) has proven very effective at relieving arthritis pain. The Journal of Osteoarthritis Cartilage reports Israel's Tel Aviv University studied 29 patients suffering from osteoarthritis of the knee, half received ginger extract, the other half a fake placebo. At the end of 12 weeks, the ginger group showed knee pain reduced significantly and joint mobility increased significantly.

Another study at University of Miami enrolled 247 subjects with severe osteoarthritis of the knee. Subjects were divided into ginger group and placebo group for six weeks. Sixty-three percent of the ginger extract group improved significantly while the placebo group showed no improvement. The Ginger group showed twice as much improvement in pain after a walking test. Journal of Arthritis and Rheumatism Nov 2001.

Dr. Patrick Nassey, MD, reported in the Chicago Daily Herald on 3/15/04 that Ginger may be the alternative approach to reduce arthritis of the knee.

At a University study in Denmark, Dr. Srivastava reported on 56 patients who suffered from Rheumatoid Arthritis, Osteoarthritis and muscle spasm pain. Using Ginger, 75% of the arthritis sufferers experienced relief of pain and swelling. All of the patients with muscular pain experienced relief and most importantly, no side effects were reported after several months to several years of consumption. Med Hypothesis Dec 1992.

Grape Skin –

This unique supplement is very misunderstood. Magazines and catalogs try to sell you a lower quality grape seed for its content of the active ingredient Resveratrol, but scientific evidence disputes this kind of salesmanship. Research performed on quantitative analysis by Xingjian Medical School, one of the great medical schools in Asia, clearly shows that contents of Resveratrol are much higher in the grape skin of grapes from wineries, followed by fresh grape skin, and lastly, the Resveratrol content in grape seeds. Published by Dr. Xiang on Sept 2003. This research was confirmed Dr. Careri, Published in Journal Agricultural Food Chem Aug 2003. University of Parma, Italy. Resveratrol is particularly able to neutralize the destructive COX-2 enzyme that causes inflammation and pain of the joint and muscle. (From research by Michigan State University and published in Journal of Agricultural Food Chemistry Jan 2004.)

This unique ingredient is very rarely used in pain formulation because the research and information has just become available to the public. It will take some time for the copy cats to catch up here.

Quercetin –

This very rare ingredient and even more unusual usage is the "ultimate weapon" against inflammation. Quercetin is the champion of anti-inflammation, as reported by Dr. Morikawa from Sagami Women's University in Japan. Wonderful laboratory cell microscopy demonstrates proof of Quercetin suppression of inflammatory response in animals studies published in Life Science Dec 2003.

An even greater technological breakthrough reported by Dr. Woo from Chubu University is that Quercetin is able to suppress bone loss which may stop cartilage degeneration published in Biological & Pharmaceutical Bulletin 2004.

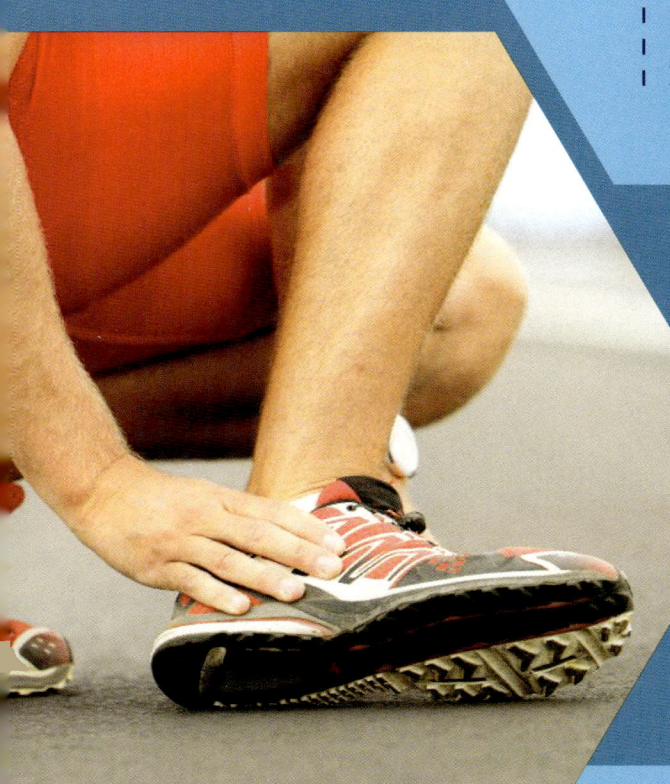

Boswellia Serrata –

This ancient Ayuverdic herb of Frankincense has been used as anti-inflammatory for a thousand years. Boswellia acid, the active ingredient, has been found to block the destructive leukotrienes enzyme which trigger painful inflammation.

Recently at University of Poona, India, researchers report that 42 severely arthritic patients failed to respond to prescription medication. After 3 months of Boswellia extracts, they experienced significant decrease in joint pain, joint swelling and stiffness. They began to have improvements in the first 2 to 4 weeks. J. Ethnophama 91:33.

Dr. Kimmatkar reported in J. Phytomedicine Jan 2003, that in his clinical study (double blind and placebo controlled) 30 patients showed 100% success in the decrease of knee pain, increased knee flexibility and increased walking distance. Dr. Amon of University Tubingen, Germany went even further to report Boswellic acid improved not only rheumatoid arthritis, but also chronic colitis, ulcerative colitis, Crohn's disease and even bronchial asthma. The famous Dr. Andrew Weil, MD, recommends Boswellia herb for inflammatory conditions such as chronic fibromyalgia and Prostatitis.

Curcumin –
It is one of the finest anti-inflammatory herbs in the natural arsenal. Curcumin is very special because of its unique ability to inhibit and neutralize both the destructive enzyme the 5-LO from Leukotrienes as well as COX-2 who are the main culprits causing inflammation and pain. J. Ethropharmacology March 1993.

Dr. Kaug, J., Pharmacol. March 2004 confirms that curcumin indeed "significantly inhibits" destructive enzyme COX-2 which produces further prostaglandins during episodes of inflammation. Curcumin even protects against colon cancer, according to Dr. Goel's published Cancer Letter 2001. According to Dr. Susan Lark, in a study published by the American J. of Natural Medicine, curcumin was able to reduce morning stiffness and swelling as comparable to cortisone and phenylbutazone, without the side effects.

White Willow –
Centuries old, this natural remedy provided pain relief for all conditions. It is the grandfather of all analgesics and pain pills with a number of strong clinical and proven efficacies as reported by Dr. Chrubasik in his research on Pain Management published in German Wein Med 2002.

In Summary:
The bad enzymes causing inflammation and pain are COX-2 and Leukotrienes (5 LO). Good enzymes, COX-1, protect your stomach from ulcers and normalize and balance body functions.

- Pinpoint & Eliminate Destructive causes of joint pain
- May restore joint flexibility
- Stop your dependence on Dangerous Pharmaceutical Drugs
- May provide relief from pain & inflammation
- Halt the destruction of your joints
- Start Enjoying Life Again!

Directions:
Take 1 capsule three times daily as needed. For additional pain control, take 2 capsules. The improvements will reach the best potential after taking for 1 or 2 months. Keep out of reach of children.

Ingredients:
White Willow, Quercetin, Boswellia Serrata, Curcuma Longa, MSM, Glucosamine Hcl, Ginger Extract, Grape Skin, Corydalis Yahusa, Peonia Lactifora, Angelica Sinensis, Panax Notoginseng, Schefflera Arbor, Angelica Deharica, Glycyrrhiza Uralensis, Piperine Longa, Cetyl Myristoleate, Dl Phenylalanine, Gelatin Capsules,

These statements have not been reviewed by the FDA. This product is not intended to diagnose, treat, cure, or prevent any disease.

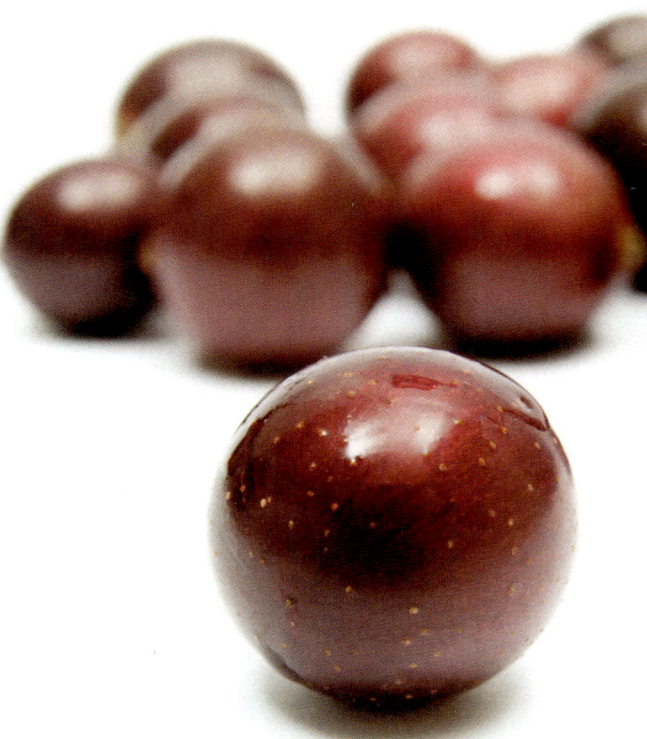

Dr. Tai's Pearl

Very few countries do extensive research on natural supplements and ingredients except for India and China, where universities still support natural scientific studies. We are very grateful for the knowledge, as well as TCM ingredients and history, and for the science that has been published throughout the centuries. Using the accumulation of all the great scientific breakthrough from the past 4,000 years, this formula has very deep roots into the traditional Chinese medicine as well as ancient secrets from India. Rarely do you see so many scientifically proven ingredients working together to solve the problems of inflammation by neutralizing the inflammatory enzymes which cascades towards pain and disability. Doctors from all around the world have relied on Max Pain for its significant efficiency to provide relief for pain and inflammation throughout the body.

Side Effects:
When using large doses, some G.I. tract upset has been reported. There have been positively mitigated by taking Max Pain with food and after meals.

Contraindications:
Patient should not be taking Max Pain with active stomach ulcers, IBS and diarrhea. Do not take product if you are allergic to any of its ingredients.

Clinical Cases:
Betty, 36-year-old nurse and physician assistant suffering from severe arthritis in both hands. She was having difficulty doing physical therapy in the clinic for patients. She has tried many prescription medications which created many complications for her immune system, as well as swelling and even numbness of the extremities. Max Pain, together with Max Arthro, was used in order to facilitate her transition. She found the treatment highly effective and slowly progressed within six weeks of having larger dosages, finally adjusting to lower dosage in order to maintain progress. She is now relatively 90% pain-free and able to perform most of her activity with full range of motion of the hands and wrists, without any significant side effects.

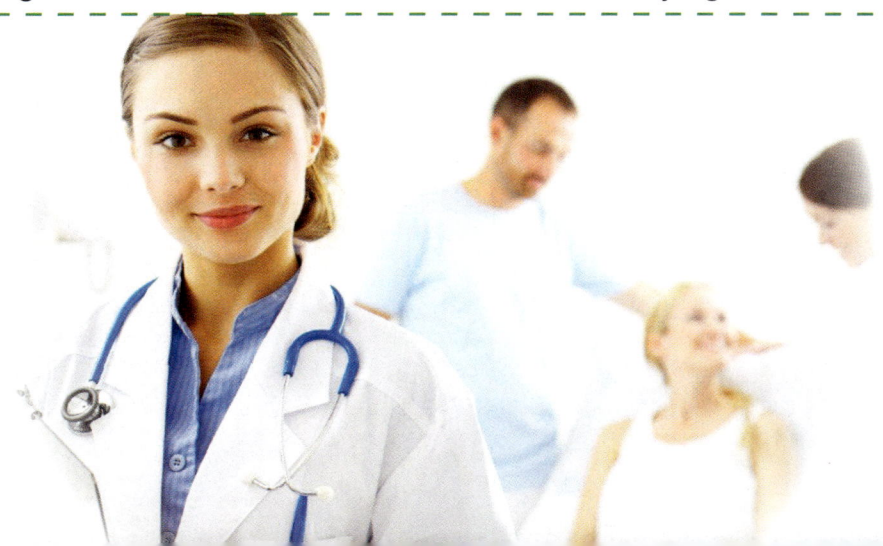

Max Performance Specialist

The First Anti-Aging Supplement Known to Mankind

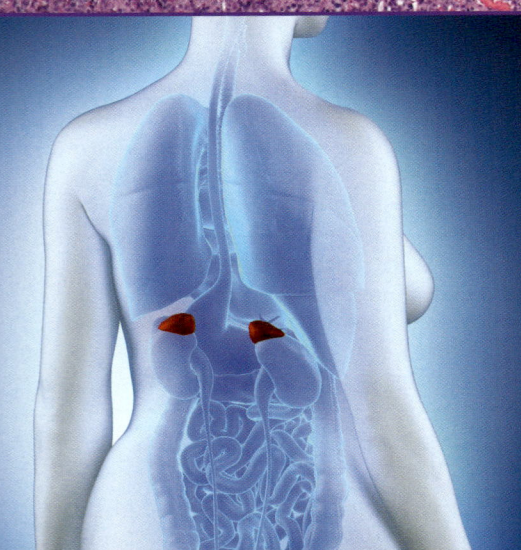

STOP ADRENAL FATIGUE – Improve Adrenal function, control stress and depression.
IMMUNE SYSTEM – Increases NK cell activity (makes more)
MUSCLE – Increases Power, builds better/younger cells.
ENDURANCE & STAMINA - Reduces muscle Soreness, Enhances Recovery, Promotes Better Oxygen efficiency, Improves Hormones, Adrenal, Thymus, Mitochondrial energy, supports lung disease, up to 30% increase in bioenergy.
BLOOD CELLS – Improves Blood Cell Viability & Function. 40% more Oxygen.
LIVER – Improves Liver Functions, helps with Hepatitis and Cirrhosis.
FITNESS – Increases ATP Synthesis, Promotes Faster Energy Recovery, Reduces Fatigue, Improves Physical Function, Provides More Stamina.
SEXUAL FUNCTIONS – Improves Libido and Quality of Life in Men & Women, Fights infertility, Increases Sperm Count, Increases Sperm Survival.

CORDYCEPS The mushroom of world records

Cordyceps mushrooms come from the small Southwestern regions of China in Tibet, Nepal and nearby provinces in the high Himalayas. The altitude extremes, (over 11,000 feet) together with the isolated and severe habitats, made the natural gathering and harvest of this amazing mushroom rare, difficult and very expensive. Available only to the Chinese Emperors and the very wealthy for over 5,000 years it is prized as the most expensive herb in the world. The traditional Chinese doctors would use Cordyceps mushroom to energize, improve health and treat many ailments. It was classified as a "Life Extender" and was designated as the first anti-aging supplement in history to be enjoyed in royal courts by the Kings and Queens of ancient dynasties.

Unique Scientific Breakthroughs Revealed here!

This new organic growing method produces a pure 100% cordyceps mushroom product with no foreign contamination of any kind (even the wild harvest has soil and other organic remains) and 1500% higher HEA and cordycepin than the best wild collected samples.
• Cordyceps radically increases cellular energy by 30%, which is also known scientifically as the ATP/IP ratio. Cordyceps has been clinically proven to increase cellular Bio-Energy by as much as 30% (Reported XU C.F et al in ZHU J-S, Halpern GM, Jone,s K. The Scientific rediscovery of a precious ancient Chinese herbal regimen: Cordyceps sinensis: Part I. J Alt Comp Med 1998;4(3):289-303.)
• Cordyceps increases cellular Oxygen Absorption by up to 40% (Lou Y, Liao X, Lu Y. Cardiovascular pharmacological studies of ethanol extracts of Cordyceps mycelia and Cordyceps fermentation solution. Chinese Traditional and Herbal Drugs 1986;17(5):17-21,209-213)

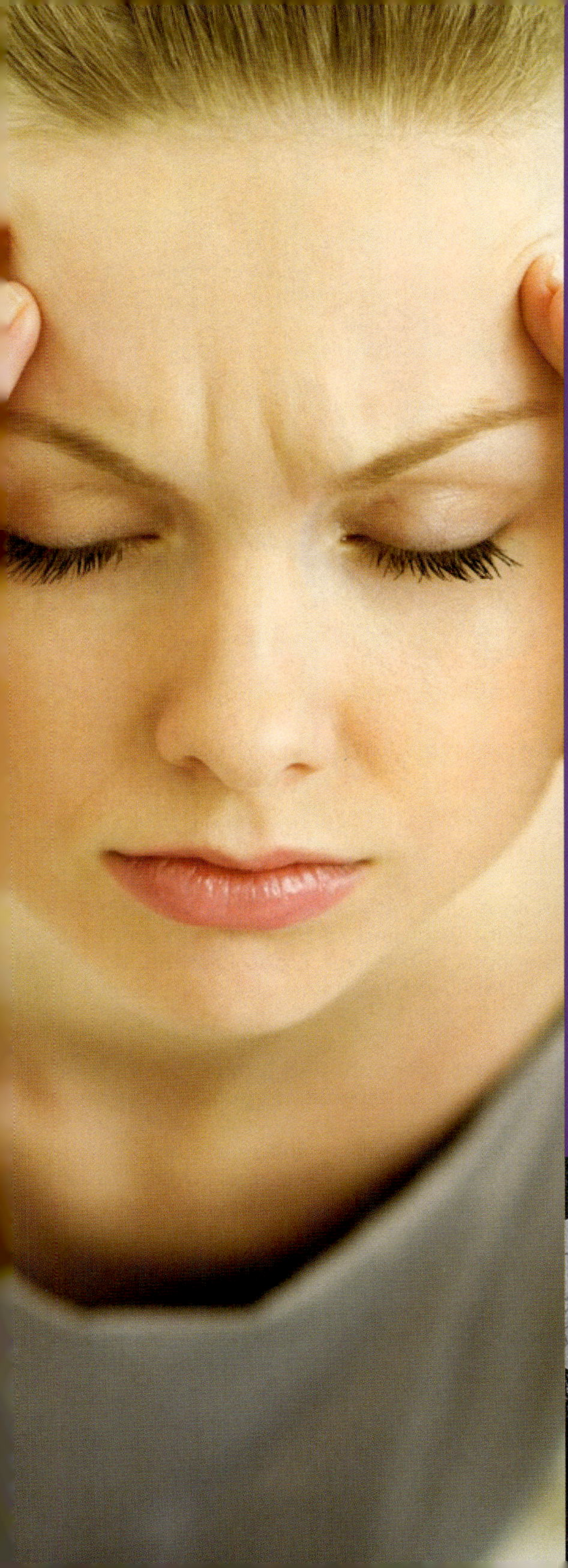

STOP ADRENAL FATIGUE - Clinical research proved in controlled studies, that elderly patients suffering from fatigue and some senility related symptoms reported improvement.

(1) Improvements in the reduction of fatigue 92%, of feeling cold 89%, in dizziness 83%, after taking Cordyceps for 30 days. Patients with respiratory/breathing problems felt physically stronger and some were able to jog for 600 ft. (Cao A, Wen Y. J Applied Traditional Chinese Med 1993;1:32-33)

(2) Chronic obstructive pulmonary diseases improvement of 40% after Cordyceps supplement. (Wang WQ. J. Administration Traditional Chinese Med 1995;5(supp;):24)

(3) Chronic kidney diseases improvement of 51% after only one month with Cordyceps supplement.(Jiang JC, Gao YF. J Administration Traditional Chinese Med 1995;5(sup pl):23-24)

Dramatic Natural Improvements are seen in endocrine hormone levels, in fertility and in Sexual Libido for men and women.

(1) Research on animal studies shows cordyceps increases natural sex hormones (Wan F, Guo Y, Deng X. Chinese Traditional Patented Med 1988;9:29-31) (2) Prevention and improvement of adrenal glands and thymus hormones, and infertile sperm count improve by 300% after cordyceps supplement.(Huang Y, Lu J, Zhu B, Wen Q, Jia F, Zeng S, Chen T, Li Y, Xheng G, Yi Z.. Zhongchengyao Yanjiu 1987;(10):24-25)(3) Human clinical studies involving both men and women of 189 patients with decreased libido and desire showed improvement of symptoms and desire of 66% (Wan F, Guo Y, Deng X. Chinese Traditional Patented Med 1988;9:29-31) and (4) Another double blind study by the Institute of Meteria Medica in Beijing, China showed women's improvement of libido and desire at 86%. (JIA-SHI ZHU, M.D., Ph.D. The Journal of Alternative & Complementary Medicine, Vol.4, Number 3, 1998, pp.289-303) (5) The most dramatic physical proof came from a Fertility Study (Guo YZ. J Modern Diagnostics Therapeutics 1986;(1):60-65) involving a clinical research of 22 males. It showed clear evidence that cordyceps supplements increased sperm counts by 33%, decreased incidences of sperm malformations by 29% and a 79% increase in survival rate after 8 weeks of using a cordyceps supplement.

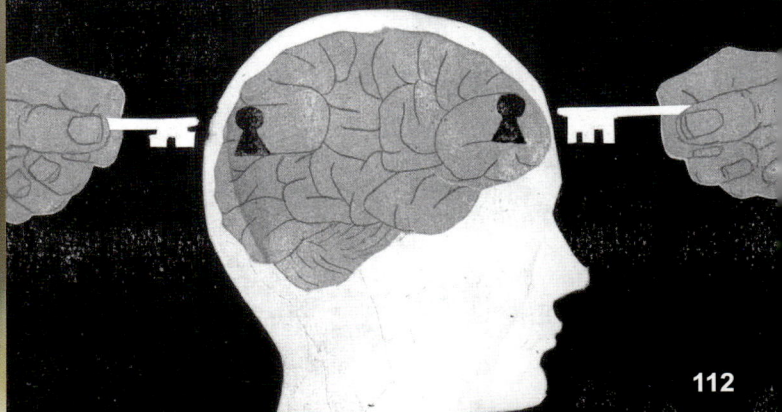

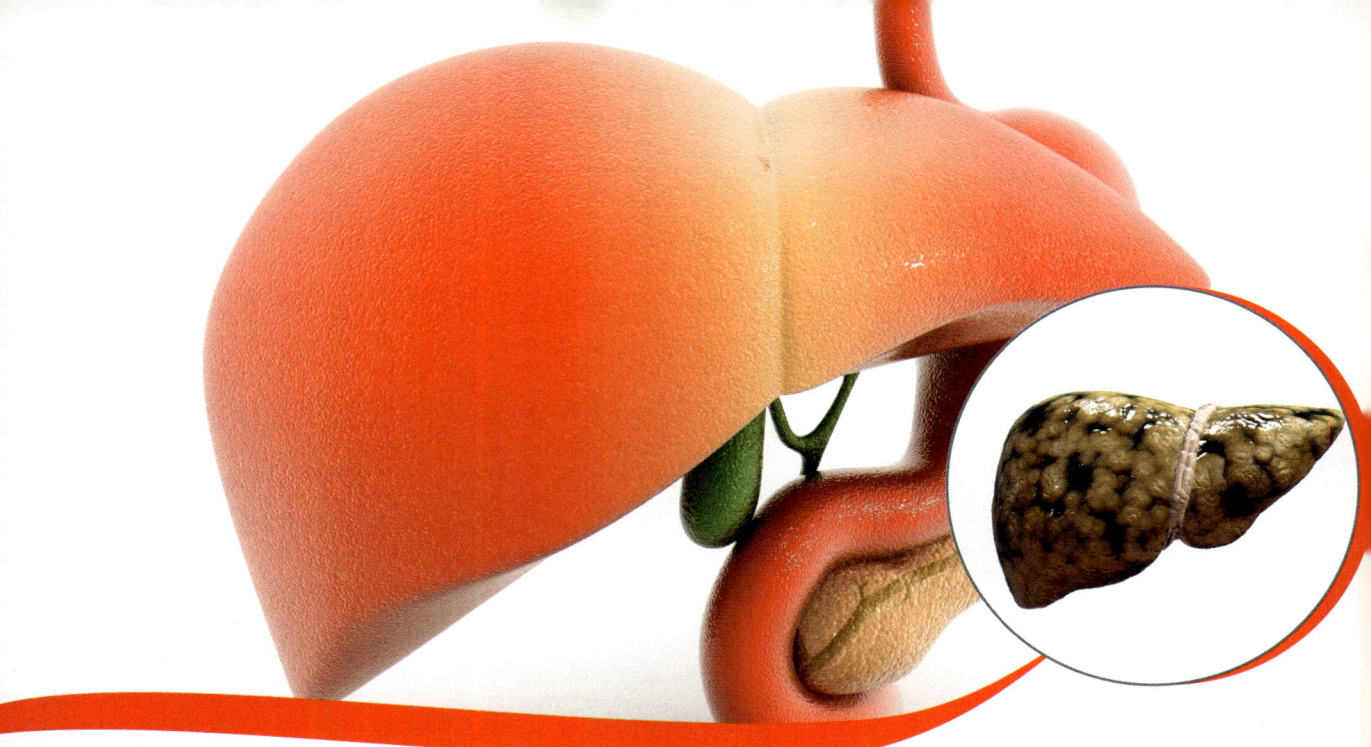

Liver Protection – Sub chronic and chronic hepatitis on related liver diseases are more prevalent than most people think. Liver is the living filter of the human body, cleaning the blood and all other fluids of impurities. There is no way for you to survive, much less feel healthy, without a functioning liver.

Research clinical trials on 33 patients with Hepatitis "B" and on another 8 patients with cirrhosis taking Cordyceps supplement showed 71.9% improvement on "Thymol Turbidity Test" and 78.6% improvement in" SGPT Test" both of these are enzyme tests which show improving functions of the liver. (Zhou LT, Yang YZ, Xu YM, Zhu QY, Zhu YR, Ge XY, Gao JD. Short term curative effect of cultured Cordyceps sinensis (Berk.) Sacc. Mycelia in chronic hepatitis B. China J Chinese Materia Medica 1990;15(1):53-55)

Recharge the Protective Army of NK cells – Your body's ability to fight infections and tumors depends on the availability of Natural Killer (NK) Cells. These are the essential first lines of defense for our body's protection mechanisms commonly known as the Immune System.
Several scientific studies of Cordyceps have especially focused on Natural Killer (NK) cells and Cordyceps effect on them and cancer formation. One such in-vitro study demonstrated Cordycep adding significant enhancement of NK cell activity in normal individuals as well as leukemia stricken individuals. (Liu C, Lu S, J MR, Xie Y. effects of Cordyceps Sinensis on in-vitro natural killer cells.) Chinese J Integrated Traditional Western Med (Chung-Kuo Chung His I Chieh Ho Tsa Chih) 1992;12(5):267-269) showed that natural Cordyceps enhanced the NK cell activity of normal patients by 74% and increased the NK activity of leukemia patients by 400% and similar improvements of NK cell activities was found in melanoma cancers (Xu RH, Peng XE, Chen GZ, Chen GL. Effects of Cordyceps Sinensis on natural killer activity and colony formation of B16 melanoma Chinese Med J 1992;105(2):97-101)

The improvements in the Immune System were so impressive that Dr. Zhu at the Journal of Alternative and Complementary Medicine 1998 stated: "Because of the above profound influence on immune functions, natural Cordyceps products have been used in many clinical conditions in patients with altered immune functions.

Directions:

Take 1 capsule 3 times daily with food. Higher or more frequent dosages may be taken as needed or recommended by your health practitioner. Keep out of reach of children.

Ingredients:

Cordyceps Sinensis, C- Militaris, C-Ophioglosoides, Epimedium Extract, Tribulus Extract, Notoginseng Extract, Eurycoma Ext. Cnidium Monier Ext. Panax Ginseng Ext., Piperine Longa Ext, Cellulose, Silica, Dicalcium Phosphate, Cross Caramellose.

These statements have not been reviewed by the FDA. This product is not intended to diagnose, treat, cure, or prevent any disease.

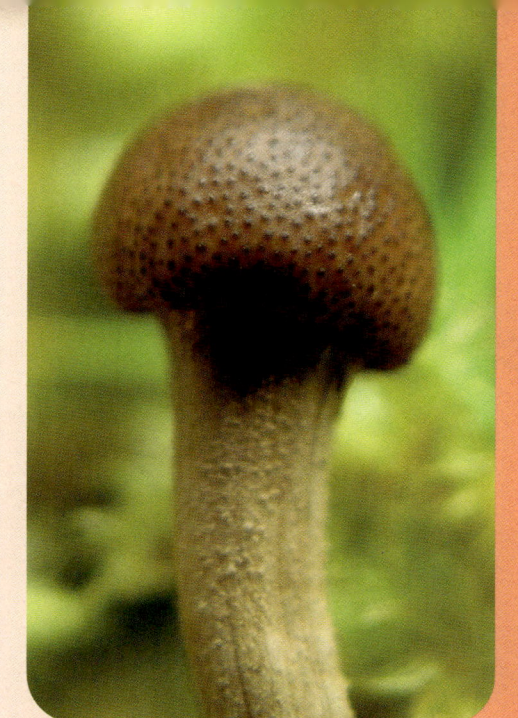

Dr. Tai's Pearls

There is just so much to say about cordyceps, that I actually wrote a book called "The Cordyceps Miracle", where we tell the stories from ancient Chinese emperors to the modern day research – every single article published was actually summarized and the data and statistics given in the book. Copiously illustrated with clinical stories. It's difficult to talk about a particular ingredient that is so versatile and extraordinary in its qualities. This is truly one of the first ancient "anti-aging" supplements that has survived thousands of years of scrutiny by trillions of families who have benefited from this incredible, natural ingredient.

Clinical Case:

Marcy, 78-years-old, not as much energy as she used to have for her daily schedule of activities. She always wanted to learn how to use a computer – only to participate for about 15 minutes before she would begin to tire mentally. She started using cordyceps on a daily basis and can now stay on the computer for 6 – 8 hours at a time. She says her mind is much sharper and that she is astounded with the fact that her body is less fatigued.

Side Effects: None

Contraindications:

Do not take product if you are allergic to any of its ingredients.

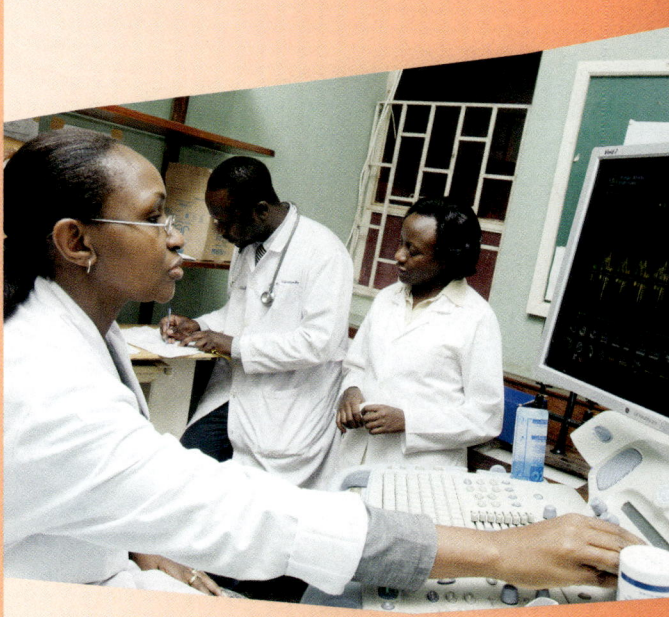

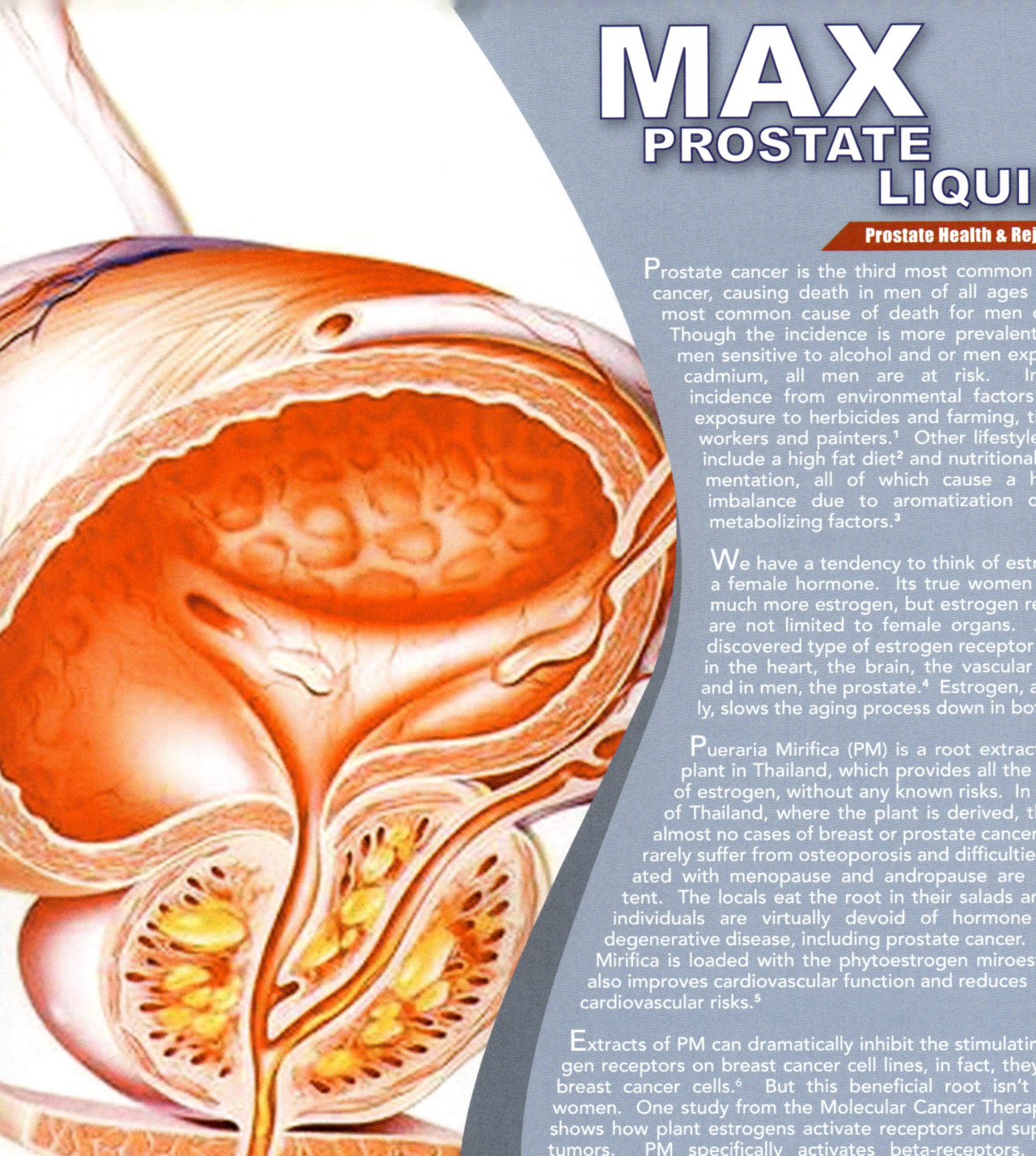

MAX
PROSTATE
LIQUID

Prostate Health & Rejuvenati

Prostate cancer is the third most common form o cancer, causing death in men of all ages and th most common cause of death for men over 75 Though the incidence is more prevalent amon men sensitive to alcohol and or men exposed t cadmium, all men are at risk. Increase incidence from environmental factors includ exposure to herbicides and farming, tire plan workers and painters.[1] Other lifestyle factor include a high fat diet[2] and nutritional supple mentation, all of which cause a hormon imbalance due to aromatization or othe metabolizing factors.[3]

We have a tendency to think of estrogen a a female hormone. Its true women posses much more estrogen, but estrogen receptor are not limited to female organs. A newl discovered type of estrogen receptor is foun in the heart, the brain, the vascular system and in men, the prostate.[4] Estrogen, amazing ly, slows the aging process down in both sexe

Pueraria Mirifica (PM) is a root extract from plant in Thailand, which provides all the benefit of estrogen, without any known risks. In the are of Thailand, where the plant is derived, there ar almost no cases of breast or prostate cancer, peopl rarely suffer from osteoporosis and difficulties assoc ated with menopause and andropause are nonexis tent. The locals eat the root in their salads and thes individuals are virtually devoid of hormone relate degenerative disease, including prostate cancer. Puerari Mirifica is loaded with the phytoestrogen miroestrol tha also improves cardiovascular function and reduces cardiovascular risks.[5]

Extracts of PM can dramatically inhibit the stimulating estro gen receptors on breast cancer cell lines, in fact, they can k breast cancer cells.[6] But this beneficial root isn't just fo women. One study from the Molecular Cancer Therapy stud shows how plant estrogens activate receptors and suppresse tumors. PM specifically activates beta-receptors, in fac miroestrol is about 3,000 times more active on these benefici receptors than soy phytoestrogens. We know isoflavon phytoestrogens of the soy variety are associated with les prostate cancer, implicating PM can help the prostate bette than soy and Pueraria Mirifica is a more potent, more effe tive, more beneficial stimulator than isoflavones is soy.[7]

115

Butea Superba extract is also a beneficial ingredient included in the Max Prostate Specialist which naturally reduces prostatic hypertrophy and carcinoma health issues. In addition to it benefiting the prostate, Butea Superba also enhances sexual performance and sexual interest in men. [8]

Recent studies have indicated Aloe Vera as having anti-tumor properties and it seems active against stomach and colon cancer cells as well as leukemia.[9] Aloe Vera contains anti-tumor agents, including emodin and lectins. According to Cancer Cover-Up by Kathleen Deoul, Aloe Vera boosts the immune system, giving a promising contribution to cancer treatment.[10] Aloe Vera's Extract can help the body heal itself from cancer and damage done during conventional cancer therapy. In a past study, lectin from aloe caused the immune system to attack cancer. It seems aloe activates macrophages, the white blood cells that eat antigens, causing release of immune-boosting and anti-cancer substances such as interferons, tumor necrosis factor and interleukins.[11]

Directions: Shake well. Take on an empty stomach one (1) dropper full by mouth. May increase dosage as needed by condition. See your Health consultant.

Ingredients: Aloe Vera Extract, Sterol, Pueraria Mirifica Extract, Butea Superba Extract and Distilled Water

These statements have not been reviewed by the FDA. This product is not intended to diagnose, treat, cure, or prevent any disease.

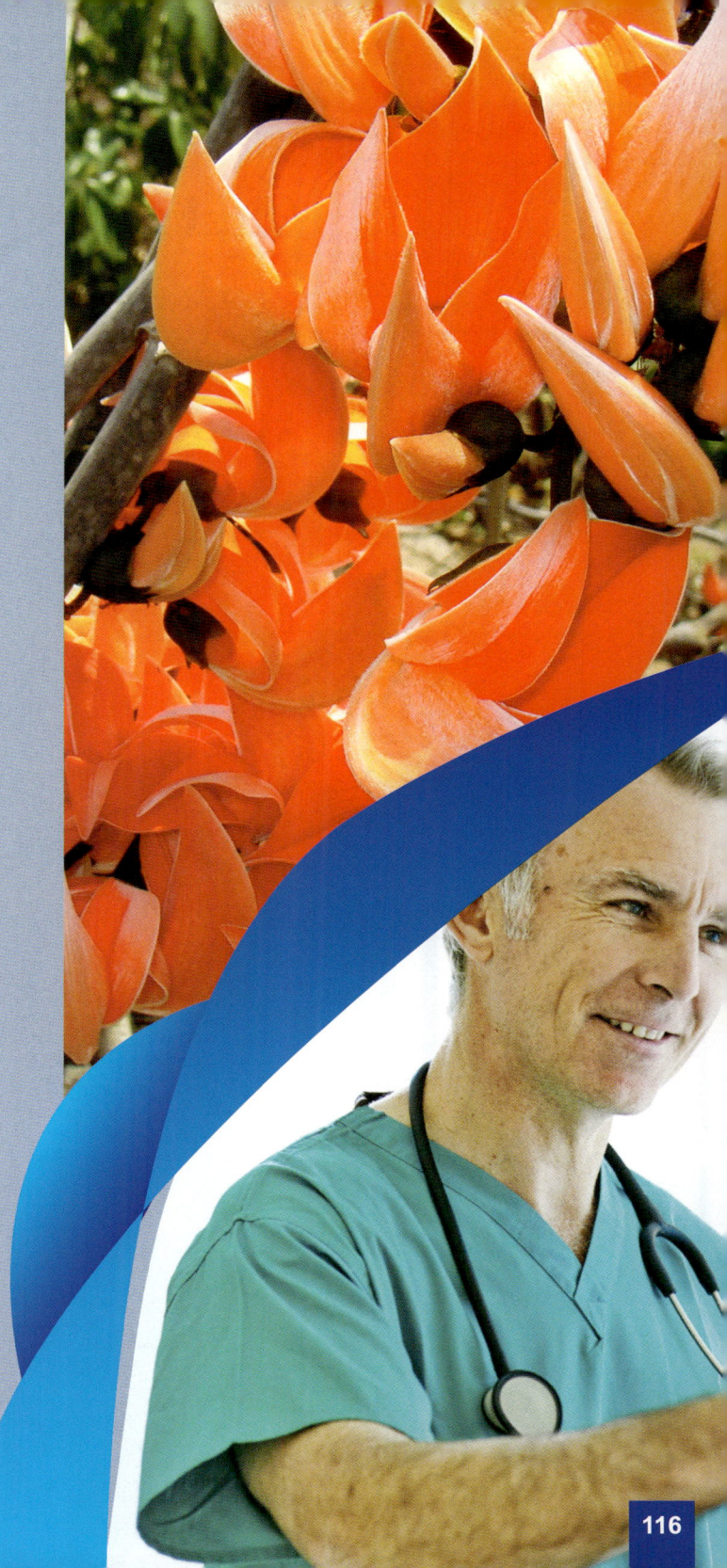

References

1. National Institute of Health. A.D.A.M. Medical Encyclopedia. Prostate cancer. September 23, 2010.

2. Vainio H, Bianchini F. IARC handbooks of cancer prevention. Volume 6: Weight control and physical activity. Lyon, France: IARC Press, 2002.

3. Longcope C. Methods and results of aromatization studies in vivo. Cancer Res. 1982;42:3307s–3311s. PMID: 7083191

4. Chansakaow S, Ishikawa T, Seki H, Sekine (née Yoshizawa) K, Okada M, Chaichantipyuth C. Identification of deoxymiroestrol as the actual rejuvenating principle of "Kwao Keur", Pueraria mirifica. The known miroestrol may be an artifact. J Nat Prod. 2000 Feb;63(2):173-5. PMID: 10691701

5. Wattanapitayakul SK, Chularojmontri L, Srichirat S. Effects of Pueraria mirifica on vascular function of ovariectomized rabbits. J Med Assoc Thai. 2005 Jun;88 Suppl 1:S21-9. PMID: 16862667

6. Cherdshewasart W, Panriansaen R, Picha P. Pretreatment with phytoestrogen-rich plant decreases breast tumor incidence and exhibits lower profile of mammary ERalpha and ERbeta. Maturitas. 2007 Oct 20;58(2):174-81. Epub 2007 Sep 17. PMID: 17870258

7. Stettner M, Kaulfuss S, Burfeind P, Schweyer S, Strauss A, Ringert RH, Thelen P. The relevance of estrogen receptor-beta expression to the antiproliferative effects observed with histone deacetylase inhibitors and phytoestrogens in prostate cancer treatment. Mol Cancer Ther. 2007 Oct;6(10):2626-33. Epub 2007 Oct 3. PMID: 17913855

8. Cherdshewasart W, Nimsakul N. Clinical trial of Butea superba, an alternative herbal treatment for erectile dysfunction. Asian J Androl 2003;5:243-6.

9. El-Shemy HA, Aboul-Soud MA, Nassr-Allah AA, Aboul-Enein KM, Kabash A, Yagi A. Antitimor properties and modulation of antioxidant enzymes' activity by aloe vera leaf active princi ples isolated by supercritical carbon dioxide extraction. Curr Med Chem 2009 Nov. 24.

10. Deoul K. Cancer Cover-Up. Cassandra Books, 2001.

Dr. Tai's Pearls:

Pueraria Mirifica is significantly different in its approach to settle the complications of hypertrophy of the prostate, as well as prostate cancer. Right at the center of the problems of the prostate, is the presence of receptors that are very sensitive to hormones, both testosterone as well as estrogen. While many times misunderstood, the latest publications from Harvard Medical School show that testosterone is actually good for the healthy physiology of the prostate. That is not true of estrogen. Estrogen has a prolific effect on the receptors of the prostate, making them grow and enlarge just as estrogen does for the breast and the uterus of the woman. In fact, from a rigidal embryo layer the uterus and the prostate are organ twins of each other. Pueraria works so well because the estrogen-like effects are really strong affinities to the estrogen receptors that are present in the prostate. This creates an occupation of the pueraria on the receptors, without having the negative estrogen effects of enlargement. Secondly, it occupies the receptors so no other estrogen hormones can occupy it at the same time. Therefore, it makes the receptors unavailable to the estrogens that are present in the blood of the individual. This is a very novel approach to combating the BPH problem – simple, yet effective. It is quite remarkable in its results. In fact, we see many bonuses because the active phytoestrogen, miroestriol actually helps with cardiovascular help, as well as preventing other cancers.

Clinical Case:

47-year-old construction worker, slightly overweight; however, moderately good health. Complaining of persistent pain in the rectal area and behind the pubis. He states that the discomfort is cyclical, appearing most severely during the early morning hours. He does not have any symptoms or discomfort at night. The complaint is that around 4 – 6 o'clock in the morning, he gets up with severe pain, and has difficultly urinating. He actually said that it is his personal secret that he sits down for urination, just like a woman – and he laughed. He has tried different prescription medications from his physician, but stated that they made him ill and didn't seem to help. His PSA appears to be within high-normal limits. His family physician spoke with him about potentially doing a needle biopsy, but patient refused. Running a salivary hormone test showed his testosterone was normal in the lower range, DHEA was also normal in the lower range; however Estrone was high, above normal range and Estradiol was also in the high normal range. Patient chose to take anti-aromatization supplements, such as Estrogen DeTox and Estrogen Defense and began supplementing with liquid pueraria. He started originally with a double-dose, until the discomfort started to subside. When his condition was normalized, he adjusted to a maintenance dose of 1 dropper full per day. Now, after three years, he is still symptom free and has no more complications.

Side Effects: None

Contraindications:
Do not take product if you are allergic to any of its ingredients.

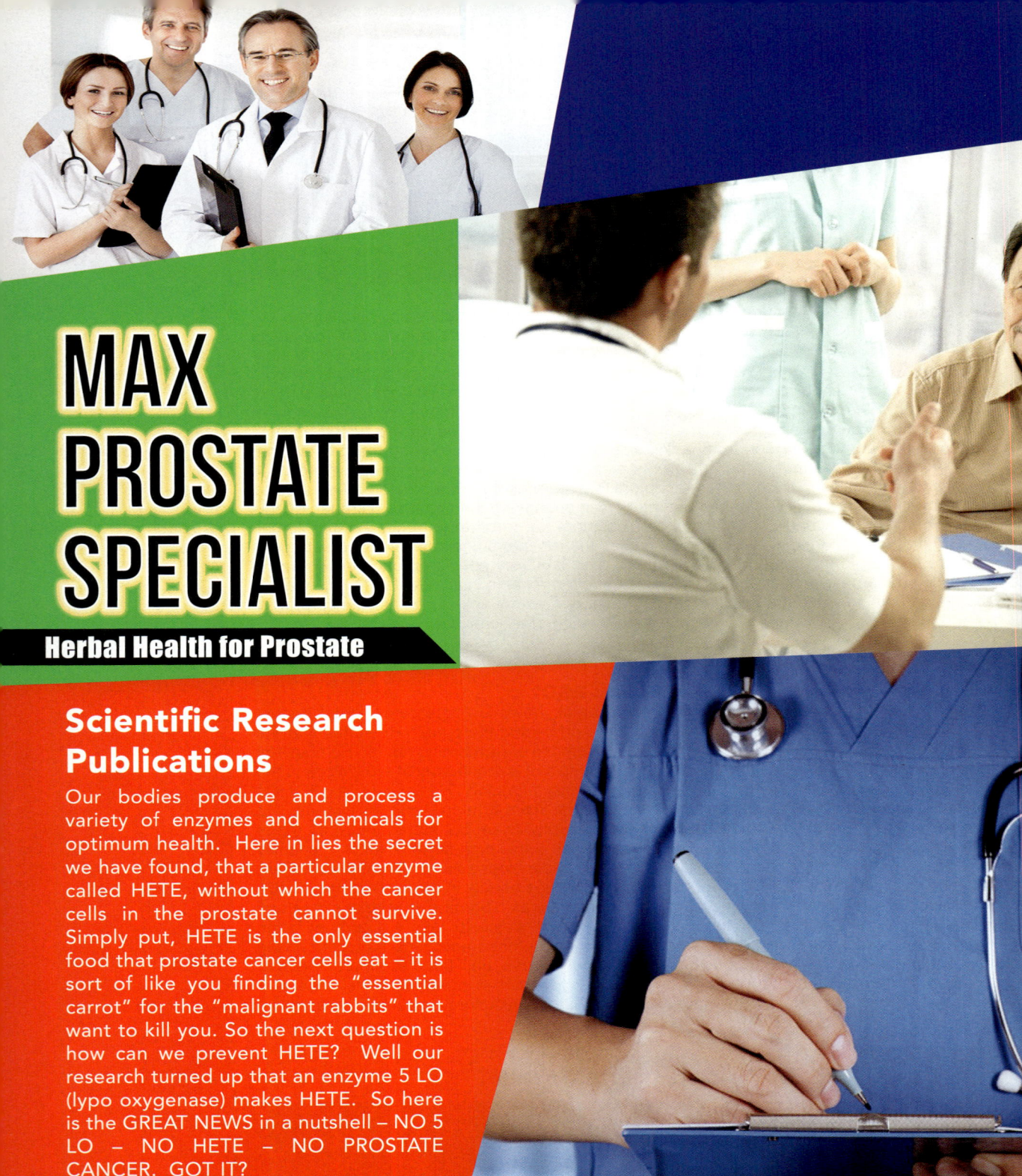

MAX PROSTATE SPECIALIST
Herbal Health for Prostate

Scientific Research Publications

Our bodies produce and process a variety of enzymes and chemicals for optimum health. Here in lies the secret we have found, that a particular enzyme called HETE, without which the cancer cells in the prostate cannot survive. Simply put, HETE is the only essential food that prostate cancer cells eat – it is sort of like you finding the "essential carrot" for the "malignant rabbits" that want to kill you. So the next question is how can we prevent HETE? Well our research turned up that an enzyme 5 LO (lypo oxygenase) makes HETE. So here is the GREAT NEWS in a nutshell – NO 5 LO – NO HETE – NO PROSTATE CANCER. GOT IT?

Published Medical Journal Research:

A. BETA-SITOSTEROL- is a standardized combination of plant phytosterols found in vegetables and herbs.

1. **Dr. Klippel et al**, University Dresden, Germany
This double blind study involving 177 men with BPH ran for 6 months, quite a substantial research with 32 references concluded "These results show that Beta Sitosterol is an effective option in the treatment of BPH". Brit.J. Urol 1997 Sept. '80: 427-32

2. **Dr. Bernges et al**, University of Bochum, Germany
This large double blind, 200 men, 1 year study said "significant improvement and urinary flow parameters show effectiveness of Beta Sitosterol in BPH" By far one of the BEST research published. Lancet 1995 Jun 17. 354 1929-32.

3. Veteran Hospital of Minneapolis, USA Reviewed 30 years and 32 researches and concluded that beta Sitosterol was "The greatest efficacy among phyto therapeutic substances" and "Beta Sitosterol improves urological symptoms and flow measures.

B. ZINC- This is a crucial and vital micronutrient for a healthy prostate because zinc has its highest concentration in the prostate on a human being. And yet our diet is sorely deficient in zinc causing terrible tissue damage to the prostate. Zinc has been widely studied and published in research in Journal of Steroid Biochemistry, and Kliniche Endokninologya (Germany).
1. Dr. Chang G.T. et al "Characterization of a zinc hunger protein and its association with Apoptosis in prostate cancer cell". J. Nati Lancer list Sept 6, 92:1414-21. Shows zinc and protein's effect on prostate cancer cell natural death.

C. GREEN TEA – A special catechin compound bio-active called Epigallocatechin Gallate (EGCG for short) has been found to be a new herbal polyphenol extract break thru.
1. Dr. Pashce et al "Induction of Apoptosis in prostate cancer by green tea ECGC". Cancer letter 1998:130:1-7
2. Dr. Hilpakka R.A. et al "Structure Activity Relationship for inhibition of human 5- alpha-Reductase by polyphenol" Biochem Pharmacol 2002 Mar 15; 63:1165-76
3. Dr. Gupta S. "Inhibition of prostate carcinogenesis in TRAMP mice by oral infusion of green tea polyphenols" Proc Nat'l Acad. Science USA 2001 Aug 28:98:10350-5
4. Dr. Lyn-Cook B.D. "Chemo preventive effect of tea extract and various components on human pancreatic and prostate tumor cell in vitro" Nutr. Cancer 1999; 35:80-6

D. SAW PALMETTO - Known by its Latin name (Serenoa Repens) is a small palm tree native to Florida. The fruits and berries were eaten by the Seminole Indians and have been used since the 1800's by physicians to treat various kinds of urinary problems.

1. Dr. Mark L.S. "Tissue effects of Saw Palmetto and Finasteride: Use of Biopsy cones for in situ Quantification of Prostatic Andro gen" J. Urology 2001; 57:999-1005. This study showed a double blind clinical result of men taking Saw Palmetto had 32% less DHT- a hormone associated with BPH- in 6 months treatment concluding that Saw Palmetto may be an effective treatment for reducing the symptoms of BPH", said Dr. Mark's director of Urological Sciences Research Foundation. "This is a very important study", said Dr. Blumenthal, founder of American Botanical Council, a non profit organization.
2. Dr. Wilt T.J. et al, Saw Palmetto extract for treatment of benign Prostatic Hyperplasia: A systemic Review. JAMA 1998:280 (18):1604-1609

E. BOSWELLIA SERRATA - Frankincense used to be more expensive than Gold. It is the same as one of the gifts from the 3 Kings of the Orient to pay homage to Jesus when he was born. It was prized for thousands of years in herbal medicine Boswellia Serrata Inhibits 5 LO.
1. Dr. Safayhi H et al Boswellia acids, novel, specific, redox inhibitors of 5-lipoxygenase. J. Pharmacol Exp Ther 1992 Jun:261(3) 1143-6 shows specifically a new Boswellia to inhibit 5-LO.
2. Dr. Ammon H.P. et al Mechanism of anti inflammatory actions of curcumina and boswellic acid. J. Ethno pharmacol (993 Mar; 38 (2-3):113-9
3. Dr. Huang M.T. et al Anti tumor and anti-carcinogenic activities of triterpenoid, beta-boswellic acid. Biofactors. 2000:13:225-30 this research narrowed a specific molecule of triterpene in the boswellic acid that stops cancer.
4. Dr. Jakoksson P. et al On the expression and regulation of 5-Lipoxygenses (5-LO) in human Lymphocytes. Proc Natl. Acad Sci USA 1992 April 15 89 (8):3521-5
5. Dr Gosh, J (Univ Virginia Cancer Ctr) Dr. Herzenber LA (Stanford Univ. Med School) Inhibition of arachidonic 5-Lypoxygenese triggers massive apoptosis in human prostate cancer cells. Proc Nat'l Acad Sci USA 1998 October 27; 95 (22) 13182-13187 report said that inhibition of 5 LO completely blocks 5 HETE production and induces massive cancer cell death to hormone responsive as well as hormone non-responsive human prostate cancer cells. It continues "the critical role of 5 LO in prostate cancer cell life". Dr. Zhang confirmed the study at Nat'l Acad Sci 1992, Dr. Stockton et al also confirmed likewise on Mol Bio/Cell 2001.

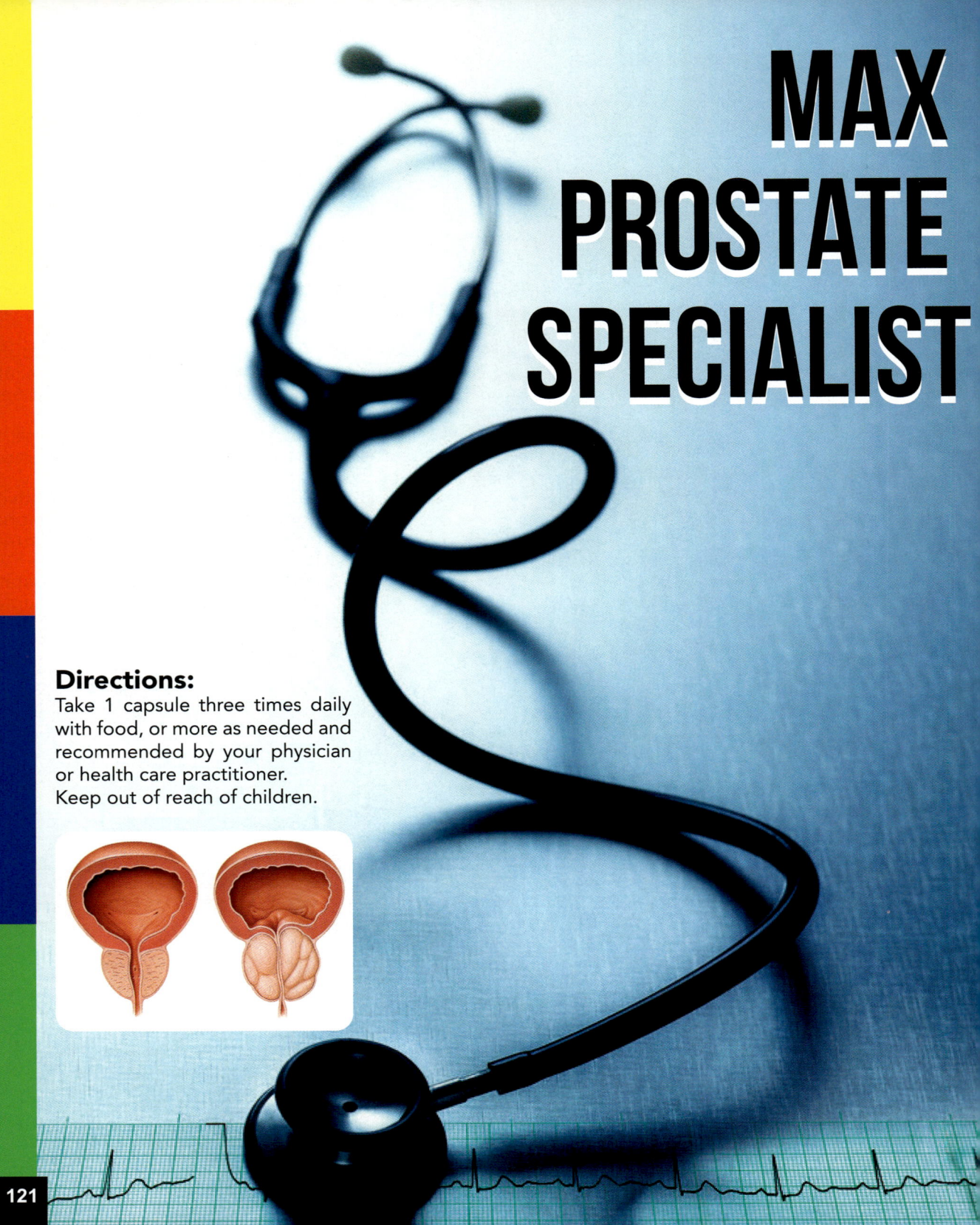

MAX PROSTATE SPECIALIST

Directions:
Take 1 capsule three times daily with food, or more as needed and recommended by your physician or health care practitioner.
Keep out of reach of children.

Dr. Tai's Pearls:

The key element for the Max Prostate is herbal ingredients that work synergistically by neutralizing the enzymes that creates the inflammation, as well as many of the herbs which support the synergistic lowering of the levels of inflammation, in the body as well as the prostate. By stopping the 5-LO, therefore neutralizing the HETE, you prevent the hypertrophy and growth of the prostate cells. This is, of course, one of the main pathways which helps having beta-sytosterol, lowering the hypertrophy of the prostate. No other compound has this variety of ingredients all synergistically working together to enhance the anti-inflammation of the prostate cells.

Clinical Case:

56-year-old wood and tree cutter does a tremendous amount of physical activity, pretty healthy for most of his life. He started to have discomfort upon urination. His stream was very low and the volume of urination was very low by his standards, compared to previous years. He had increased frequency and often urinated without completely emptying his bladder. His supplementation with Max Prostate Specialist started with a higher dosage until the symptoms started to subside, within three months. After that, he was able to lower the dosage to a maintenance level. He did comply that frequent ejaculation did seem to help keep the prostate hypertrophy under control and provide better results overall.

Side Effects: None

Contraindications:
Do not take product if you are allergic to any of its ingredients.

MAX RECEPTOR E DEFENSE

Protect Estrogen Receptors against TOXINS!

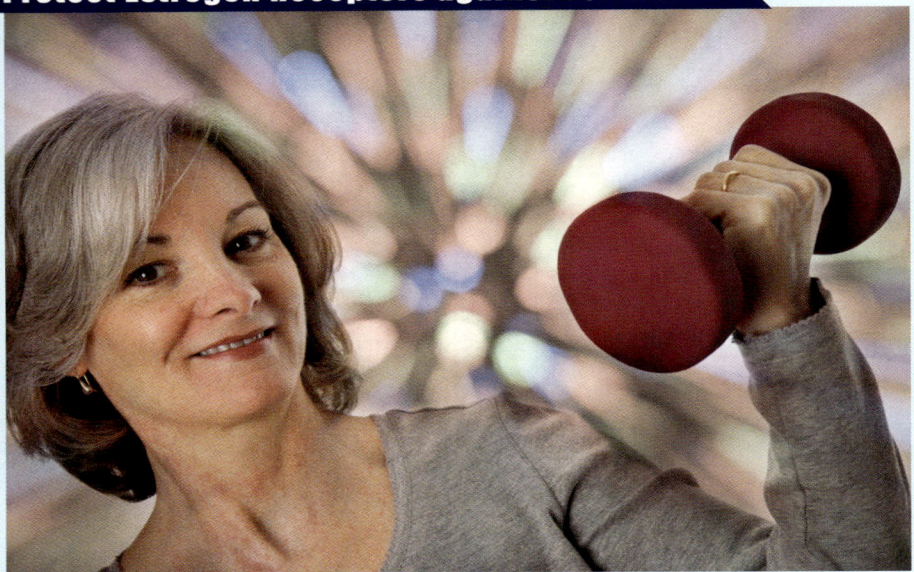

The human body produces its own estrogen; part of this process is called Aromatization. After the age of 50 years old, this process is more accelerated and becomes even more prominent, setting up potential major problems for women with a familial history of Breast Cancer, Uterine and Ovarian Cancer. For men, Aromatization exacerbates prostate hypertrophy and increase risk of Prostate Cancer due to increased levels of estrogen. Did you know that a man at the age of 55 has as much or even more estrogen than a woman of 55 years old??? Yes, this is a fact.

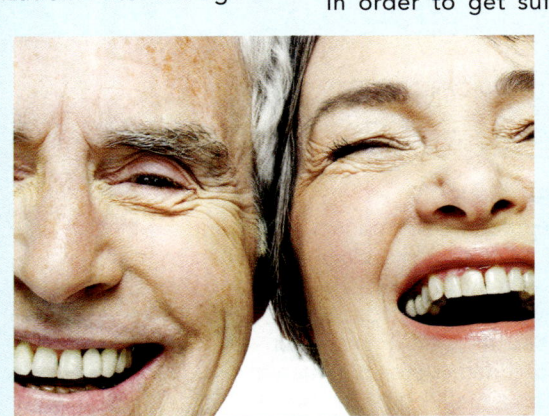

An article published by Osborne CK, et al, "Estrogen self proliferation and implication for treatment of breast cancer" Cancer Treatment Research 1988, reported that the increase of estrogen levels for women leads to a potential increase in cancer particularly in cervical, ovarian, breast and endometrium.

Extensive research confirmed recent studies that Brassica vegetables have a strong active ingredient in the form of Indol-3-Carbinol (I3C). I3C shows promise in Cancer prevention as well as an estrogen hormone modulator as reported by Vonpoppel GFO, et al, "Brassica vegetables and cancer prevention". Adv Exp Med Bio 1999. Terry P, et al. "Brassica vegetables and breast cancer risk" Jama 2001.

When I3C is ingested in the stomach and mixed with the stomach acid, another very active and more powerful ingredient Diindolylmethane (DIM) is produced, which is a vital natural compound known to have potent anti-cancer and anti-tumor properties. Both I3C and the converted DIM have proven to lower the circulating estrogen, estradiol (E2), by quickly neutralizing and excreting it out the body by the liver. Benabadji SH et al., Anti estrogenic and antioxidant diindolylmethane. Octa pharmacol sin 2004.

In order to get sufficient amounts of I3C and DIM, a person has to eat very large quantities of vegetables such as broccoli, 103 pieces of Brussel sprouts or a ¼ head of raw cabbage in order for it to do any good. Many people find these dietary requirements impossible to meet on a daily basis, therefore, the National Cancer Institute and the National Cancer Prevention Center have shown interest in the natural cancer prevention agents for breast, cervical, endometrial, colorectal cancers as well as prostate cancers, I3C and DIM, Balk JL et al., Indol-3-Carbinol for cancer prevention. Alt. Med. Rev. 2000 and Wong GY et al Indol-3-Carbinol for breast cancer prevention J. cell biochem 1997.

In males, the aging problem of hypertrophic of prostate and prostate cancer becomes more severe as we advance in age, because the level of estrogen rises from the aromatization of testosterone into estrogen. It is believed by many researchers that both I3C as well as DIM has an important part to play in mitigating the effects of estrogen on prostate cancer and prostate

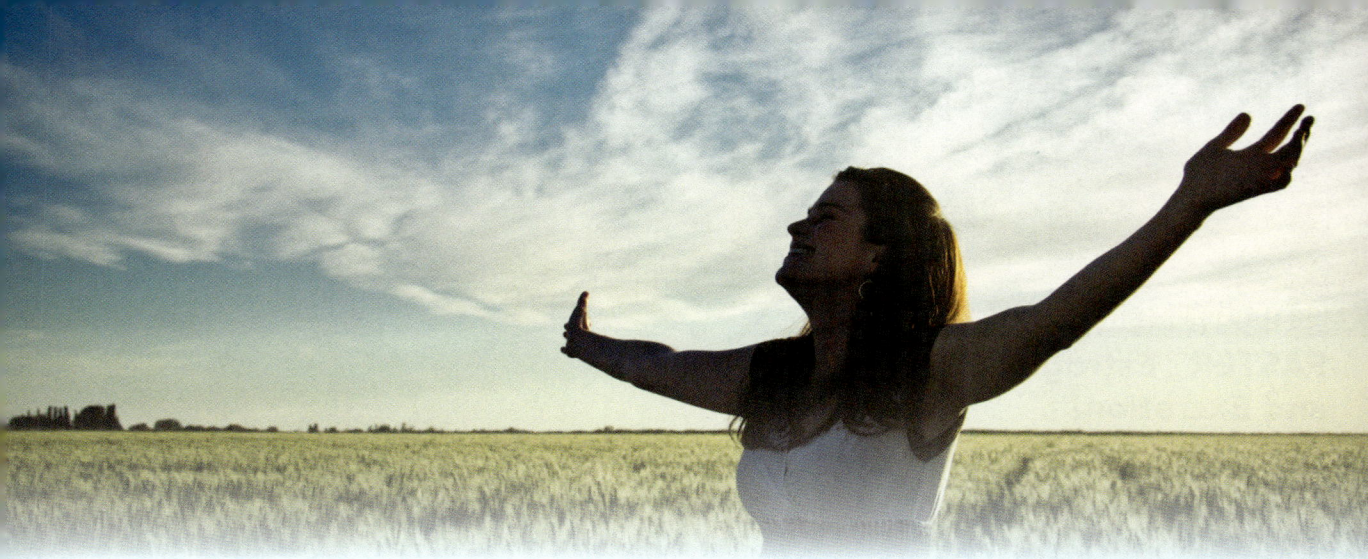

hypertrophy. These compounds are used in prevention as well as treatment. Nachshonketmi M et al. I3C and DIM induced apoptosis in human prostate cancer cells. Food Chem Toxic 2003. Beyond cancer, I3C and DIM also play an important beneficial part on all immune diseases and other abnormalities. McAlidon DE et al. I3C effect in women with SLE (Systemic Lupus) on estrogen metabolism. Lupus 2001. Other additional powerful anti-estrogen ingredients contained in this proprietary formula are Fermented Grape Skin and Seed containing an extraordinary active ingredient called Resveratrol as well as the natural Chrysin (an extract from vegetables) and a long respected Asian extract, Evodia. These ingredients work synergistically as an anti-estrogen through different pathways and mechanisms. This balanced formulation is not available anywhere else in the world.

Directions: Take one capsule twice daily or more as needed. Adjust dosages per your special condition or as instructed by your health care practitioner.

Ingredients:

Indole-3 Carbinol (I-3-C) Diindolymethane (DIM), Evodia, Resveratrol, Fermented Grape Skin & Seed, Chrysin, Piperine Extract

These statements have not been reviewed by the FDA. This product is not intended to diagnose, treat, cure, or prevent any disease.

Dr. Tai's Pearl

I use Max Receptor E Defense myself. You cannot help it because at a certain age, generally 50 or older, or at a certain body weight, with excess fat cells, the CYP genes start to go into hyperdrive. This is the problem of aromatization for both men and women. A lot of the complications of aromatization, I discovered, are more local to the tissues that are in the gastrointestinal tract. In women's breasts, research shows that local breast duct tissues actually convert testosterone into high levels of bad estrogen – primarily Estrone, that create the possibilities of increased incidence of cancer of the breast. Estrone is the main culprit because the breakdown metabolite constitutes mostly of 4, and 16-hdyroxy Estrone, which research shows related to an increased incidence of cancer. This estrogen occurs in a much higher rate as you become older and accumulate more body fat.

Side Effects: None

Contraindications:
Do not take if you are allergic to any of the ingredients.

Max Receptor E Detox

EXCRETE Excess Estrogen for Natural Levels!

FASTER Estrogen Metabolism and Excretion!

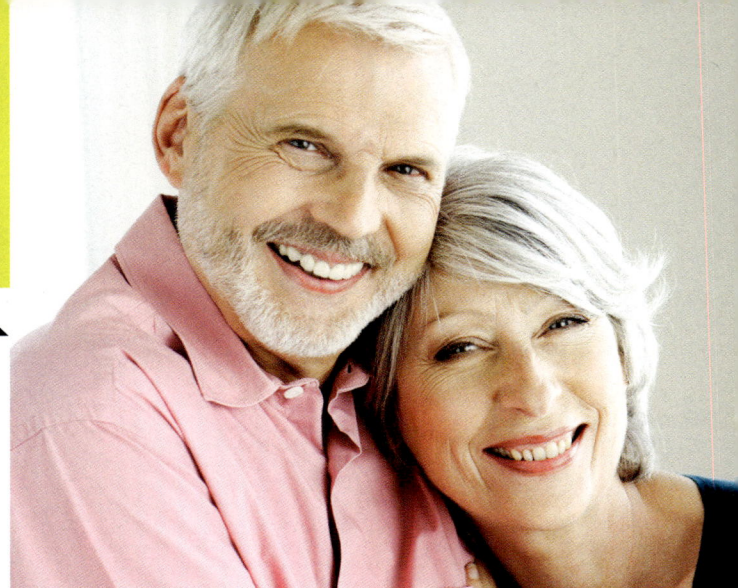

MAJOR MISCONCEPTIONS OF ESTROGEN

Is Estrogen bad for you?
Absolutely not. Natural estrogen is essential to our bodies and provides all of the important functions for a woman's health including the formation of strong bones, a healthy heart and the menstrual cycle. All the reported negative side effects come from pharmaceutical synthetic estrogen that is not natural to our bodies, increasing the incidence of strokes, Cancer and Heart Disease. A Natural Bioidentical Hormone in physiological doses is essential for the replacement of natural estrogen loss from menopause.

Is estrogen a woman's hormone?
Absolutely not. Both men and women have estrogen. As men grow older the body produces more estrogen from testosterone, causing a hyper elevated estrogen condition to the male body. A male over 50 years of age may have higher estrogen levels than an average female.

When is estrogen bad for women?
When the estrogen is in excess of the optimum level for a woman. Excess estrogen increases the cell multiplication cycle, creating potential problems for breast cysts, ovarian cysts, uterine cysts, endometriosis, excess bleeding at menstrual time and PMS.

When is estrogen bad for men?
When excess estrogen accumulates in the male body causing an imbalance noted by increased proliferation of cells in the prostate leading to benign prostate hypertrophy, prostate cancer, prostate pain, decreased libido, gynecomastia, weight gain and feminization.

Am I helpless with excess estrogen?
Definitely not.

Negative effects of excess estrogen can be decreased by:

1. Protecting the estrogen receptors in tissues from the circulating estrogen. A number of clinical studies and research show that ingredients such as the ones present in Max Receptor E Defense from Health Secrets USA may be helpful.

2. Powerful, natural ingredients can diminish the half-life time of the estrogen circulating in our body. This results in greater secretion of the estrogen, which is metabolized much quicker. There is a unique process of special natural extracts from the Sarasparilla S. Officinalis, Chinensis Araliacea, Zingiberoide Curcuma and Purple Nutsedge C. Rotundus. These carefully concentrated extractions provide you with extraordinary protection from the hazards of excess estrogen.

3. Calcium D-glucarate is a mineral naturally found in nature which speeds up the metabolism of estrogen breakdown and excretion through the stomach, GI track and liver.

Where can I find these natural ingredients to combat excess estrogen?
All of these natural ingredients are available in a "one of a kind formulation". Max Receptor E Detox, created by Dr. Paul Ling Tai for Health Secrets USA.

How should I take Max Receptor E Detox?
Max Receptor E Detox is a natural formula with no known side effects. Take (1) or (2) capsules, two or three times a day depending on your excess estrogen. Estrogen Detox can be taken in higher doses depending on your condition and lower doses for maintenance. Max Receptor E Detox may address and target the excess estrogen metabolism in the body by protecting the tissues from the negative effects of estrogen and increasing the estrogen metabolism excretion. Max Receptor E Detox is a powerful natural aromatase inhibitor.

What does research reveal about Calcium D-Glucorate?

Calcium D-glucorate is a natural extraction from fruits and vegetables and has no known side effects. Calcium D-glucorate has detoxifying as well as anticarcinogenic properties because of its ability to increase the glucorinidation, meaning the excretion of potentially toxic compounds from our bodies through the liver and gall bladder.

In summary, the calcium D-glucorate lowers estrogen levels in the body and lowers the level of beta-glucoronidase, which lowers the risks of various cancers of the breast, skin, liver, lung, prostate, and colon. See published research of Max Receptor E Detox.

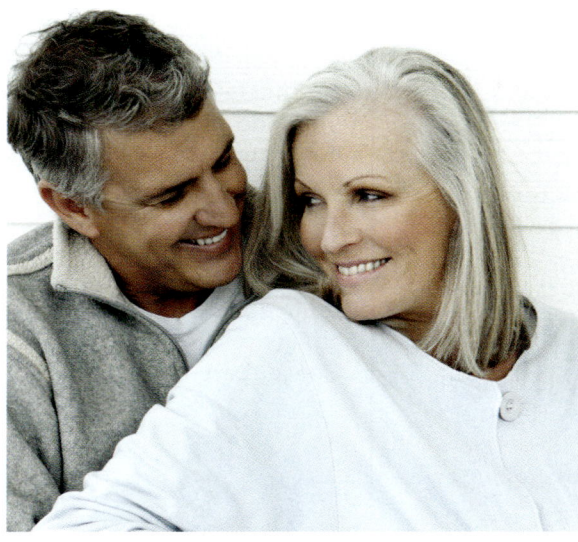

May help:
- Breast tumors
- Breast cancer
- Breast pain
- Ovarian cysts
- Endometriosis
- Prostate cancer
- Benign prostate hypertrophy
- Gynecomastia
- Feminization of men
- Male libido

Ingredients:
Proprietary Blend: Calcium D- Glucarate , Chinensis, Araliacea, Zingiberoide Curcuma, Purple Nutsedge C, Rotundus, Sarsparilla S. Officinalis

These statements have not been reviewed by the FDA. This product is not intended to diagnose, treat, cure, or prevent any disease.

References
1. Dwived C, Fleck WJ, Downie AA, et al. Effect of calcium glucarate on heta-glucuronklase activity and glucarate content of certain vegetables and fruits. Biochem Mod Metab Biol 1990:43:83-02.
2. Walasvek Z. Szemraj J. Narog M, et al. Metabolism, uptake, excretion of a D-glucaric acid salt and its potential use in cancer prevention. Cancer Detect Prev 1997;21:178-190.
3. Heerdt, AS, Young CW, Borgen Pl. Calcium glucarate as a chemopreventive agent in breast cancer, Isr J Med Sci 1905:31:101-105.
4. Horton D. Walaszek Z. Conformations of the D-glucarolactones and D-glucaric acid in solution. Carbohydr Res 1982; 105:95-109
5. Walaszek Z. Hanausek-Walaszek M. D-glucaro-1,4-lactone: its excretion in the bile and urine and effect on biliary excretion of beta-glucuronidase after oral administration in rats. Hepatology 1988:9:552-556.
6. Selkirk JK. Cohen GM. MacLeod MC. Glucuronic acid conjugation in she metabolism of chemical carcinogens by rodent cells. Arch Toxicol 1980:139:S171-S178.
7. Walaszek Z. Hanausek-Walaszek M, Adams AK. Sherman U. Cholesterol lowering effects of dietary D-glucarate. FASEB 1991;5:A930
8. Yoshimi N. Walaszek Z, Moil 1, et al. Inhibition of azoxymethane-induced rat colon carcinogenesis by potassium hydrogen D-glucarate. Int J Oneol 2000:16:43-48.
9. Schmittgen TD, Koomans-Beynen A. Webb TE. et al. Effects of 5-fluorouracil, leucovorin, and glucarate in rat colon-tumor explants. Cancer Chemother Pharmacol]992;30:25-30.
10. Walaszek Z. Hanausek-Walaszek M. WebbTE, Dietary glucarate-mediated reduction of sensitivity of murine strains to chemical carcinogenesis. Cancer Lett 1986;33:25-32.

Dr. Tai's Pearl

I am very partial to Max Receptor E DeTox because, like one of my children, this formulation is exclusive to me. I carefully chose the ingredients and then did a special cold water extraction of the active nutrients from the herbs in a very high level of 16:1 to improve its effectiveness in clinical studies. Even though many ingredients have been tested and researched to show that it works to lower aromatization or excrete excess estrogens from the G.I. tract, they don't' show very good results in clinical applications. Therefor it is often appointment of both the patient and the physician prescribing it. Max Receptor E Detox overcomes these shortcomings. It is powerful yet gentle and it increases the excretion of the excess estrogens without allowing it to be reabsorbed.

Side Effects: None

Contraindications:
Do not take if you are allergic to any of the ingredients.

Clinical Case:

56-year-old male of Eastern European decent, moderately overweight with complications of prostatitis, difficult, painful urination, difficult erection, 40" waist, noticeable gynecomastia. He noticed that breast pain was a sudden occurrence when working on trucks, leaning against the metal frames of the vehicles pressing against his breast nipple tissues causing severe pain. This concerned him and he sought help from a physician. This is a classic case of aromatization and male feminization. Saliva hormone testing confirmed high levels of both Estrone and estradiol. He began using Max Receptor E Defense, Max Receptor E Detox along with Max BioCell for a period of 2 months, dramatically reducing the discomfort in the breast upon palpation. Patient was advised to partake in a weight loss program to diminish fat and body mass. Loss of 22 lbs. helped to diminish the waist circumference to 35" and gynecomastia resolved.

Directions: Take 1-2 capsules two or three times daily or as directed by your health care practitioner.

Max Sea

Concentrated Ocean Algae – Organic Iodine

Many studies have shown that Americans are suffering from severe Chronic Thyroid Deficiency.
One of its major causes is the deficiency of balanced Iodine and Iodide due to the lack of food sources of Iodide in our Western diet.

World Health Organization studies have shown that certain world populations, principally women living in the coastal areas of Japan and China, have less Iodine deficiency, as a result, these women suffered less hormone sensitive cancers, such as ovarian, uterine and breast cancers than any other population segment of the world. Careful studies of their diet regimen showed generous portions of Sea Kelp, which is an excellent and significant source of balanced Iodine and Iodide. The net daily dietary consumption of 6 mg of Iodine and 6 mg of Iodide gives a perfect balanced overall total protection where the Iodine is supportive of the thyroid gland hormone and Iodide is supportive of the breast and ovarian tissues. Many published articles have supported the proposal that deficiency of Iodide, which is stored in the breast tissue, is the primary cause in females of fibrosis of the cystic ducts in the mammary gland (Breast).

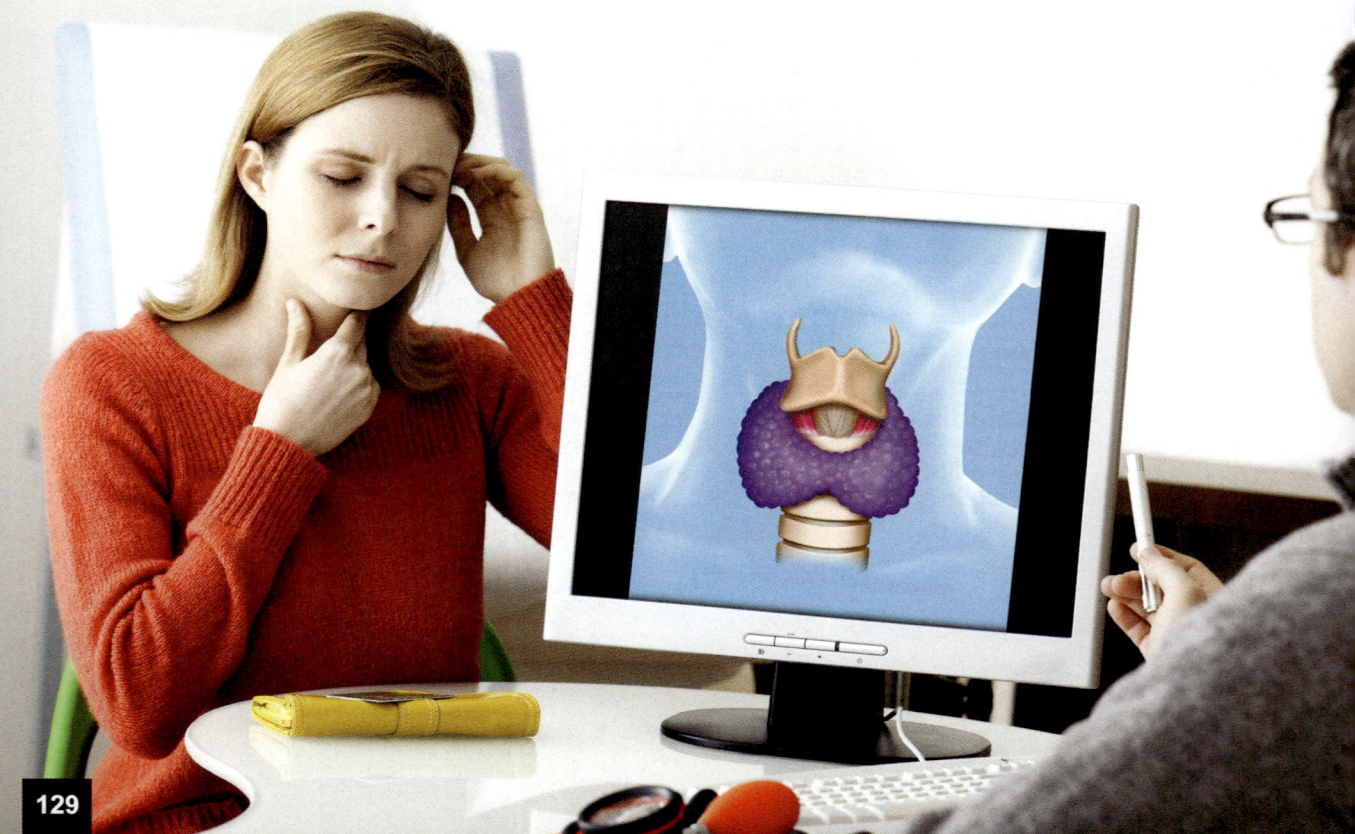

Max Sea is made of a natural herbal base called Mozuko extract which is a rare, marine sea kelp found in the coastal water of Okinawa, Japan. The Mozuko kelp is extracted with water and naturally concentrated with all the essential polysaccharides, algenate and very high fucoidan.

Max Sea has the natural properties derived from mozuko extract with all of the healthy ingredients from the ocean. Only 6 drops of Max Sea diluted in juice give you a balance of 6 mg of Iodine and 6 mg of Iodide, reflecting the daily dietary consumption of Japanese women in the coastal region.

- May support thyroid hormone metabolism
- May balance Iodine and Iodide
- May be Supportive of healthy breast tissue
- All natural Mozuko Sea Kelp extract
- High concentration of natural fucoidan
- Excellent source of Essential polysaccharides
- Daily dosing of 6 drops in diluted juice

Directions:
Take daily, 6 drops diluted in 8oz of juice or your favorite beverage.

Ingredients:
Mozuko Extract, Brown Algae Extract, Iodine, Potassium Iodide

These statements have not been reviewed by the FDA. This product is not intended to diagnose, treat, cure, or prevent any disease.

Dr. Tai's Pearls:

Understanding that man comes from the ocean where millions of years ago he walked out to the beach and began the evolution of becoming a human. We may not have the gills of our ancestors today, but within our blood, the serum still resembles the same iodine and sea water that flows within our veins, just like it did when we were in the sea. Iodine is one of those microminerals that participates in all of the major metabolism that is necessary for us to have energy and the creation of the thyroid hormone. This master hormone requires four elements of iodine to make thyroid hormone complete. Americans and Westerners do not have a high level source of iodine in our diet. The Asians, who customarily eat sea weeds, have an excellent source of organic iodine. This iodine cannot be substituted for inorganic iodine, as it has no affinity to the cellular membrane. Organic iodine from the sea was the original source and still has preferential transport from the cellular membrane into the mitochondria. Most doctors and health workers forget the biochemistry that iodine requires and active transport and cannot be carried inside the cell, only passive gradient differentiation. So our bodies prefer organic iodine and iodide for different activities in our tissues. The ingredients give this formula clear advantage benefits, making the iodine available to the cellular tissue for control of normal cellular activity and prevention of tumors and cancers.

Clinical Case:
Marianna, a 42-year-old nurse's aide, suffered for many years hard lumps and painful breast tissues. Although the right breast appeared to be more inflamed than the left, both of them gave her a very rough time, principally, she did not know if this was cancerous, even though her family physician had taken biopsies and removed some of the tissue which proved to be benign. However, she was always fearful that those hard nodules would someday become cancerous. The physician did send her to a gynecologist who treated her with birth control pills to control the pain. However, this only caused her to gain weight and proved not to work very well. In desperation, she actually contemplated having her breast surgically made smaller, as well as removing all the nodules, but the plastic surgeon would not help her fear of recurrence, even after the surgery. Salivary hormone testing was completed and showed low, but within normal range of progesterone. She had already stopped the birth control pills and started using transdermal progesterone day and night on her skin. High doses of 15 drops of Max Sea were given twice a day using a dilution in water or tea. Within six weeks, she started to have less discomfort and the rock hard nodules became softer and smaller. After one year, the breast nodules were small enough to be barely palpable and pain and discomfort had subsided completely. We did add the Melatonin Transdermal application to both breasts at night. Now the patient is even able to play sports and is no longer considering surgery.

Side Effects: None

Contraindications:
Allergy to iodine from nuclear iodine treatments. Allergies to kelp and sea weed. Do not take this product if you are allergic to any of its ingredients.

Max Sinus
Stop Congestion & Nasal Inflammation!

Sinusitis or RhinoSinusitis is inflammation of the Paranasal Sinuses. It can be due to infection, allergy, or autoimmune problems. Most cases are due to a viral infection and resolve over the course of a few weeks. It is a common condition, with over 24 million cases annually in the U.S.[1]

Symptoms of Sinusitis may include any combination of the following: nasal congestion, facial pain, headache, night-time coughing, thick green or yellow discharge, feeling of facial 'fullness' or 'tightness', and/or Halitosis.[2] Sinusitis can also lead to a reduced sense of smell.[2] Occasionally Acute or Chronic Maxillary Sinusitis is associated with a dental infection.

Chronic Sinusitis is caused by allergy or environmental factors such as dust or pollution, bacterial infection, or fungus. Chronic RhinoSinusitis represents a multifactorial inflammatory disorder.[3] To combat it we must be focused upon controlling the inflammation and reducing the incidence of infections. There are several paired Paranasal Sinuses, including the Frontal, Ethmoidal, Maxillary and Sphenoidal Sinuses surrounded in the front of your face.

Acute Sinusitis is usually precipitated by an earlier Upper Respiratory Tract Infection, generally of viral origin, mostly caused by Rhinoviruses, Coronaviruses, and Influenza Viruses, others caused by Adenoviruses, Human Parainfluenza Viruses, Human Respiratory Syncytial Virus, Enteroviruses other than Rhinoviruses, and Metapneumovirus. If the infection is of bacterial origin, the most common three causative agents are Streptococcus Pneumonia, Haemophilus Influenza, and Moraxella Catarrhalis.[3] It is thought that nasal irritation from the pressure of nose blowing leads to the secondary Bacterial Infection.[4]
Chemical irritation can also trigger Sinusitis, commonly from cigarette smoke an chlorine fumes.[5]

COMPLICATIONS

Stage	Description
I	Preseptal Cellulitis
II	Orbital Cellulitis
III	Subperiosteal Abscess
IV	Orbital Abscess
V	Cavernous Sinus Septic Thrombosis

Biofilm Bacterial Infections may account for Chronic Sinusitis.[6][7][8] Biofilms are Aggregates of the Extracellular Matrix and Microorganisms from multiple species, many of which may be difficult or impossible to isolate using standard clinical laboratory techniques.[9] Bacteria found in Biofilms have their antibiotic resistance increased up to 1,000 times when compared to free-living Bacteria of the same species. A recent study found that Biofilms were present on the Mucosa of 75% of patients undergoing surgery for Chronic Sinusitis.[10]

Directions:
Spray twice in each nostril. Wait 5 minutes & clear nose. Repeat as often as necessary.

Ingredients:
Arnica 3C, Sea Salt, Aloe Water

These statements have not been reviewed by the FDA. This product is not intended to diagnose, treat, cure, or prevent any disease.

References
1. Anon JB (April 2010). "Upper respiratory infections". Am. J. Med. 123 (4 Suppl): S16–25. doi:10.1016/j.amjmed.2010.02.003. PMID 20350632.
2. Christine Radojicic. "Sinusitis". Disease Management Project. Cleveland Clinic. Retrieved November 26, 2012.
3. Leung RS, Katial R (March 2008). "The diagnosis and management of acute and Chronic Sinusitis". Primary care 35 (1): 11–24, v–vi. doi:10.1016/j.pop.2007.09.002. PMID 18206715.
4. Gwaltney JM, Hendley JO, Phillips CD, Bass CR, Mygind N, Winther B (February 2000). "Nose blowing propels nasal fluid into the paranasal sinuses". Clin. Infect. Dis. 30 (2): 387–91. doi:10.1086/313661. PMID 10671347.
5. Mucormycosis at eMedicine
6. Palmer JN (2005). "Bacterial biofilms: do they play a role in Chronic Sinusitis?". Otolaryngol. Clin. North Am. 38 (6): 1193–201, viii. doi:10.1016/j.otc.2005.07.004. PMID 16326178.
7. Ramadan HH, Sanclement JA, Thomas JG (2005). "Chronic rhinoSinusitis and biofilms". Otolaryngol Head Neck Surg 132 (3): 414–7. doi:10.1016/j.otohns.2004.11.011. PMID 15746854.
8. Bendouah Z, Barbeau J, Hamad WA, Desrosiers M (2006). "Biofilm formation by Staphylococcus aureus and Pseudomonas aeruginosa is associated with an unfavorable evolution after surgery for Chronic Sinusitis and nasal polyposis". Otolaryngol Head Neck Surg 134 (6): 991–6. doi:10.1016/j.otohns.2006.03.001. PMID 16730544.
9. Lewis, Kim; Salyers, Abagail A.; Taber, Harry W.; Wax, Richard G., ed. (2002). Bacterial Resistance to Antimicrobials. New York: Marcel Decker. ISBN 978-0-8247-0635-7.
10. Sanclement JA, Webster P, Thomas J, Ramadan HH (2005). "Bacterial biofilms in surgical specimens of patients with Chronic rhinoSinusitis". Laryngoscope 115 (4):578–82. doi:10.1097/01.mlg.0000161346.30752.18. PMID 15805862.

Dr. Tai's Pearl

Using this special formulation, Max Sinus removes the Biofilm as well as heals the Inflammation of the Nasal Passages – the red, swollen, and painful tissues quickly and naturally return to its resting calm state. Countless patients share their enthusiasm and happiness when using Max Sinus. Made of all Natural & Homeopathic Ingredients, Max Sinus cannot cause side effects due to its very mild nature, yet is still highly effective in resolving the issues that plagues Millions of people suffering from Chronic & Acute Nasal Congestion. Frequent use prevents infections, Sinus irritations and may stop severe Sinus pain

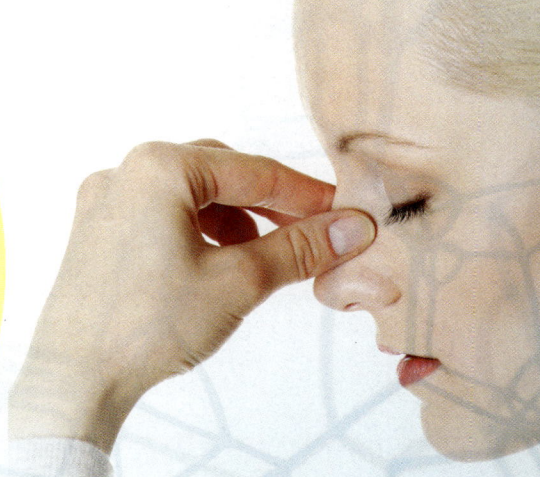

Side Effects: None

Contraindications:
Do not take if you are allergic to any of the ingredients.

132

Melatonin Transdermal
Direct Melatonin for Skin & Tissues

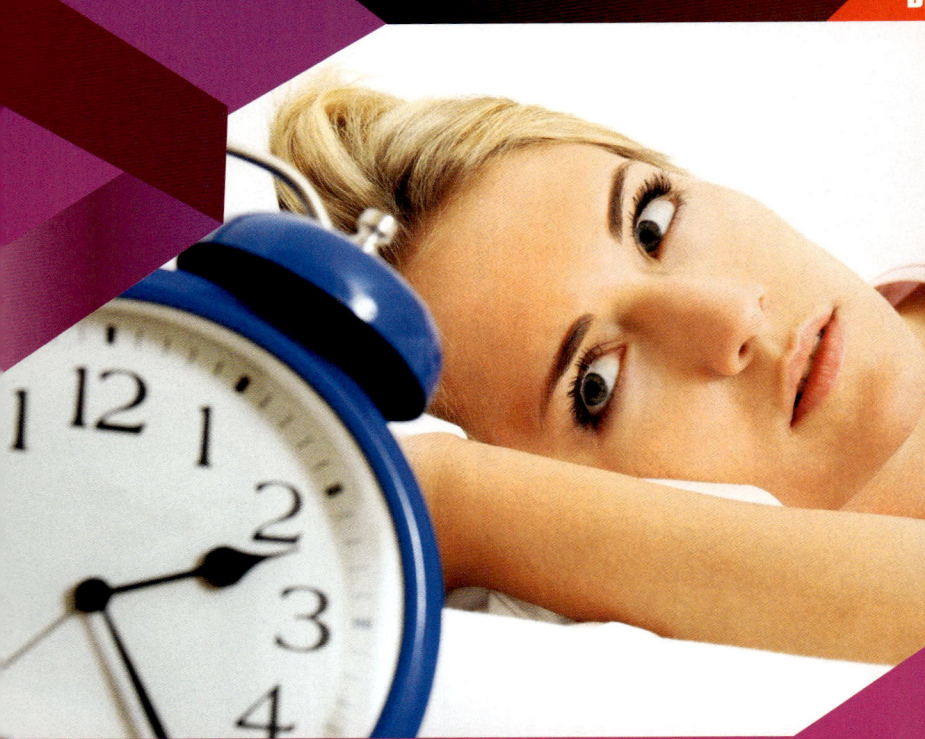

Melatonin is a 3 billion year old molecule, dating back to the beginning of life on Earth[1], which is found in every human, animal, and plant. It is an essential hormone and powerful antioxidant with a vast array of biological functions, from the promotion of restful sleep to the improvement of memory and mood to the enhancement of immune function.

Production of Melatonin

Melatonin is produced by the pineal gland, a small gland, once thought to be useless, located near the center of the brain. It is synthesized from tryptophan, first into serotonin, then finally into melatonin.[2] Its production, dependent on the presence of darkness, peaks at approximately 3 AM and begins its gradual decline once the sun rises again. In many of today's modern cities, work doesn't stop when the sun goes down and the lights don't dim, which can cause significant reduction in the nighttime production of melatonin. Studies show that as little as 500 lux of light suppresses melatonin production; people with the lowest levels of melatonin, being the most vulnerable to the suppressive effects of light.[3-4]

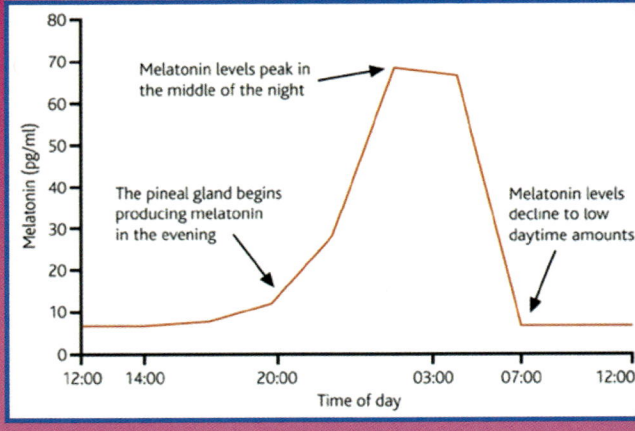

This circadian melatonin rhythm is generally established by 9 months of age and reaches its lifetime peak between 3 and 5 years of age, subsequently declining to adult amounts by the onset of puberty.[5] This amplitude remains relatively stable until old age, at which point a marked decline is reported.[6]

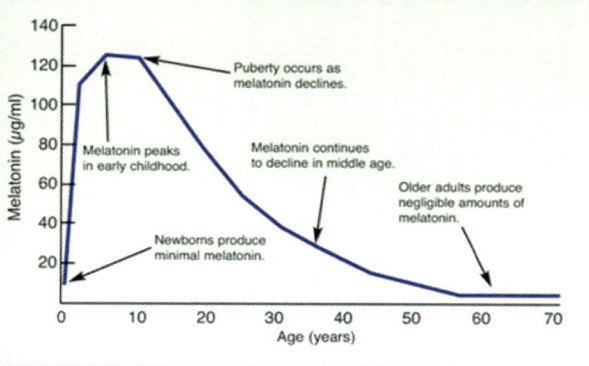

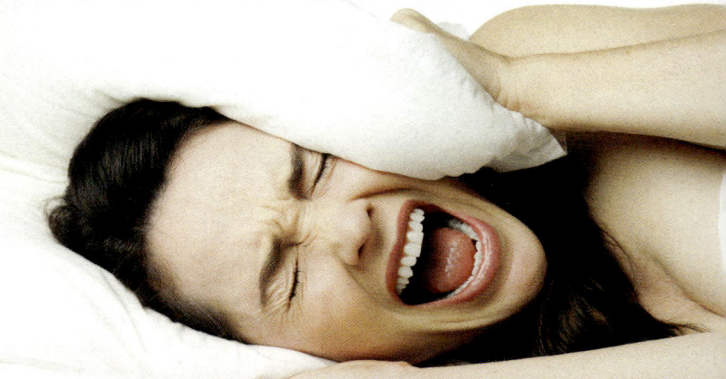

Functions of Melatonin
Besides regulating the circadian rhythm of the sleep/wake cycle, melatonin is also responsible for a wide range of other biologic activities including:[7]
- Assistance of immune system function
- Powerful antioxidant effects
- Prevention and improvement of cancer
- Improved mood
- Improved memory
- Improved stress response
- Induction of sleep

Melatonin: A Powerful Antioxidant

Melatonin is the most efficient and versatile antioxidant known – it is twice as effective as Vitamin E and five times more efficient as glutathione. Melatonin supplementation may prove to be a valuable tool in the fight against free radical damage, believed to be evident in diseases such as Alzheimer's.[8]

Melatonin Supplementation
A Good Night's Sleep
Melatonin is a powerful anti-aging supplement, offering protection to cells and organs throughout the body. It has been found quite helpful in those who have trouble sleeping (blind persons, those with jet lag, insomnia, and the elderly). The general public first learned of melatonin as a remedy for insomnia in 1993, after the publication of a sleep study conducted at the Massachusetts Institute of Technology. It was revealed that a mere trace of melatonin, 0.1 mg, enhanced sleep in young, healthy volunteers.[9] Subjects reported supplementation of melatonin made them feel relaxed and sleepy, a feeling people with sleep disorders long for.

Don't Be Sad
People suffering from some kinds of depression have low melatonin levels. Studies show stimulating melatonin production may play a role in the relief of depression.[10]
- Some antidepressant drugs increase melatonin levels
- Some drugs that increase melatonin levels relieve depression
- Taking melatonin itself has improved the mood of some people

In one study, in particular, Johan Beck-Friis and his colleagues noted that depressed adults who were separated from a parent before the age of 17 had very low levels of melatonin. In some cases, levels were undetectable.[11] This leads to the belief that production of melatonin could be influenced by strong emotional experiences prior to the completion of puberty.

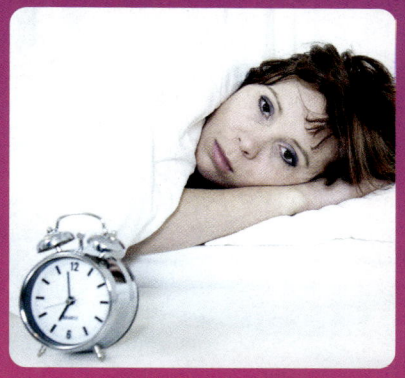

The Fight Against Cancer
In 1987, Paolo Lissoni conducted the first melatonin clinical trial for cancer.[12] His study involved giving melatonin injections to 19 cancer patients, none of which reported any toxic effects. In a subsequent study, melatonin was combined with Interleukin-2, in hopes of requiring a much lower dose of IL-2 without compromising its effects. After one year, 46% of the patients involved were still alive compared with only 15% of the patients receiving only IL-2. It was concluded that adding melatonin to IL-2 greatly increased the types of cancer that responded to the treatment.[13] The types of cancers involved were:
- **Lung**
- **Endocrine gland**
- **Brain**
- **Colon**
- **Stomach**
- **Liver**
- **Pancreas**

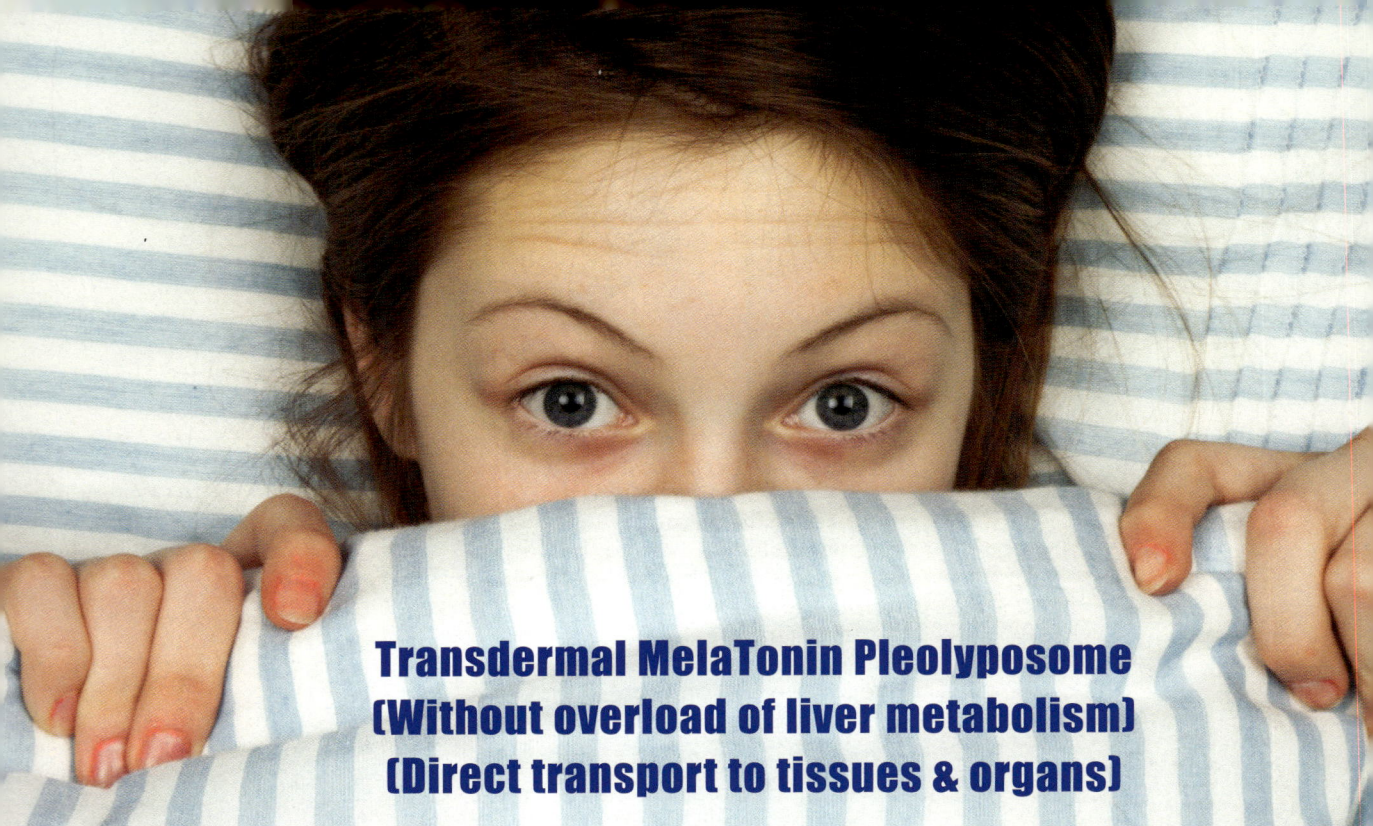

Transdermal MelaTonin Pleolyposome
(Without overload of liver metabolism)
(Direct transport to tissues & organs)

References

1. Kolaf J and Machackova I. "Melatonin: Does it Regulate Rhythmicity and Photoperiodism Also in Higher Plants?" Flowering Newsletter 1994; (17): 53

2. Arendt, J. Melatonin. Clin Endocrinol (Oxf). 1988; 29(2(:205-229

3. Lewy AJ, Wehr TA, and Goodwin PK. "Light Suppresses Melatonin Secretion in Humans." Science 1980 Dec; 210

4. Murphy DG, Murphy DM, Abbas M, Palazidou E, Binnie C, Arendt J, Campos Costa D, and Checkley SA. "Seasonal Affective Disorder: Response to Light as Measured by Electroencephalogram, Melatonin Suppression, and Cerebral Blood Flow." The British Journal of Psychiatry 1993; 163: 327-331

5. Cavallo A. "Melatonin and Human Puberty: Current Perspectives." Journal of Pineal Research. 1993; 15: 115-21

6. Arendt, J. "Melatonin and the Pineal Gland: Influence on Mammalian Season al and Circadian Physiology." Reviews of Reproduction 1998; 3, 13-22

7. Reiter RJ et al, Crit Rev Oncogen, 2007

8. Reiter RJ, Poeggeler B, Chen LD, and Barlow-Walden LR. "Melatonin as a Free Radical Scavenger: Theoretical Implications for Neurodegenerative Disorders in the Aged." Unpublished

9. Dollins AB, Wurtman RJ, and Deng MH. "Effect of Inducing Nocturnal Serum Melatonin Concentrations in Daytime on Sleep Mood, Body Temperature, and Performance." Proceedings of the National Academy of Science 1994; 91: 1824-28

10. Stanley M and Brown G.M. "Melatonin Reduced in the Pineal Glands of Suicide Victims." Psychopharmacology 1988; 24(3): 484-87

Directions:
Apply to soft skin 1 to 3 pumps at bedtime. Adjust dosage to your individual needs.

Ingredients:
Essential Phospholipids, Glycerin, Aloe Vera, Acrylate Crosspolymer, Melatonin

These statements have not been reviewed by the FDA. This product is not intended to diagnose, treat, cure, or prevent any disease.

Dr. Tai's Pearl

Proably the single most useful natural antioxidant in the human body. Just imagine every single living cell in the entire universe must have production of melatonin. That means that from the early single-cell amoeba and even microscopic organisms, such as bacteria, fungus, all the way to every single vegetable, plant, flower, and animal, from dogs, to chickens, to humans, produce melatonin in a very specific cycle of day and night. It is melatonin that allows bears to hibernate in the winter. And it is during this period of time that our body recuperates. We show clearly that there are cycles of growth in cancer and cycles of cancer control in our body. It is the melatonin cycle that controls the cancer significantly. As you lose the production of melatonin from the pineal gland during your older age, that cancer, Alzheimer's, cardiovascular disease, etc. occurs more frequently.

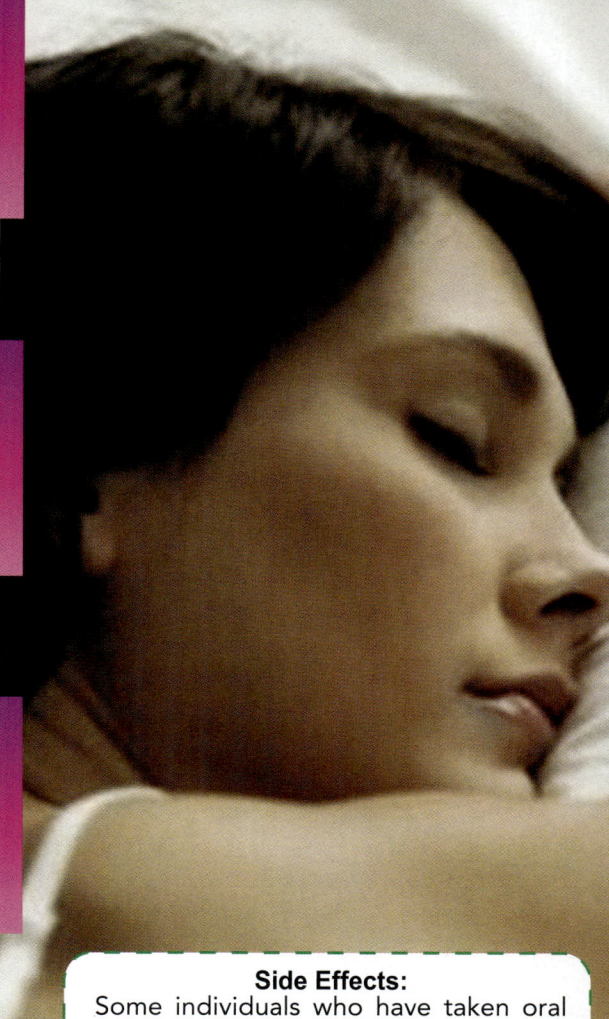

Clinical Case:

Marcia, a 39-year-old furniture sales person, working in a large department store. Experienced severe problems with falling and staying asleep. Her problems started when her mother, an Alzheimer's patient, during the last few years of her life suffered from complications, where Marcia had to be one of her primary caregivers. She stayed with her mother during very odd hours, staying with her very late, but still having to return to her normal job during the day. She said that it made her sleep patterns very irregular and created this habit of staying up late and not being able to sleep soundly. All the different tests showed that Marcia's cortisol levels were irregular, with fairly low cortisol in the morning when it should have been high and high at night when it should have been low. Her melatonin levels were also very low at night. Melatonin Transdermal application of three pumps on the face nightly, helped to restore the cycle of natural sleep. After three months of supplementation she was much improved. She stayed on the Melatonin Transdermal at a lower dose for maintenance.

Side Effects:

Some individuals who have taken oral melatonin have noticed that their dreams were more vivid and sometimes had nightmares. On careful examination, we do not know whether it is the melatonin that has been the reason for these symptoms or if it is the carrier and fillers of those tablets. These occurrences are rather rare. Another thought is that these side effects are more from the individual remembering a memory rather than melatonin causing these effects. However, the vast majority of individuals taking melatonin have not had any side effects.

Contraindications:

Do not take this product if you are allergic to any of its ingredients.

136

MEMORY SPECIALIST

Protect & Rejuvenate Brain Cells

Do you ever suffer from one of those "Blank-Out" Senior Moments where you can't remember words, places, dates or names?

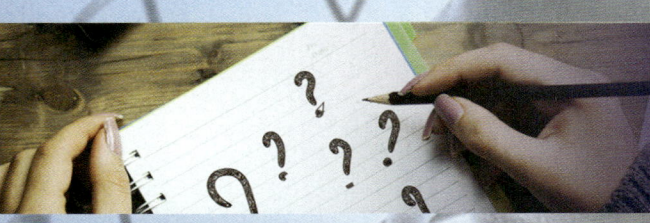

Are you over 40 and you're having problem concentrating, focusing on solutions, and remembering that telephone number that someone just gave to you?

Are you having problems driving? Couldn't see the car that was beside you before you changed lanes? Can't remember where you're going? Can't remember where you are?

Have you ever walked into another room in your home and can't recall why you're there? What was the purpose? What did you come to do? It's not until you go back to your original place and that is when you remember what you were doing!

I remember my mother always having problems with her memory. She could never remember where she put her glasses despite their usual spot on her forehead; or even where she left her house keys, even though they were in her handbag. I always laughed at her when I was younger, thinking how ridiculous she was and not realizing that I was also going to be a victim of these same lapses in memory.

I started having subtle memory problems at a very early age, but it became pretty obvious that I was about to embark on a very difficult and depressing journey on one Sunny Sunday…

On this particular day I went to do several errands, including light grocery shopping and picking up a rather large, antique Chinese scroll. This scroll, a rare remnant of the Quan Ying Collection, was being cleaned and restored due to being attacked by fungus in its old age. I paid out of pocket for the professional restoration that was under the watch of museum curators. One small fortune and several months later, the scroll had finally been brought back to perfection. I was beyond happy to be reunited with this large, full size painting after a long absence. Having finished my shopping and picked up the painting, I returned to my car to finally go home and cook dinner. Of course, I was already thinking about the elaborate recipe and the intricate cooking techniques it would require to master this new short-rib dish. Driving down the freeway at 70mph, I was concentrating hard on conquering this dish to prepare for my inevitable fantasy battle with Bobby Flay in a once in a lifetime showdown.

By the time I had gotten home, fumbled for my keys and taken my grocery bags into the house, I began to worry. I knew that something was missing, but I wasn't quite sure. I definitely have always had a worry-wart personality to begin with, making me more uptight than necessary at any given moment. I brushed this feeling aside and continued to put away my groceries and pull my apron on. As I started to sharpen the knife, the impending doom became too much to bear. Slowly, I came to realize that the rare, antique scroll of Quan Ying, the very scroll that I had so carefully and expensively repaired and restored, is MISSING!!! Quicker than the thought could sink in, I ran back to the car to look for it – Nowhere to be found. I couldn't understand!! I looked around the house frantically for what felt like an eternity, only to confirm what I already knew. My irreplaceable scroll was gone…Forever!

When my panic attack subsided, I realized that I had placed the scroll on "Top of my Car" while I put grocery bags in my trunk. Without thinking, I drove off down the freeway, leaving the manuscript in the dust on US M-14. Somewhere, some Michigander is enjoying a very rare, full-sized, centuries old Chinese Scroll from a bygone Dynasty and here I was sick to my stomach and ill for having lost it. This all came from one of those nearly fatal "Senior Moments," and to make it worse, I was only in my early 50's. I knew for the rest of my life, from that point forward, I had many more scrolls to lose and many more "Senior Moments" to agonize over…

What Do I Do?

Statistics show that many of us, 50% in fact, over the age of 70 will start to have some form of Dementia. By the time we are in our 80s, the Dementia will have set in and Alzheimer's is full blown. The memory loss and lack of focus will start earlier in life for some, and things only get worse from here. Please, go ahead… Enjoy laughing away at my sad story. Oh, you're approaching 50 and not experiencing these problems? Don't worry! Pretty soon you'll be relating your own tales just like mine! You too will have your own "Scroll Stories" to tell!

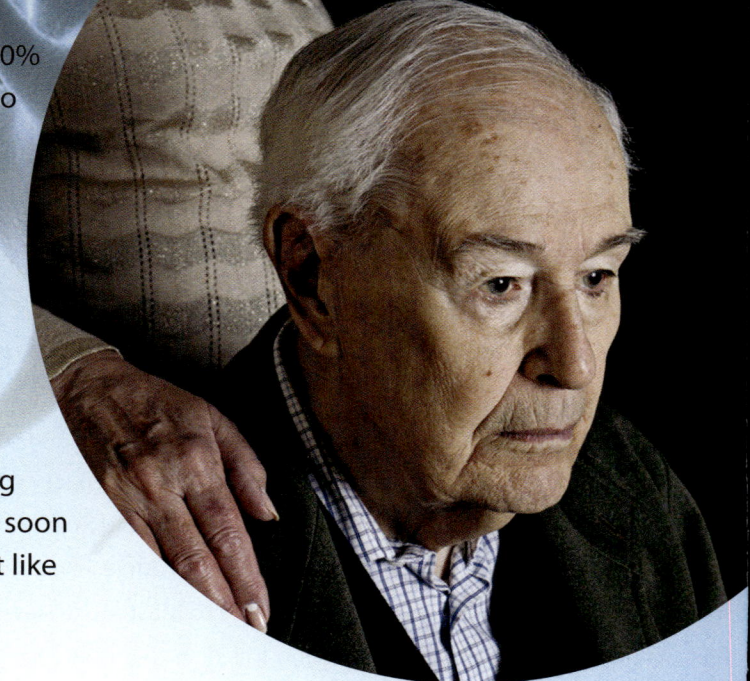

4th Century, BC. The Greek philosopher Aristotle spoke of memories as making impressions of the moment in the wax of our mind. These impressions are long-lasting copies of all your experiences. Our minds are a digital photo album of sorts, storing those pictures that we've collected all the way from our childhood. We carry these memories closely in our hearts, as they are the most precious jewels in our life. When we talk about going back into our memory, we are searching this digital catalogue in the computer of our brain. The stories of days passed have been encoded and stored in our memory tank for future use, able to be retrieved at any time and brought back to life just as vivid as when we stored it. These recalled memories are just as colorful and sensory rich as they were when we lived the moment, filled with the same sights, smells, sounds, and even feelings from the time we stored it.

There is no doubt that we lose the ability to retrieve this information as we get older. Much like an old Polaroid picture, your memory starts to fade and the image, once crisp and exact, becomes more and more blurred and faint until it reaches the point where you can barely make out what it was. I am horrified at this prospect as a physician, a surgeon, a researcher who has studied, investigated and attempted to cure mental deterioration as well as the "Old Man" who has suffered the most as I enter into my 70s.

As a writer, a speaker, and inventor, I have noticed a severe decline in my personal work. The productivity of my work has gone down as well as my mental energy. Thinking, focusing and understanding and solving problems have become increasingly more difficult. Actually finalizing and finishing my work became a rare occurrence. Even mundane things such as driving were affected by this cognitive decline. For some odd reason, people blare their car horns at me now more than any time in my life! What's worse is that sometimes I don't even know why they're so mad at me! It is very scary when someone had just given you their name and telephone number only for you to forget it just ten minutes later. As he talks, I do not have the foggiest idea as to who this person is, what the heck we were talking about, or why I stopped to greet him. I found myself dwelling, crying and being mad, shouting "WHY ME!?" I even at times denied that I had any problems, but finally came to the conclusion that I had to do something about it or just accept the fact that I was going to be dragged kicking and screaming out to the pasture to stop living the life of a productive individual.

I only found the answer I was searching for after trying what seemed to be endless numbers of products, ingredients and methods. I have tried multiple electronic frequencies, putting lasers through my nose and ears before inserting all sorts of lights and probes in every orifice of my body. This did very little besides making me look like a human disco ball. I attempted meditating, yoga and all sorts of humming, but it didn't help my memory. As a last resort I tried every conceivable potion, lotion, supplement, and, yes, even drugs, but none showed any benefit. Then again, would I be able to tell if they had? Maybe my Dementia and Alzheimer's had become too severe to notice it??? I became sick and depressed just thinking about it.

Then one day... EUREKA!!! I came across an ancient story of Chinese Monks using Green and Yellow Moss growing off tiny little Evergreen Shrubs in China. This particular species of Topezia Serrata has been used by these monks for many centuries for the treatment of Brain Injury, Neuropathy, Inflammation, Fatigue, even Male Declining Hormone and Sexual Performance. The moss, containing a special extract called Huperzine A, had been revived in modern Chinese Universities through multiple studies. Researchers produced prolific results in the treatment and care of Memory Loss and Diabetic Neuropathy. Several Double-Blind, Randomized Cross-Over trials have shown in both China and the United States that Huperzine has an amazing capacity to facilitate neurons in the brain. Those specialized nerve cells will grow and in turn become more active before going on to initiate transmissions and improve memory and focus lost to old age.

It was revealed by these careful, rigid studies that there was a secret to the Huperzine A Extract. In studies of both animals and humans, this natural compound was capable of inhibiting the powerful enzyme that destroys and breaks down Acetylcholine. Acetylcholine is a chemical neurotransmitter used by our nerves and brain cells to pass on information from one nerve to another. This also creates thoughts, words and memories. Think of Acetylcholine as the proverbial 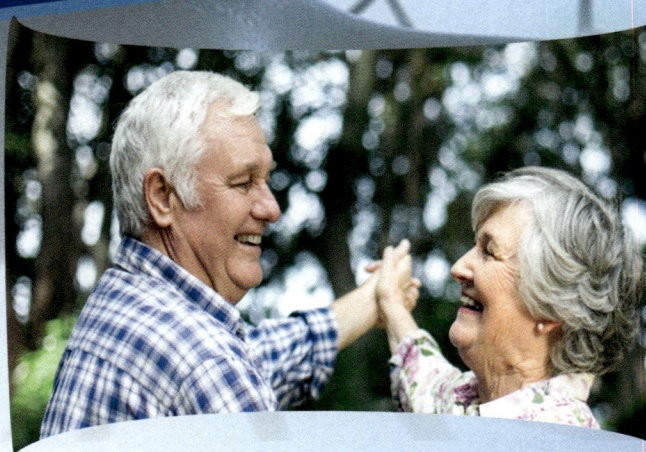 golden chalice of brain and memory that actually makes everything function. When you lose Acetylcholine, you also lose the ability for your nerves to function to transmit thought and memory. We now believe that as you become older, you have a shortage of both Pregnenolone, the main hormone to keep brain cells alive and well, and Acetylcholine, the main electrical conduit for all nerves to communicate. The presence of Acetylcholinesterase, the Acetylcholine-destroying enzyme discovered by "Cheng 1996," guarantees a shortage of Acetylcholine. Nerves in the brain, even in close proximity, will not be able to speak to each other. Picture holding the newest iPhone in your hands. You have the latest and greatest technology and a 64 GB memory card, to boot. You attempt to use it and all its endless wonders but you can't – there is no cellphone signal and no Wi-Fi. There will be no Facebooking, Instagramming or Tweeting for you just like there will be no focusing, recollection or retention for your brain.

Scientists at the Zhejiang Medical University in Hangzhou China performed double-blind studies with Alzheimer's Patients, giving them Huperzine A over the course of 8 weeks before comparing them to patients receiving placebo pills (Xu 1995). This study resulted in 58% of the patients treated with Huperzine A experiencing improvements in the memory, cognition and behavior functions while suffering no severe side effects. All physiological parameters (Blood Pressure, Heart Rate, Electrocardiogram, Electroencephalogram, Liver and Urine analysis) showed no abnormalities from taking this special kind of natural Huperzine A.

Not every Huperzine A is made equal!

Huperzine A is a Special Sesquiterpene Alkaloid that naturally inhabits this club moss. This means there's no chemical meddling apart from the extraction. Huperzine A naturally has the ability to protect neurons and nerves as well as lower inflammation, swelling, and other properties of Acetylcholinesterase. In turn, this will help to retain Acetylcholine function that will help memory and brain functions. The pharmacokinetics of this wonderful club moss is truly amazing when in special formulation, making it it is very bioavailable - meaning it does not require for you to take injections. You can take it by mouth and your stomach will still be able to absorb it. More importantly, it is amazing in its ability to penetrate the blood-brain barrier that normally stops anything from crossing its giant physiological walls. This makes Huperzine A available to the brain for immediate use.

Studies on both animals (dogs) as well as humans show that once supplemented, Huperzine A is distributed widely throughout all the tissues in the body and brain, keeping it in our system at a very moderate rate. This slow and prolonged release keeps Huperzine A working with our brain for longer periods of time. The Clinical Trials have been able to ascertain that the benefits are astounding by reversing and improving the cognitive deficits in humans and a broad range of animals. These findings have demonstrated that Huperzine A is capable of helping with the forgetfulness, mild Alzheimer's Disease and Vascular Dementia that is often seen with aging.

In my desperate search for and study of natural ingredients that successfully improve memory, I came across the perfect mate to go along with Huperzine. The wonderful amino-acid that is naturally in our body called Acetyl L-Carnitine. We now know that memory loss is due in part to the decay of those nerve cells and interference or loss in nerve conduction. What one has to ask, "What is the Primary Cause for such a decay and such a loss? Why does it happen with Aging and not when we are younger?" Upon careful research we have noted that these memory losses are based on the accumulation of the damage created by oxidative changes and attacks to our cellular membrane, which is made of fatty acids, lipids, and proteins. The Membranes of these nerve and brain cells are the essence and heart to all the activity that occurs within the cells. What would we do without these membranes? Well, what would you do if your home had no walls? You'd have to bear the attacks of the environment and wild animals. You'd constantly wake up in the middle of the night to some burglar trying to snatch your television or have to repair your home that was ravaged by the weather.

The membrane is what protects the cells of the brain. It is made of a double-wall from two layers of lipid fatty acids and sandwiched in the middle of water and protein. There are constantly trillions of attacks to our cell membranes every minute of the day for our whole entire lifetime. These oxidative attacks and damages are created by the normal function of oxygen, byproduct of our metabolism. Oxidation, or free radicals from oxygen, are the bane of our existence. Eventually your body will give in and these attacks finally break through, bringing down the walls of the cell membrane, creating havoc with our memory, and disrupting the neuro function of our brain.

People often hope to protect against such attacks and eat antioxidant-rich foods and take supplementation. This is done in vain as these forms of antioxidants cannot cross the Blood-Brain Barrier. All of the nutrients and protection are delivered to the other tissues in the body, but is unable to help with memory. This is the unfortunate truth of Human Brain Physiology. The Blood-Brain Barrier is the proverbial Chinese Wall that protects the brain from the outside.

The Carnitines are classified as Betaine, primarily used in the essential transport of the long-chain fatty acids to our cellular wall. They are also used as the essential battery and energy in the mitochondria for the processes and production of ATP along with cleaning up and removing excess trash such as short-chain fatty acids. Acetyl L-Carnitine is the most efficient of the Carnitines, which is well-recorded in rigid Clinical Studies and Research showing it efficiently crossing the Blood-Brain-Barrier. , University Clinical Studies have shown that when you administer small amounts of Acetyl L-Carnitine to patients with Alzheimer's disease, there's marked improvement in the spatial orientation of their surroundings as well as their short-term memories. , Other studies supplemented Acetyl L-Carnitine for one year, which helped to improve the mild cognitive emphasis and stabilize the global neuro psychological test scores in actual human subjects as reported by Hager et al. in 2001.

The understanding of its mechanism is primarily because of the improvement of the mitochondrial loss and decay, which obviously if there is no energy within the cells there is no activity that can take place creating the memory, concentration and focus. Greater activity may be because it decreases the damage created by this Oxidation to the neurons and the resulting cognitive dysfunction. It is essential that the reader understand the importance of the mitochondria which is the battery of the brain and the battery of each cell. If you lose the battery as well as destroy the activity, you have, in essence, Advanced Aging as well as Loss of Function of that cellular activity in the brain. This point was made plentifully clear from the research of the University of California in Berkley, Published by Gen Ken et al in February 19, 2002. Although I can't stop being old (or "Demented" if you ask my family), I am still able to work, produce, perform research, speak and write. I am totally aware that further research is needed, but at least for now this combination of Memory Specialist has made an enormous difference to not only myself, but to many people who have seen its immediate result. In as quickly as 48 hours people have seen a positive change in their total body performance and, for sure, memory and focus.

Dr. Tai's Pearl

"Excuse me… what's your name again?"
This is my awful opening line in a typical social party.
I just have TERRIBLE memory… but then again, I AM old – what's YOUR excuse?
I created Memory Specialist for ME!
I need help!
Super-fast combination of green-yellow moss with Acetyl-L-Carnitine for the brain is like Super Duo Batman & Robin. Not only makes my brain Super Charged, but the formula is great for prevention of Alzheimer's plaques. I LOVE **Memory Specialist**!

Directions:
Take 1 Capsule at A.M. & Noon

Ingredients:
Proprietary Formulation: Acetyl L-Carnitine, Huperzine A

These statements have not been reviewed by the FDA.
This product is not intended to diagnose, treat, cure, or prevent any disease.

Summary of Memory Specialist

- Improving the Focus, Thinking, Problem Solving, Memory of Anyone from Young as well as Elderly.
- Improvement in individuals who have had damage and loss from Alcoholism and Alcohol-related nerve and brain-cell death in Memory as well as Solutions and Focus.
- Improvement of slowing down the aging process and the decay of the brain cells and nerve cells.
- Slowing Down of Mitochondrial loss and increase energy of the brain cells.
- Prevention and treatment of Inflammation and loss of Circulation of Vascular and Neurologic to the brain.
- Improved activity and efficiency of the brain muscles and reaction times of athletes.
- Immediate & continuing improvement in long term of Memory, Mental Function, Behavior function and Thinking as well as Solution skills for mental tasks.

Clinical Cases:

Maria, a Post-Menopausal elderly woman, who had a long history of working with her famous husband, a physician of international stature, finally broke down and cried in our meeting that she could no longer help her husband and felt useless. Maria confided in me that she used to handle all of his scheduling and trips and functioned as his right hand helper. She was able to travel with him effortlessly with the "energy of a young woman." Maria not only kept up with him, she was extraordinarily affective at preparing and putting on large conferences for his medical teaching. Before long she was missing appointments, forgetting to write down schedules and leaving event planning until the last second if she remembered it at all.

Maria finally came to the point where she thought her life had ended. She no longer could help her husband! She had forgotten her tasks on more than one occasion and jeopardized all their plans more than once with her absent-mindedness. All the problems that came with conferencing proved to be too much for her, but even more so she was burned out and tired. Maria was completely tapped out of all her mental and physical energy to keep up with the rigors of her once daily-grind. She is tired and finds herself unable to grasp all of the facts to make their important decisions – always saying she'll "think about it," but by the time she tries she can't even comb through the mess in her head. This caused Maria to keep postponing, unable to admit that she didn't know what was going on. Instead of being part of the solution, she quickly became part of the problem. Maria was ready to give up her professional and social life when she decided to try a new protocol.

We began with a Salivary Hormone Test to determine what deficiencies Maria was encountering with Menopause and her inability to deal with stress. We provided a complete protocol, starting with Super B12 Liposome and Max Performance to elevate the energy level and get the Adrenals working. This was combined with Memory Specialist and Max Brain to increase brain activity, prevent further loss and damage of brain cells, and improve memory. The supplements helped to delay any mitochondrial damage and act as a super antioxidant for the free radical attacks that caused the Accelerated Aging in her brain. Maria recently called me and she was ebullient in her praises. She never thought that these supplements would work for her, but tried them out of pure desperation. She's now embarrassed to say that it only took her 4 weeks to experience a major improvement in her ability to think, work and remember. She's a brand new woman. Congratulations, Maria!! You are Back! We wish you and your husband a long productive and professional life.

Contraindications:

Do not take if you are allergic to any of the ingredients.

Although Huperzine A and Acetyl L-Carnitine have shown to be exceedingly safe in both Clinical Studies on Animals as well as Humans, there are some side effects that one should watch out for, although they are rare: Potential Nausea, Loss of Appetite and High Blood Pressure

The ingredients Huperzine A and Acetyl L-Carnitine have not been studied for pregnancy or women who are breastfeeding and should not be used by those individuals.

As a precautionary note, we do not suggest that these ingredients should be used on children with a history of Epilepsy, as it may affect their brain activity

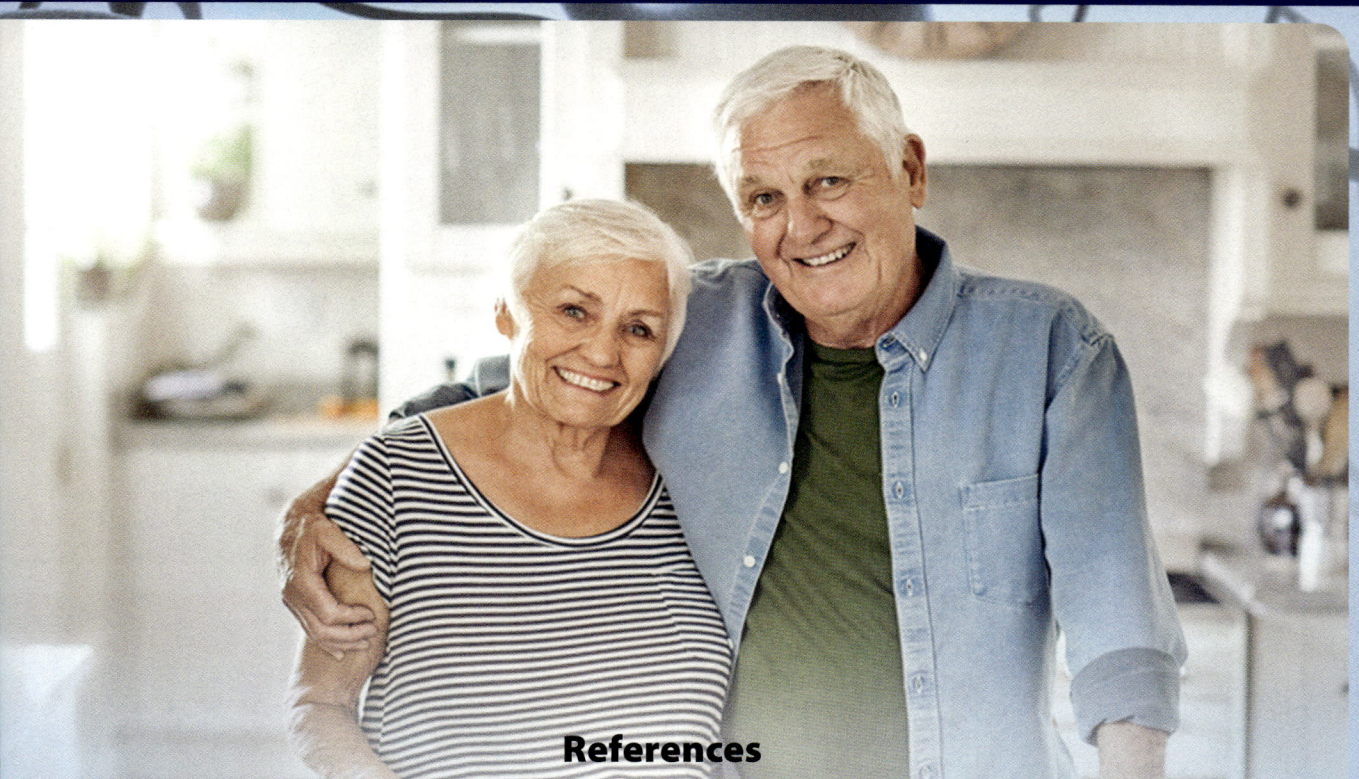

References

1. Brooks JO 3rd, Yesavage JA, Carta A, Bravi D. Acetyl L-carnitine slows decline in younger patients with Alzheimer's disease: a reanalysis of a double-blind, placebo-controlled study using the trilinear approach. Int Psychoger 1998;10:193-203.
2. Bai, D. L., Tang, X. C., and He, X. C. Huperzine A, a potential therapeutic agent for treatment of Alzheimer's disease. Curr.Med Chem 2000;7(3):355-374
3. Cheng, D. H., Ren, H., and Tang, X. C. Huperzine A, a novel promising acetylcholinesterase inhibitor. Neuroreport 12-20-1996;8(1):97-101.
4. Chen M, Gao Z, Deng H, and et al. Huperzine A capsules vs tablets in treatment of Alzheimer disease: multicenter studies. Chinese Journal of New Drugs and Clinical Remedies 2000;19(1):10-12.
5. Aisen, P. A Multi-Center, Double-Blind, Placebo-Controlled Therapeutic Trial to Determine Whether Natural Huperzine A Improves Cognitive Function. Georgetown University Medical Center, Memory Disorders Program 2004
6. Pettegrew JW, Levine J, McClure RJ. Acetyl-L-carnitine physical-chemical, metabolic, and therapeutic properties: relevance for its mode of action in Alzheimer's disease and geriatric depression. Mol Psychiatry 2000;5:616-32.
7. Cucinotta D, Passeri M, Ventura S, et al. Multicenter clinical placebo-controlled study with acetyl-L-carnitine (ALC) in the treatment of mildly demented elderly patients. Drug Development Res 1988;14:213-6.
8. Hudson S, Tabet N. Acetyl-L-carnitine for dementia. Cochrane Database Syst Rev 2003;2:CD003158.
9. Bonavita E, Bertuzzi D, Bonavita J et al: L-Acetylcarnitine (L-Ac) (Branigen) in the long-term symptomatic treatment of senile dementia. Clin Trials J 1988; 25(4):227-237.
10. Mayeux R, Sano M. Treatment of Alzheimer's Disease. N Engl J Med 1999;341:1670-9.
11. Rosadini G, Marenco S, Nobili F, et al. Acute effects of acetyl-L-carnitine on regional cerebral blood flow in patients with brain ischaemia. Int J Clin Pharmacol Res 1990;10:123-8.

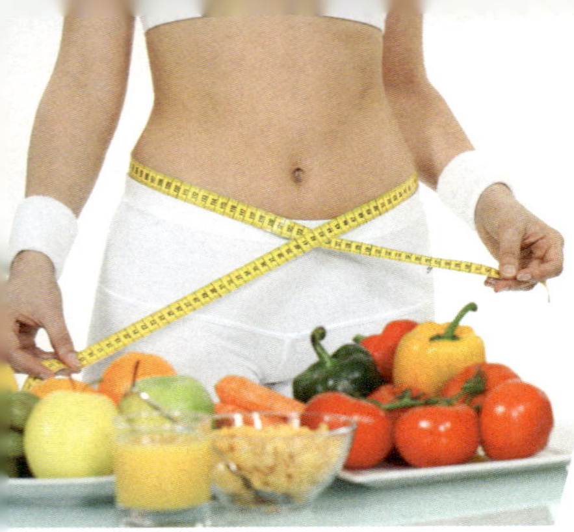

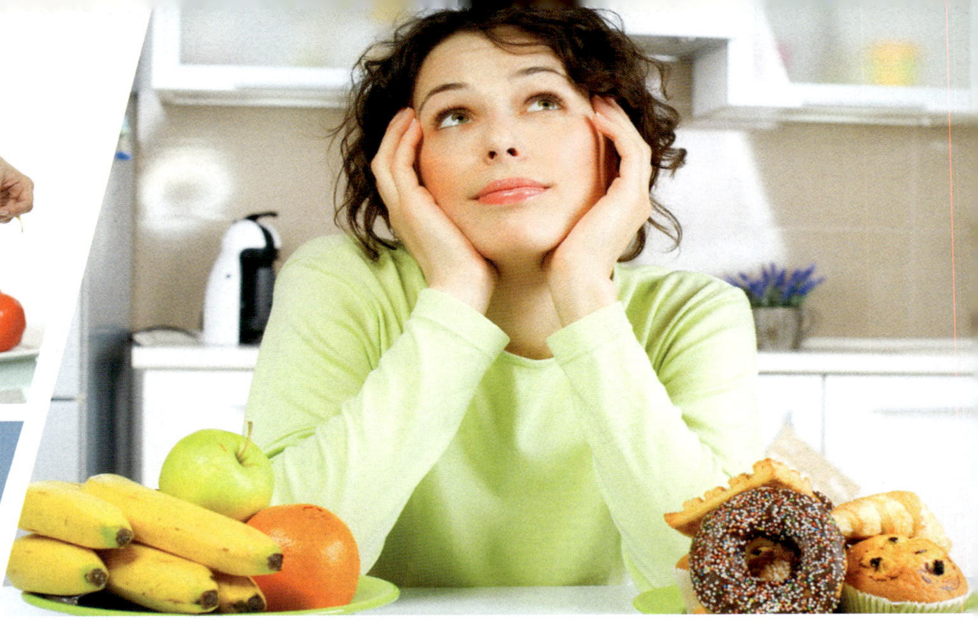

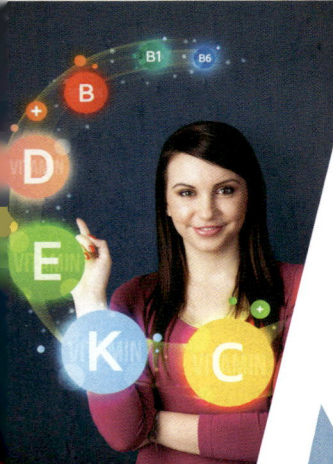

Directions: Take 3-6 tablets daily with food

Is your diet lacking Essential Nutrients?

Are you on a Detox Program and losing Minerals?

MINERAL PAK
Powerful Combination of Vital Macro Minerals

No time for a balanced diet?

The Complete Mineral Pak was designed with you in mind. The lack of essential mineral nutrients is the single most common mistake in their supplement program. Sometimes we overlook the most important and yet the simplest of all the nutrients.

Minerals are essential for powerful bio-chemical reactions in our body, and essential to millions of enzymatic processes that occur throughout the day.

Complete Mineral Pak is chockfull of special "Chelated minerals and micro-nutrients for quick and effective absorption". It is a powerful combination of Calcium, Iron, Phosphorus, Iodine, Magnesium, Chromium, Potassium and Boron.

MINERAL PAK

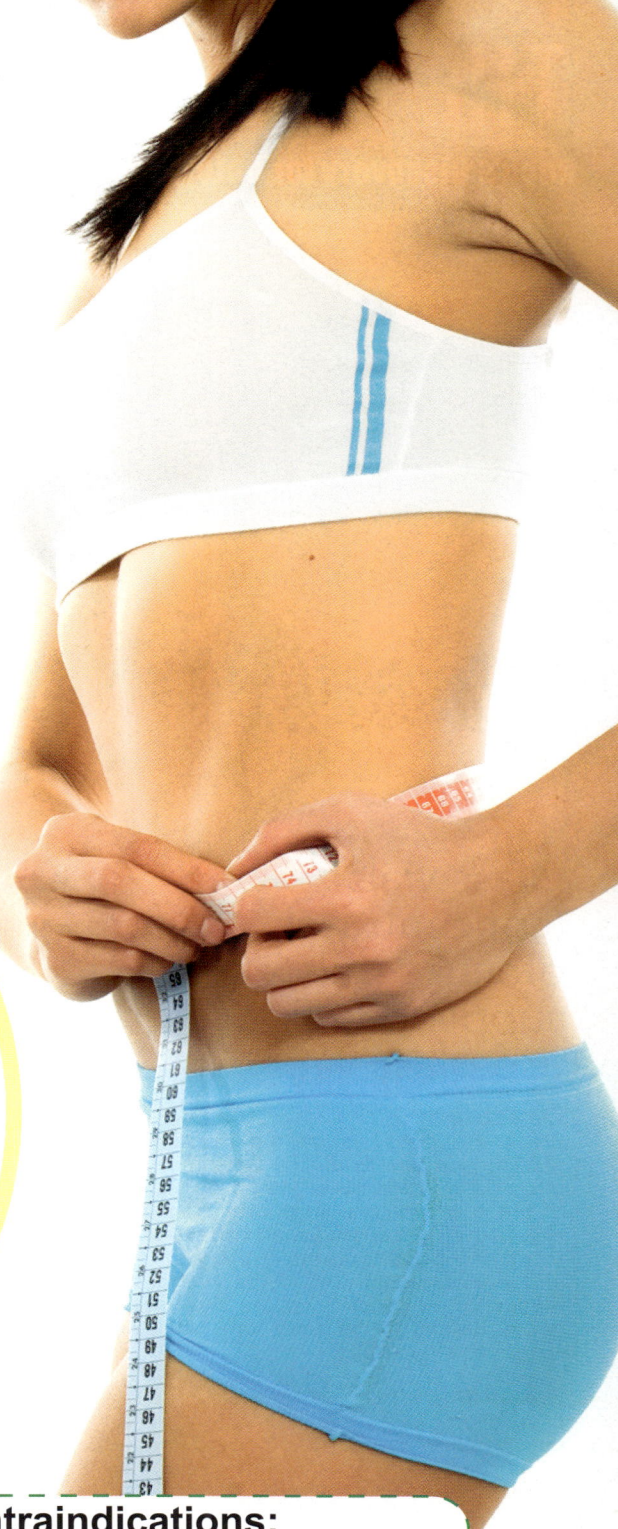

Ingredients:

Calcium, Iron, Phosphorus, Iodine, Magnesium, Zinc, Selenium, Copper, Manganese, Chromium, Potassium, Boron

These statements have not been reviewed by the FDA. This product is not intended to diagnose, treat, cure, or prevent any disease.

Dr. Tai's Pearl

Mineral Pak was made with careful attention to the fact that all living animals are electrical beings. Every activity that allows us to run, move, think, digest, and breathe and your heart to beat all comes form the electrical activity that passes from nerves to muscles. Without minerals, both macro and micro, we are as good as dead. Without these minerals we have NO ELECTRICITY. No Electricity means No Life. Make sure your body is full of minerals in order to have a healthy life.

Side Effects: None

Contraindications:
Do not take if you are allergic to any of the ingredients.

THE MOLECULAR THERAPY (TMT)
Koch's Discovery for Detoxification & Cancer Cells

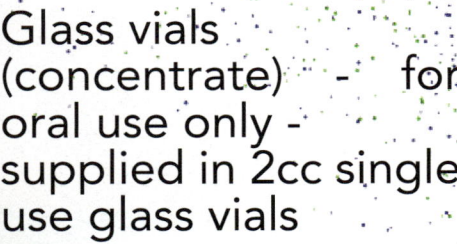

Glass vials (concentrate) - for oral use only - supplied in 2cc single use glass vials

Directions:
Break the glass vial at the neckline by placing one thumb on the bottom of the glass vial and the other thumb on the top of the glass vial and snap open the glass vial. Use a mini-straw (small coffee stirrer) to sip all of the contents in the vial. Hold and swirl contents around the wall of the mouth for 30 seconds before swallowing. Avoid Eating for at least one-half hour before or after taking.

Recommended dosages:
First: Use one (1) vial each day for ten (10) days. You may repeat this process if needed or as directed by your health care practitioner.
After 10 days: Use one (1) vial once a week for ten (10) weeks. You may repeat this process if needed or as directed by your health care practitioner.
After 10 weeks: Use one (1) vial once a month thereafter for maintenance or prevention.

In spray or dropper bottle - (multi-dose) - for oral use only - supplied in 2oz spray bottle

Directions: Spray or place drops of the contents directly into mouth, hold and swirl contents around the wall of mouth for 30 seconds before swallowing. Avoid Eating for at least one-half hour before or after taking.

Recommended dosages:
First: Apply five (5) sprays or ten (10) drops, twice every day for 1 week.
You may repeat this process if needed or as directed by your health care practitioner.
After 1 week: Apply two (2) sprays or four (4) drops once every day for two months.
You may repeat this process if needed or as directed by your health care practitioner.
After 2 months: Apply one (1) spray or two (2) drops once every day thereafter for maintenance or prevention.

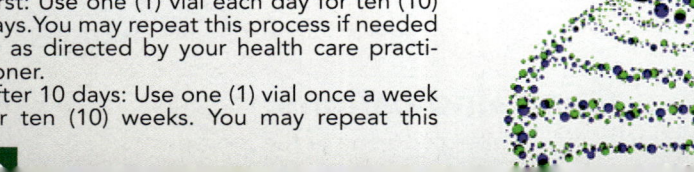

TMT Dosage Information

You may experience a "Healing Reaction" flu-like symptoms – slight fever or chills and muscle spasms that may last up to 3 days. This is a "welcome" healing reaction and there is no need to be concerned. However, DO NOT TAKE The Molecular Therapy while these symptoms are present. You may continue with the dosage after the symptoms are gone. (Only 25% of cases may experience this reaction). Good results can be still be achieved even if you do not experience this healing reaction.

Important

- Stay on a vegetarian diet: lots of juices, beans, nuts and vegetables. Stay away from sugar, meat, and dairy products. No soft drinks! Only natural drinks such as green or herbal tea.
- Stay on a vegetarian diet for a minimum of one week or longer, if possible.
- No Sugar, Beer, Liquor or Wine.
- It is preferable to monitor your body's acidity/alkalinity (pH) level. The ideal pH level is 7.0 pH (neutral)

These statements have not been reviewed by the FDA. This product is not intended to diagnose, treat, cure, or prevent any disease.

Do not take The Molecular Therapy as a substitute for medical treatment.

Always follow the advice of your personal physician.

Ingredients:
Glyoxal, Methyglyoxal

These statements have not been reviewed by the FDA. This product is not intended to diagnose, treat, cure, or prevent any disease.

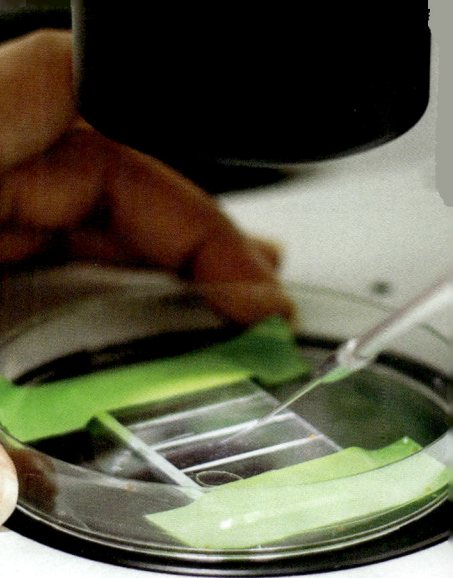

Dr. Tai's Pearls

This homeopathic formula was created by Dr. Cooke, M.D., Ph.D. He left the United States to live abroad and continue his work. When he died, he left the laboratory with a mother tincture of the homeopathic Cooke formula. This is a German formula, sold and approved in Germany. Patients have had excellent results using this formulation for normalizing cellular growth in various tumors, as well as controlling severe herpes outbreaks, including Herpes Zoster, when there is pain along the nerve. When no other treatment is available, TMT has stepped up and provided the relief the patients appreciated.

Contraindications:
Do not take this product if you are allergic to any of its ingredients.

Clinical Cases:
Dr. Neal, a physician in northern Canada, silently suffered from herpes zoster, neuralgia pain on the left lower quadrant of his chest. This was a leftover from the herpes zoster that he contracted ten years prior, without full remission. He has continued a prescription medication for nerve pain and has suffered silently and bravely his condition. One day, using the TMT, he was able to treat the remnant neuralgia. Within one week, he wrote to me with an optimistic outlook that the pain has now vanished and he was without symptoms. He was elated by the results and dumbfounded by the quickness of which TMT worked to resolve the neuralgia. The last report, two years hence, Dr. Neal still continues to be symptom-free.

Side Effects:
On occasion, patients have reported that using TMT when actively getting results for improving the cellular rejuvenation, there are detox symptoms such as high fever, a sense of tired, malaise, similar to symptoms of flu. When this happens, it is often times important not to continue active treatment until symptoms reside. These are called Hexheimer reactions.

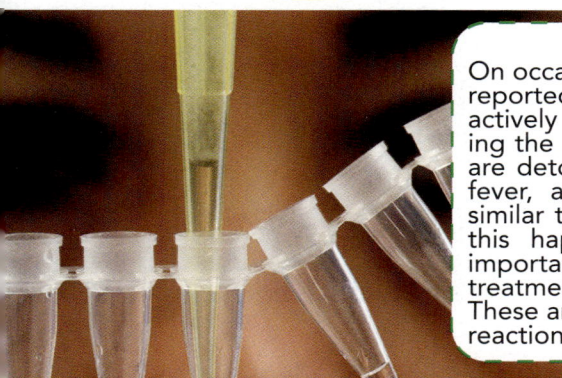
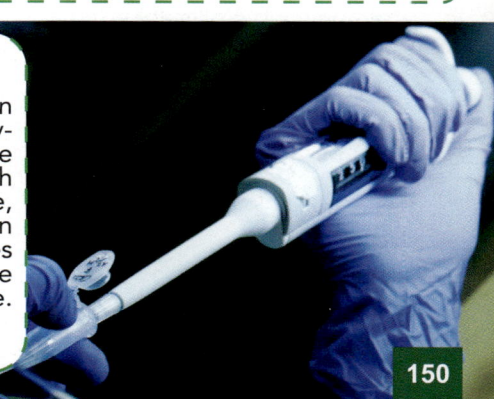

Muscle Specialist
Stop Muscle Pain Today!

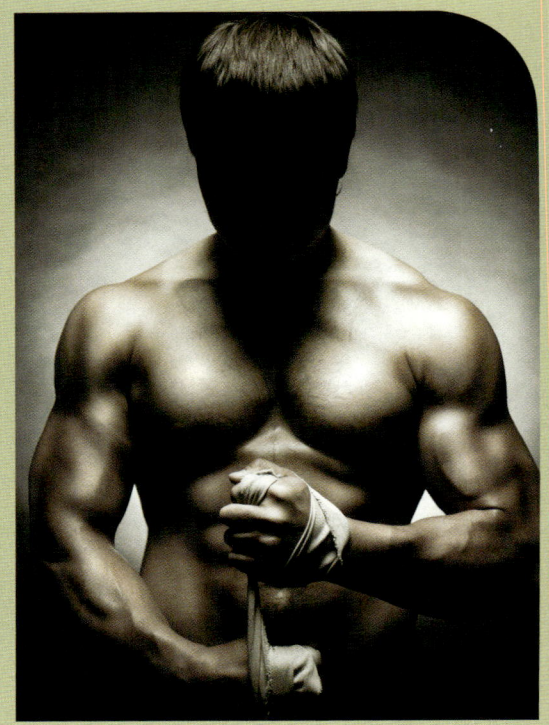

Exercise got your muscles sore and stiff? Woke up with severe neck pain? Back pain?

If your problem is muscle pain, muscle soreness or muscle stiffness, we have the answer!
No! Prescription muscle relaxants do not work very well. They make you drowsy and sleepy. Most muscle pain with critical sensitive trigger points are more than a localized problem. Ancient Chinese herbalists describe this kind of pain as stagnant circulation affecting the liver for poor filtration. Therefore, simple massage and heat serves only as a limited "partial" treatment to muscle pain and soreness

This ancient formulation dates back hundreds of years. The secret formula was found hidden within the sacred walls of old Buddhist temples, which means it has worked for centuries, and it has proven to be effective.

Doctors in ancient times trusted this formula so much they used it as part of the "differential diagnosis". If the Doctor did not know if the origin of the pain was from bone, nerves or muscle, they used Muscle Specialist. If after 5 days, no improvement was noticed, they knew the cause was not muscle related. The pain stemmed from some other cause.
But... if in 5-7 days, major improvements are noticed, you can be sure the cause is muscle related.

Direction: Take 2 pills in the morning, 2 pills in the afternoon and 4 pills at bedtime on an empty stomach. Take for 5-7 days for initial evaluation.

Ingredients: Angelica, Sinensis, Cinnamon, Frankincense, Myrrh, Curcuma, Morinda, Eucommia, Carthami

These statements have not been reviewed by the FDA. This product is not intended to diagnose, treat, cure, or prevent any disease.

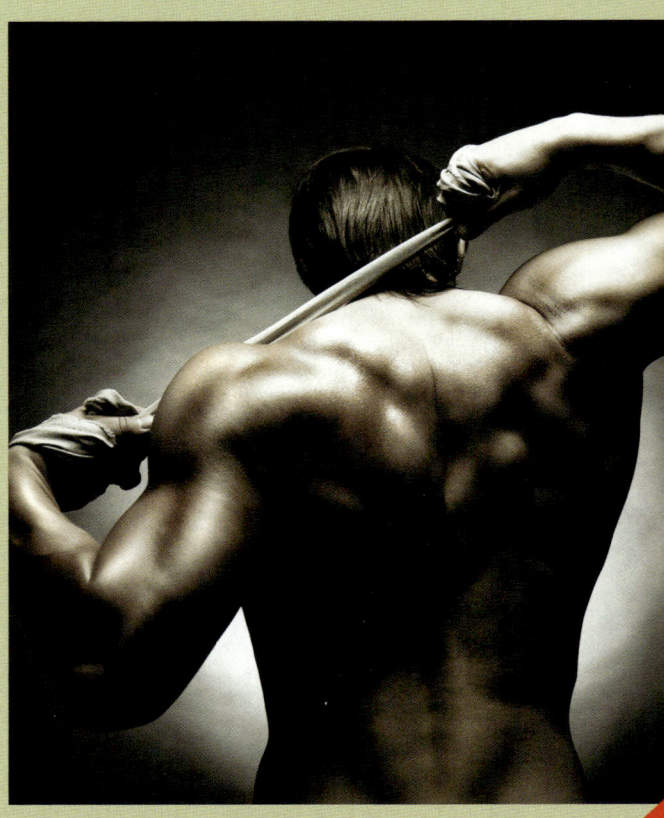

Dr. Tai's Pearl

There are only a few supplements that I actually cannot leave home without – like the commercial from American Express. It is so important when you are being stuck on an airplane seat 18 inches wide, for you to have a supplement that will actually provide relief when you arrive at the other end of your destination, after four, five, or even twelve hours. Muscle Specialist works by eliminating the pain and the muscle spasticity. It is not a muscle relaxant. It is however a supplement that returns your muscle to normal function. Nothing I have ever come across has worked as well, as predictably, or as quickly as muscle specialist in normalizing muscle pain. In fact, I use Muscle Specialist as a differential diagnosis tool to rule out any of the complex issues of muscle pain, some from nerve, some from bone, others from soft-tissue cartilage, causing the discomfort; however, Muscle Specialist only works on muscle. If it relieves more than 50% of the discomfort after three days then you know the problem and pathology you are dealing with is specifically muscle. If you don't get any relief at all, you know the problem you're dealing with is something else. Muscle Specialist is a very helpful tool for those of us who are trying to help patients pinpoint the cause of the pathology.

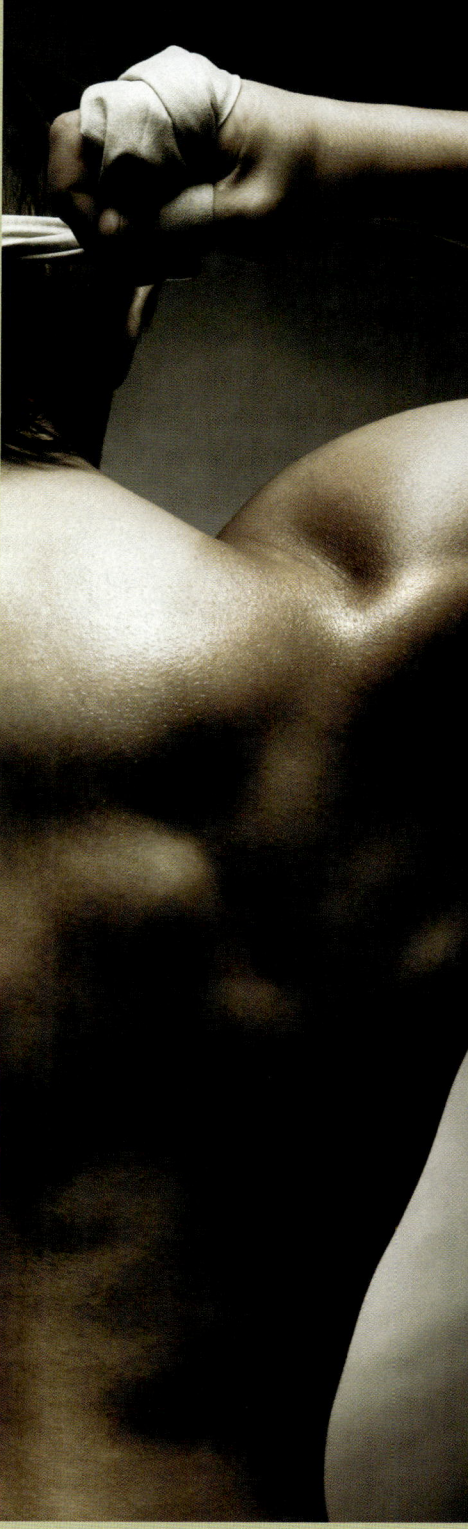

Clinical Cases:

Carla, a sales clerk at a department store, age 52, was suffering from severe neck pain for a number of years. She had been diagnosed with chronic fibromyalgia. The long search and trials of different supplements to no avail, she almost gave up. She began using Muscle Specialist and within two days, 90% of her discomfort around the cervical neck area and shoulders disappeared. Totally in awe of the relief, she told everyone she met about the wonderful results she got and how excited she was after such a long time to be able to move her neck without any pain and enjoy her life with full range of motion without any complications.

Side Effects: None

Contraindications:
Do not take if you are allergic to any of the ingredients.

NEURAL SPECIALIST

Protect & Rejuvenation of Neuropathy

One of the horrible nightmares of suffering from Diabetes Mellitus is the complications that result from this abnormal sugar metabolism disease. The severe symptoms that diabetics experience comes from the accumulation of Advanced Glycation End-product (AGE).

These abnormalities are caused by the "carmelization" of the sugar, much like what we see when we burn sugar on the stove top to make candy. These burned deposits accumulate around all the blood vessels and nerve endings initiating the abnormal and inflammatory conditions, and accelerating the Aging process.

AGE contributes to things such as diabetic neuropathy, causing loss of sensations, or burning and painful symptoms occurring in the hands, feet and toes. Up to just recently this problem was untreatable. Patients were left with only analgesics and strong narcotics in order to fight the severe pain that would occur day and night. Now, years of research have lead to a much clearer picture of the pathology and the abnormal physiology occurring in the nerves and the nerve endings of diabetics. Recent research revealed a new technology that led to this formulation of Neural Specialist. The proprietary formulation of ingredients may support the healthy nerves and specifically may delay the Advance Glycation Endproduct that leads to neuropathy.

Neural Specialist may improve the myelin sheath which is the covering of all the nerves which are under attack by the Advanced Glycation Endproduct. Neural Specialist contains ingredients called Fulvic and Humate acids which are special extracts from mesomorphic periods of earth deposited millions of years ago. These natural extracts from Fulvic Humate contain 77 micronutrients for the proper nourishment of the nerve tissues. The formula also has the entire complex of Folic acid, B6 and B12, which are essential to proper nerve support and nourishment.

Neural Specialist may help with the following:
- **Diabetic Neuropathy**
- **Nourishment to the nerve tissue**
- **May be effective in Advanced Glycation Endproducts (AGE)**
- **Burning symptoms of the feet and toes**
- **Advanced pain from neuropathy**
- **Neurodegeneration**

Directions:
Take 2 capsules twice daily in the AM and PM.

Ingredients:
Fulvic Humate, Benzoyl Thiamin, Vitamin B6, Vitamin B12, Folic Acid Macrocrystalline, Cellulose, Dicalcium Phosphate, Magnesium Stearate

These statements have not been reviewed by the FDA. This product is not intended to diagnose, treat, cure, or prevent any disease.

Dr. Tai's Pearl

Just think of the difficulty that physicians and surgeons have to deal with when a diabetic patient complains of severe, stabbing, shooting pain, asking you to please amputate their feet. This is desperation at its worst. To most doctors the polyneuropathy or neuropathy from diabetes is a nightmare of disappointment and frustrations. No doctor wants to work on it because of unrewarding results from the treatments. Neural Specialist is a rare combination, using the latest special vitamin compounds that are formulated to repair the pathology and polyneuron of the nerve that actually causes the numbness and burning sensation. Depending on the stage of pathology, the nerves actually undergo a myriad of symptoms. These nerve saving vitamins are special compounds, designed for results.

Side Effects: None

Contraindications:
Do not take if you are allergic to any of the ingredients.

Clinical Cases:
Chandler, a 28-year-old diabetic, quite overweight with a very sedentary job working as a terminal keyboard entry clerk. He spends hours sitting in front of a computer. A few years ago, he started having slight paresthesia with pins and needles throughout the bottom of his foot. In the last year, the pain has become progressively more severe and the stabbing pains are now aggravated to the point where he has to use chronic pain medication to control it. His podiatric surgeon has attempted a number of different kinds of prescription and injection therapies. He is already wearing a pair of orthotics in order to relieve any pressure points on his shoes while ambulatory. Treatment focused for the diabetic neuropathy was using Neural Specialist together with Super B12 sublingual, Ionic Micromineral Specialist and Max Nox for nitric oxide increasing the circulation to the lower extremities. It has been now three months since the commencement of treatment and most of the stabbing pain has subsided. He is comfortable now to be able to sleep and work without taking narcotic analgesics. He appears well in the progress of conquering the pathology and putting the diabetic neuropathy to bed.

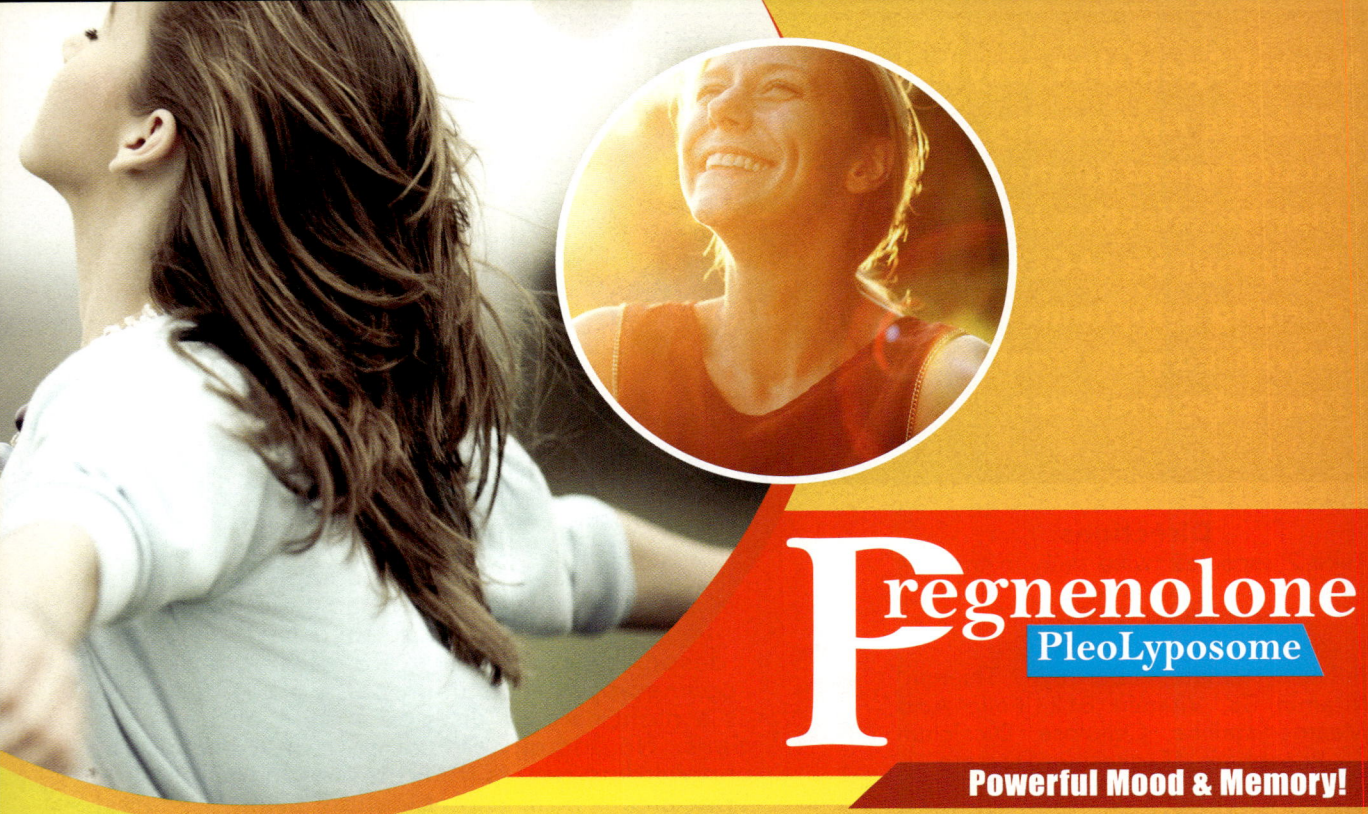

Pregnenolone PleoLyposome

Powerful Mood & Memory!

Pregnenolone is known as the "Feel Good" hormone. One doctor describes "increasing color and brightness, and that life just looks more beautiful when taking Pregnenolone." It is the first step in synthesis from cholesterol to the major sex hormones of the body. Pregnenolone is the precursor to all of the other hormones: **DHEA**, progesterone, testosterone, estrogen and cortisol. As we age pregnenolone levels decline. Physicians believe that replacement of pregnenolone to youthful levels is an important step in an anti-aging program. In published studies, pregnenolone has shown to be 100 times more effective for memory enhancement than any other hormone in laboratory animals.

If **DHEA** is known as the body energy converter, pregnenolone is known as the brain energy converter by improving the transmitting of messages from neuron to neuron and influencing positive short-term memory.

Pregnenolone, together with **DHEA** are essential members of a reverse aging program. Both are considered one of the "Parents of Hormones", Mother and Father, respectively. It is through these two very important pre-hormones that we get all of our progesterone, testosterone and estrogen. Both hormones, if used together, may help in the following areas:

1. Improves energy, vitality and youth
2. Fights osteoporosis
3. Improved depression & chronic fatigue syndrome
4. Improvement of adrenal fatigue & cortisol levels
5. Improvement of thyroid function
6. Healthy immunity – Enhance Immune System Efficiency
7. Stimulates and improves in preventing osteoporosis, cardio vascular diseases
8. Improvement of muscle mass.
9. Improves Alzheimer's diseases, mental memory and logical thinking.
10. Stress reduction, resistance to damages of stress
11. Energy improvement in meno pause
12. Repair of the nervous tissues
13. Protection to cancer
14. Protective to cardiovascular disease
15. Increases thermogenesis & burning Fat
16. Improves insulin receptor sensitivity & reduces diabetes risk

What is Pregnenolone PleoLyposome?
The latest technological advancement in anti-aging is a new delivery pathway called "First Pass Technology". It is a Transdermal Lyposome protected delivery system through the skin or sublingual mucosa, which is much faster and much more effective than anything else. It provides a direct route to the blood stream without overworking or damaging the liver.
This newer Lyposome technology delivers Pregnenolone directly to the blood stream with a lower dosage, faster results and fewer side effects.

Directions:
Apply to soft parts of skin. Females: Apply 3 pumps daily (AM). Males: Apply 5 pumps daily (AM). Adjust dosage to your individual needs.

Ingredients:

Pregnenolone, Fulvic Ext., Essential Phospholipids, Evening Primrose Oil, Shea Butter, Aloe Vera, Lavender Oil, Almond Oil, Hemp Oil, Alpha Lipolic Acid, Allantoin

These statements have not been reviewed by the FDA. This product is not intended to diagnose, treat, cure, or prevent any disease.

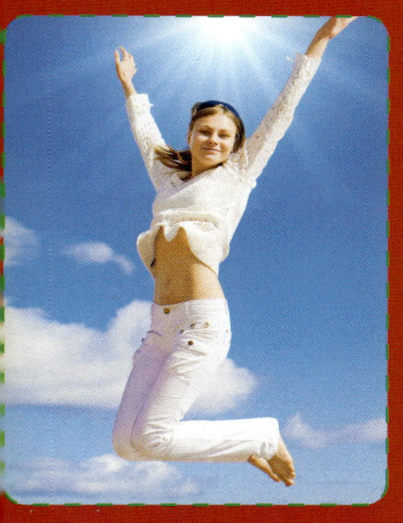

Dr. Tai's Pearls:

If you ever survey the chart of the human hormones needed for survival, you will notice that at the very top is the grandfather of all hormones – Pregnenolone. Pregnenolone is the very essence of the beginning of the cascade of hormones in humans, starting with the most important ingredient, the source of all our hormones, cholesterol. When cholesterol, under the supervision of an enzyme, converts within the cellular material, it will create pregnenolone. Pregnenolone will then be useful, providing further enzymatic changes, for just about any other hormone needed in the body. Pregnenolone was created for the specific use of helping our neural pathways and brain. As 30,000 brain cells die each day, pregnenolone is there to help you protect, regenerate, and upkeep activity within the brain for memory and mood control. Pregnenolone is the most significant change for protection of dementia into the future; as we lose the level of pregnenolone from aging. Pregnenolone also supports the normalization of mood, in the treatment of depression and tolerance of stress. In short, if you want to stay healthy in the brain and even healthy emotionally, then the hormone pregnenolone is your answer.

Clinical Case:

Dr. Jamai, a Caribbean-native physician and health worker suffering from a great deal of stress and under a lot of pressure from his new job as the director the health care services for a small university. Unaware of how he got started, he felt quite depressed as he worked throughout the day. He lacked concentration, memory and depression was completely new to this individual. Using five pumps of Pregnenolone in the morning transdermally, where he rubbed vigorously on his skin, rotating clockwise, he would do the same treatment dose at night. Additional protocol of Stress & Anxiety Specialist, he noticed that Pregnenolone was able to reverse the depression, restore a new sense of confidence, and help him to control his emotions much better.

Side Effects: None

Contraindications:

Do not take with food. Do not take if you are allergic to any ingredients.

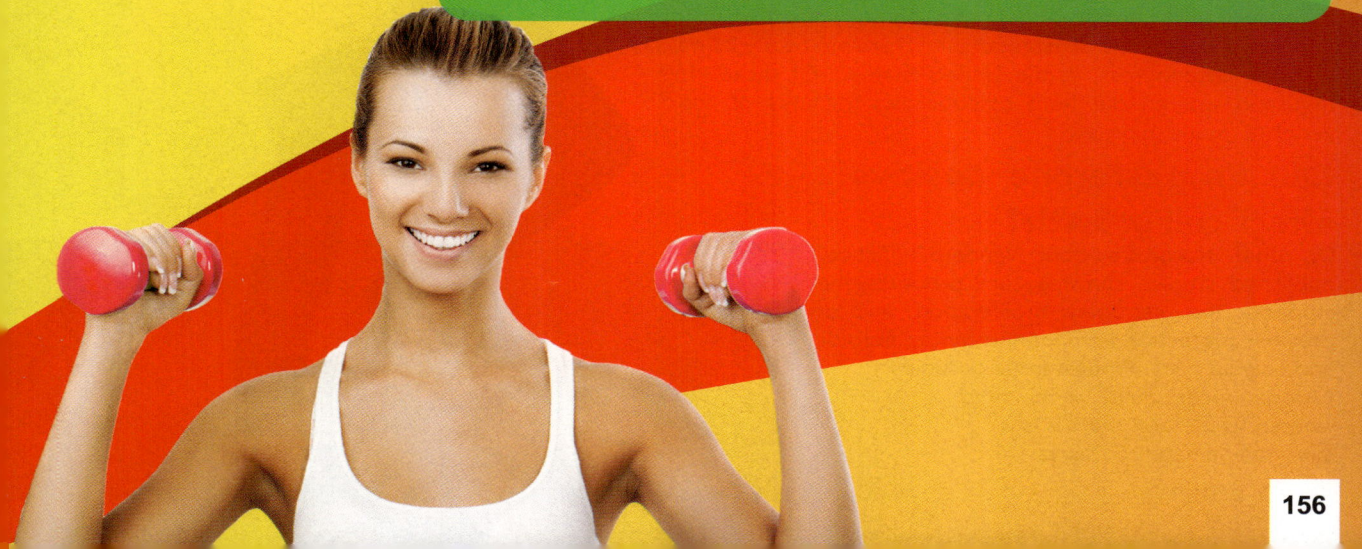

PROGESTERONE PLEOLYPOSOME

Women's Best Friend for Health During Menopause

Characteristically, women lose progesterone at a faster rate after the age of 35. In fact, when many younger women suffer from the punishment of PMS symptoms it is often due to the early lack of progesterone in their bodies. Dr. Neils Lauersen M.D. is co-author of the book titled "PMS" and a Professor of Obstetrics and Gynecology at the medical college. He claims that 90% of his patients have tried Progesterone hormone and found relief when nothing else works.

According to **Dr. John Lee, M.D.,** both men and women suffer from the excess estrogen in the body. **Dr. Lee** has written a number of books discussing the negative effects of excess estrogen in Women, which causes fluid retention, moodiness, swollen and tender breasts, increased uterine fibrosis and ovarian cysts. **Dr. Lee's** extensive research on the negative effects of estrogen was published in the National Clinical Review, a clinical report of over 100 menopausal women using natural progesterone.

The wonderful effects of natural progesterone are near "miraculous". Women rely on natural progesterone in cases of pre-menstrual symptoms as well as menopausal symptoms. Women have reported relief of their anxiety, depression, and a calming and relaxing effect on their bodies. Progesterone may also provide a good night sleep. It is a wonderful natural diuretic for water retention and bloating. It is an effective natural protector from uterine cancer, fibroids and endometriosis, as well as provides protection for breasts and helps prevent fibrocystic changes.

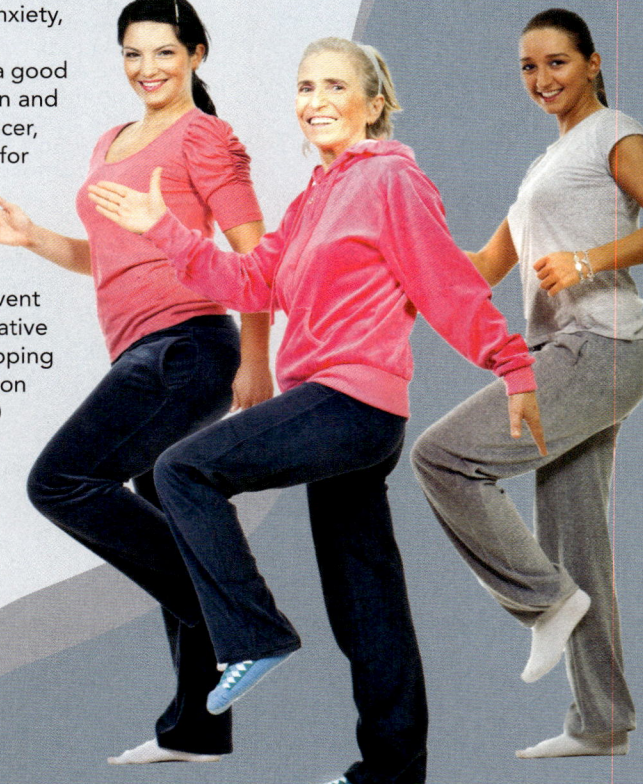

Can it help Osteoporosis?

Progesterone is one of the few natural hormones that has an Osteoblastic activity. Osteoblast cells bulid new bone to prevent both men and women's osteoporosis and prevent degenerative changes of the bones as we get older. It is truly effective in stopping this horrible epidemic of osteoporosis. There are nearly 28 million cases of osteoporosis in the United States. Of those, 150 thousand women die from osteoporosis fractures of the vertebral, spine, hips, etc.

Can Progesterone positively affect cell growth?

Dr. Joel Hargrove from Vanderbilt School published studies showing that progesterone stopped the estrogen proliferation and it provides protection from uterine cancer, fibroids and ovarian cysts. Progesterone occupies estrogen receptor sites in men and women. Therefore, there is less estrogen damage to tissues.

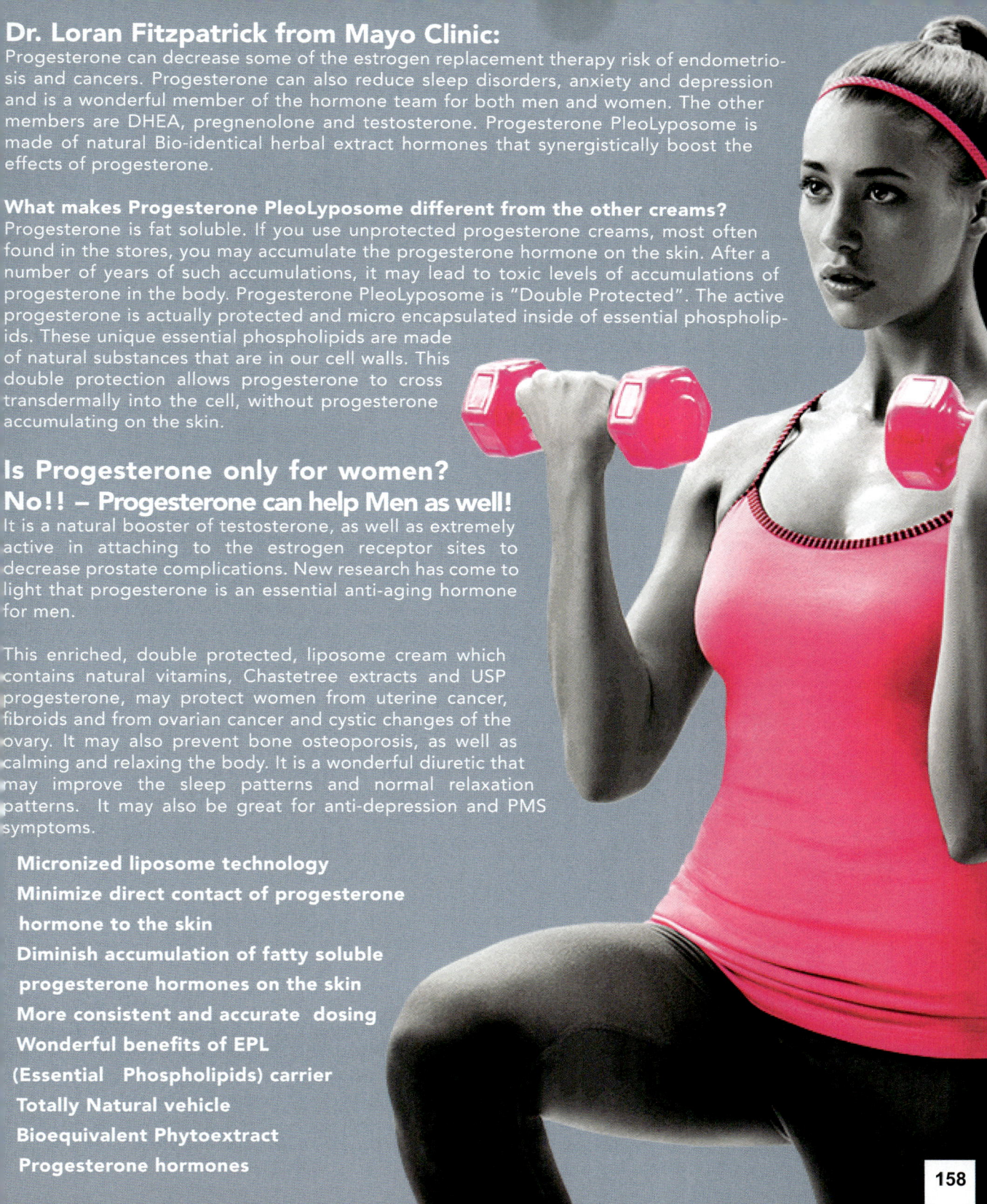

Dr. Loran Fitzpatrick from Mayo Clinic:

Progesterone can decrease some of the estrogen replacement therapy risk of endometriosis and cancers. Progesterone can also reduce sleep disorders, anxiety and depression and is a wonderful member of the hormone team for both men and women. The other members are DHEA, pregnenolone and testosterone. Progesterone PleoLyposome is made of natural Bio-identical herbal extract hormones that synergistically boost the effects of progesterone.

What makes Progesterone PleoLyposome different from the other creams?

Progesterone is fat soluble. If you use unprotected progesterone creams, most often found in the stores, you may accumulate the progesterone hormone on the skin. After a number of years of such accumulations, it may lead to toxic levels of accumulations of progesterone in the body. Progesterone PleoLyposome is "Double Protected". The active progesterone is actually protected and micro encapsulated inside of essential phospholipids. These unique essential phospholipids are made of natural substances that are in our cell walls. This double protection allows progesterone to cross transdermally into the cell, without progesterone accumulating on the skin.

Is Progesterone only for women?
No!! – Progesterone can help Men as well!

It is a natural booster of testosterone, as well as extremely active in attaching to the estrogen receptor sites to decrease prostate complications. New research has come to light that progesterone is an essential anti-aging hormone for men.

This enriched, double protected, liposome cream which contains natural vitamins, Chastetree extracts and USP progesterone, may protect women from uterine cancer, fibroids and from ovarian cancer and cystic changes of the ovary. It may also prevent bone osteoporosis, as well as calming and relaxing the body. It is a wonderful diuretic that may improve the sleep patterns and normal relaxation patterns. It may also be great for anti-depression and PMS symptoms.

- **Micronized liposome technology**
- **Minimize direct contact of progesterone hormone to the skin**
- **Diminish accumulation of fatty soluble progesterone hormones on the skin**
- **More consistent and accurate dosing**
- **Wonderful benefits of EPL (Essential Phospholipids) carrier**
- **Totally Natural vehicle**
- **Bioequivalent Phytoextract**
- **Progesterone hormones**

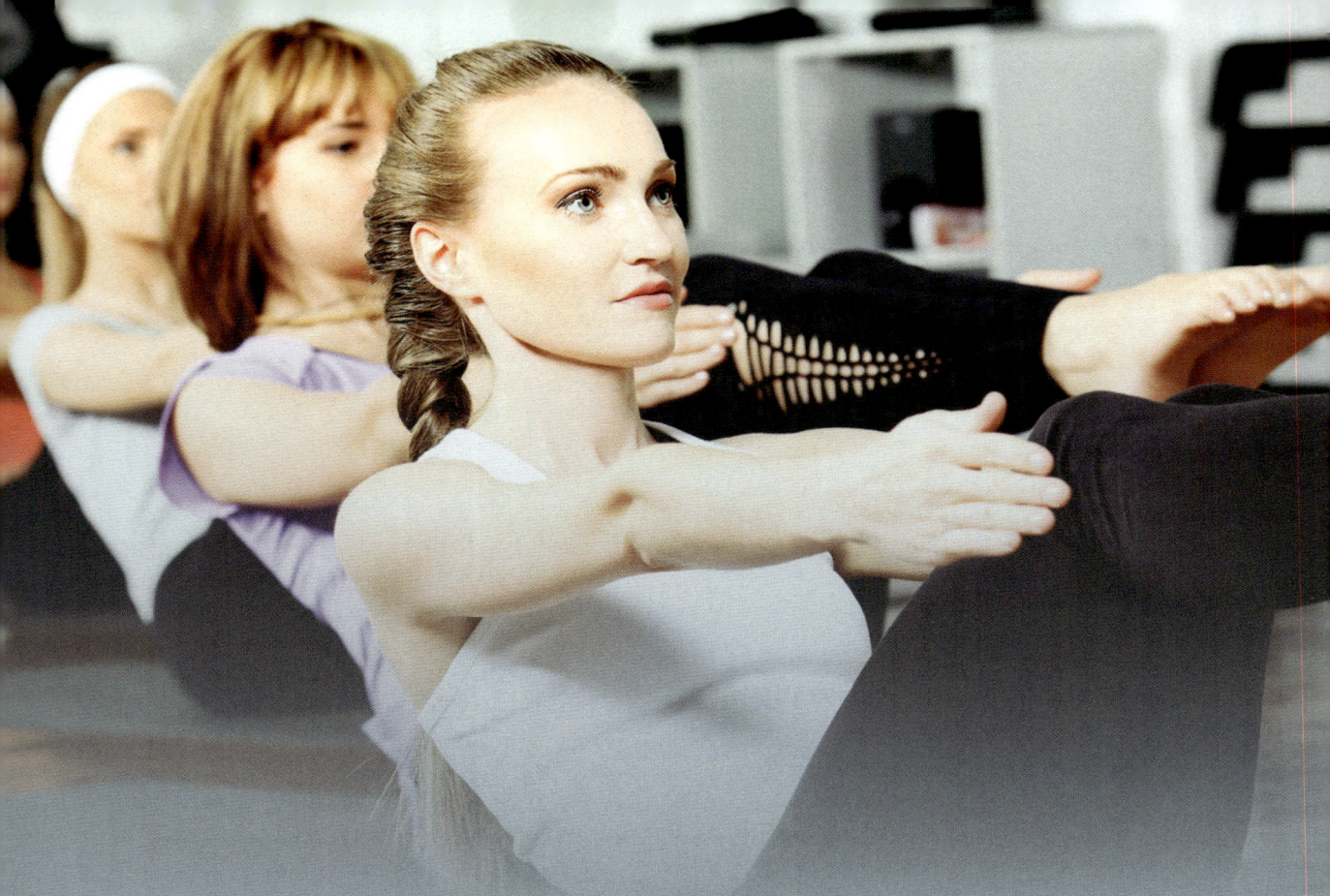

Progesterone – Clinical Applications:

Anti-Anxiety, Picaro O. Nrain Res. 1995 Anti-Osteoporosis, Lee. J. Int. Clin. Nutr. Rev. 1990; Prior J.C. Endoc Review 1999 ; Stevenson J. et al., Lancet 1990

Breast Cancer Prevention,

Cowan LD., J. Epidemiol 1981; Formby B. et al., AAnn Clin. Lab. SG 1998 HT Blockage, Lee J. Med. Letter 1999 Jan. Male Androgen, Fredricsion B., Joanorology 1989 Jan; Wammar M. Achives Addi. 1985

Directions:

Apply 2 pumps twice daily AM & PM on soft skin for 25 days. Discontinue for 5 days or if bleeding begins and then repeat cycle, adjust dosage to your individual needs.

Ingredients:

Fulvic Ext. Essential Phospholipids, Evening Primrose Oil, Shea Butter, Glycerin, Progesterone Usp, Chastetree, Dong Quai, Rhodiola Rosea, P.Ginseng, Aloe Vera, Lavender Oil, Almond Oil, Hemp Oil, Alpha Lipoic Acid, Vitamin E, Vitamin A, Allantoin, Napca, Dimethicone

These statements have not been reviewed by the FDA. This product is not intended to diagnose, treat, cure, or prevent any disease.

Dr. Tai's Pearl

Progesterone is a woman's best friend. Finding the balance and the progesterone occupy the receptors, displacing the estrogen, which may be stimulating for more growth and cellular divisions, creating possibilities of cysts, tumors, or cancers. Progesterone definitely has a calming effect, and is an excellent diuretic. For women, progesterone from days 14 – 28, will provide for excellent balance and prevention of PMS. For men, under severe circumstances of prostate hypertrophy or cancer, can use progesterone to occupy the estrogen receptors in the prostate and displace estrogen from the prostate.

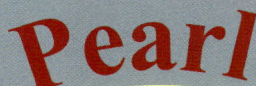

Clinical Cases:
Lillian, a 58-year-old Nigerian woman, suffering from post-menopausal symptoms – having difficulty falling asleep, anxiety at night, night sweats, and severe depression. She has attempted anti-depressants from her physician, which caused numerous side effects she could not tolerate. Using Progesterone at night, 4 pumps at bedtime and 4 pumps in the morning, she was able to, within two days, start to feel better with less of those specific symptoms. We did add Stress & Anxiety Specialist to her regimen, day and night. The relief of severe anxiety from no apparent cause she could pinpoint was a great discovery for this patient. She was amazed and grateful for this outcome – using just a simple cream for her condition.

Side Effects:
When individuals over-utilize progesterone, they may get slightly sleepy and maybe too relaxed. Further dosage can lead to these symptoms in certain individuals. In others it may lead them to a more combative, angrier reaction. This is very uncommon and very rare. Many times, lowering the dosage to a very small amount, such as 10 mg will provide all the benefits without any of the side effects.

Contraindications:
Do not take product if you are allergic to any of its ingredients.

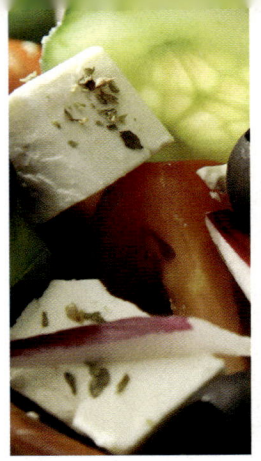 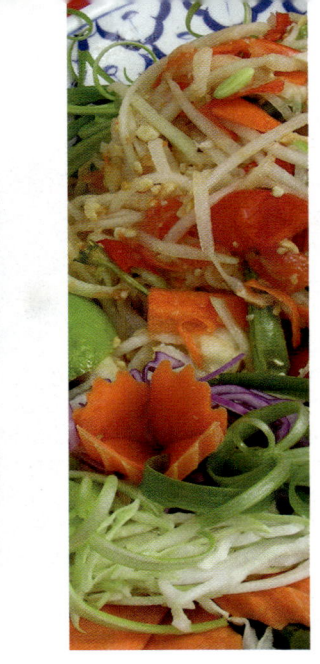 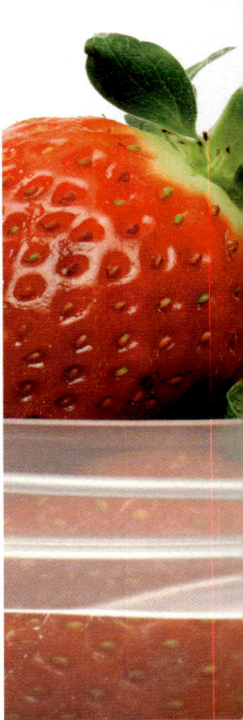

Relax Pressure Specialist

Control Destructive Forces of Blood Pressure

The destructive force of hypertension is well researched and documented. Recent publications verified that hypertension contributes to Cardiovascular Diseases, Parkinson's, Alzheimer's, and Strokes. It is said that the control of hypertension is one of the most difficult conditions to address when using herbal extracts.

Relax Pressure Specialist is a simple and yet highly effective means of supporting normal blood pressure. The dosage is highly adjustable and can be customized to meet an individual's needs by simply adjusting the number of pills taken a day.

Relax Pressure Specialist also addresses effectively the stress mechanism and anxieties often accompanying hypertension. Difficult issues such as the inability to fall asleep at night as a result of hypertension may quickly be moderated and improved, often resulting in individuals being calmer as well as lowering the blood pressure.

- All natural herbal extracts
- May lower blood pressure
- May lower stress and anxiety
- Readily available for a good night's sleep
- Fast Acting

Directions: Take 2 capsules AM & noon, take 3 or 4 capsules at bedtime until desired results are achieved then lower dosage to 1 capsule AM & noon and 2 or 3 capsules at bedtime. Take 2 capsules 1 hour before visiting your doctor. Adjust dosage for personal needs and consult your health professional for evaluation and advice. MUST BE TAKEN ON AN EMPTY STOMACH

Ingredients:
Proprietary Formulation:
S. Japonica, Panax Ginseng, Aglycon Sapogenin, Prunella, Lonicera, Hawthorne Berry

These statements have not been reviewed by the FDA.

This product is not intended to diagnose, treat, cure, or prevent any disease.

Dr. Tai's Pearl
Monitoring blood pressure is of utmost importance and the accuracy of the measurement goes without saying. Always take blood pressure measurements at the same time of day and seated in the same chair as to allow for natural variations from day to day.

Side Effects:
Over dosage may cause drowsiness. Use care when operating machinery.

Contraindications:
DO NOT take this supplement if you are taking prescription anti-hypertension medication as it may drop your blood pressure too low and cause other potential complications. Do not take if you are allergic to any of the ingredients.

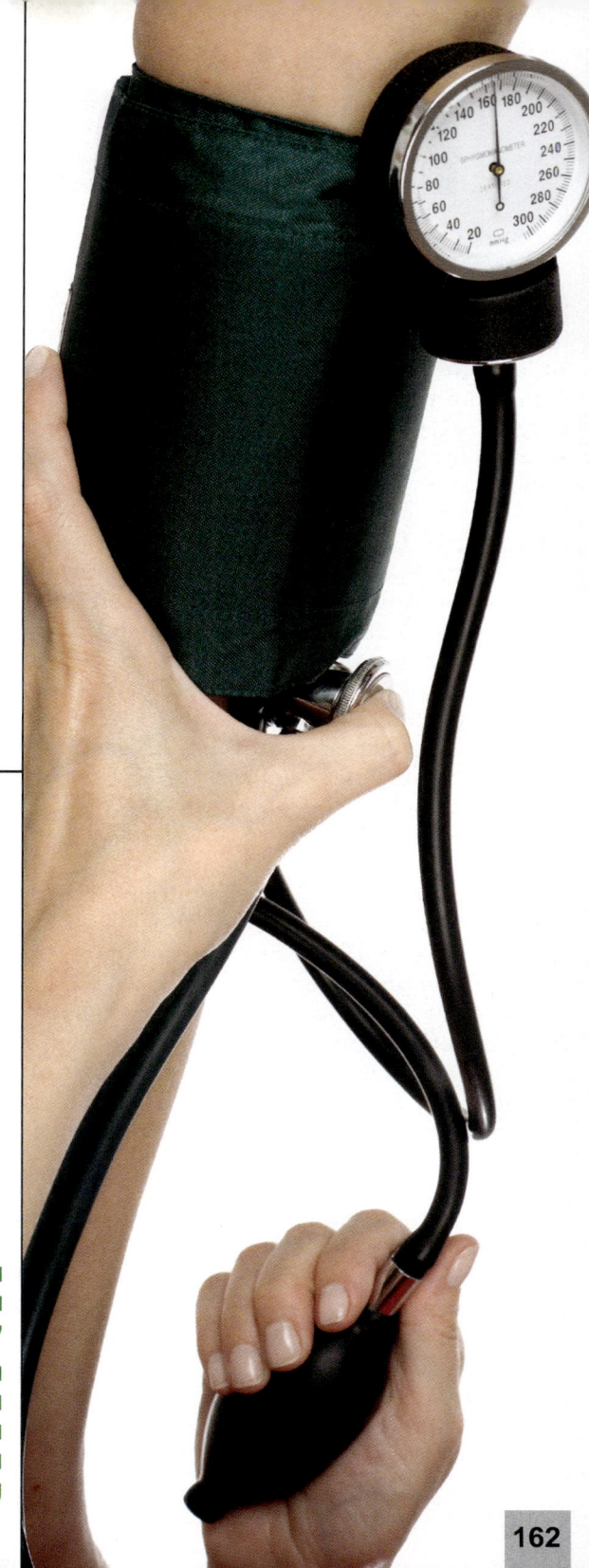

ROYAL LING ZHI MATRIX

Most Important Natural Herbs for your Body

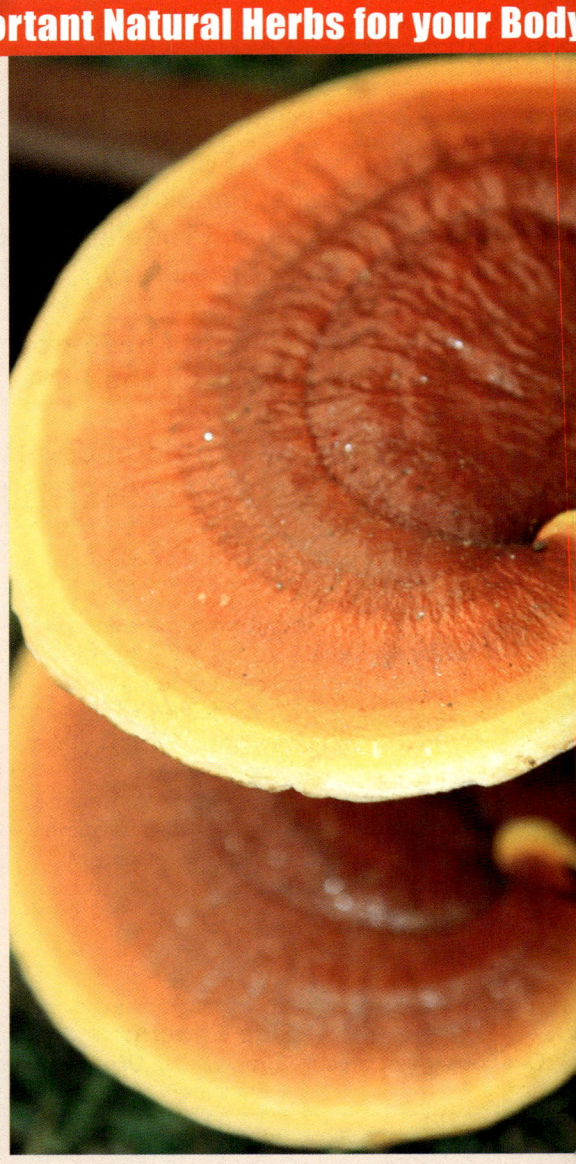

Royal Ling Zhi Matrix is a unique proprietary product which combines several essential oils to deliver incredible health benefits. Each oil has unique properties to work synergistically creating a magical formula for you to enjoy excellent health and increased energy.

Ling Zhi Oil:

The Ling Zhi mushroom, also known as 'reishi mushroom' (translated as "supernatural mushroom") is a categorical term for many mushrooms within the Ganoderma genus. The term Ling Zhi is commonly used to refer to Ganoderma Lucidum and Ganoderma Tsugae. G. Lucidum, was used as a natural medicine in Asia and now across the globe. Its use in Chinese medicine dates back to over 2,000 years ago, which puts it as one of the oldest mushrooms to ever have been used medicinally.

THE LING ZHI MUSHROOM contains 119 different triterpenoids, which provide anti-inflammatory, anti-tumor, and anti-viral effects. In fact, the vast array of health benefits associated with Ling Zhi, paired with an absence of known side effects, makes it a highly popular alternative remedy. Ling Zhi contains Ganoderic Acids which are similar in composition to steroid hormones. Ling Zhi also contains polysaccharides, such as Beta-Glucan and Coumarin, as well as alkaloids.

As with many ancient medicines, there is long history to back up the traditional usage of Ling Zhi. An ancient Chinese text speaks of the healing powers of this widely sought after mushroom, crediting it with being "useful for enhancing vital energy, increasing thinking faculty and preventing forgetfulness." It is also stated that Ling Zhi can "refresh the body and mind, delay aging, and enable one to live long"

Modern herbalists use the Ling Zhi Mushroom to treat a variety of conditions. Some of its popular uses include:

- Chronic fatigue syndrome
- Diabetes
- Detoxify the liver
- Help cure hepatitis
- Lower cholesterol
- Prevent growth of tumors (cancer)
- Prevent blood clots
- Allergy treatment
- Antibacterial
- Dementia & Alzheimer's
- Promote healthy, beautiful "baby soft" skin
- Increased oxygen to Mitochondria
- Cellular oxygen without Lactic Acidosis
- Athletic muscle energy without "Burn"
- Fast inflammatory Relief & Recovery

Sunflower Oil:

Sunflower oil has a large collection of benefits to help keep your body healthy and strong. Many people are not aware of the many natural benefits of sunflower oil because it is not the most popular oil used in cooking. It is easy to substitute into your diet and has a natural, light taste.

Benefits of sunflower oil may include:

- Improve Heart Health
- Natural Energy
- Lower Risk of Infant Infection
- Stops Free Radicals
- Natural Antioxidant
- Natural Moisturizer
- Prevents Arthritis
- Prevents Asthma and Colon Cancer
- Promotes a Healthy Nervous System
- Lowers Cholesterol
- Prevents other Cancers
- Reduces Cardiac Problems
- Repairs the Body
- Maintains Healthy Immune System
- Helps Create New Cells

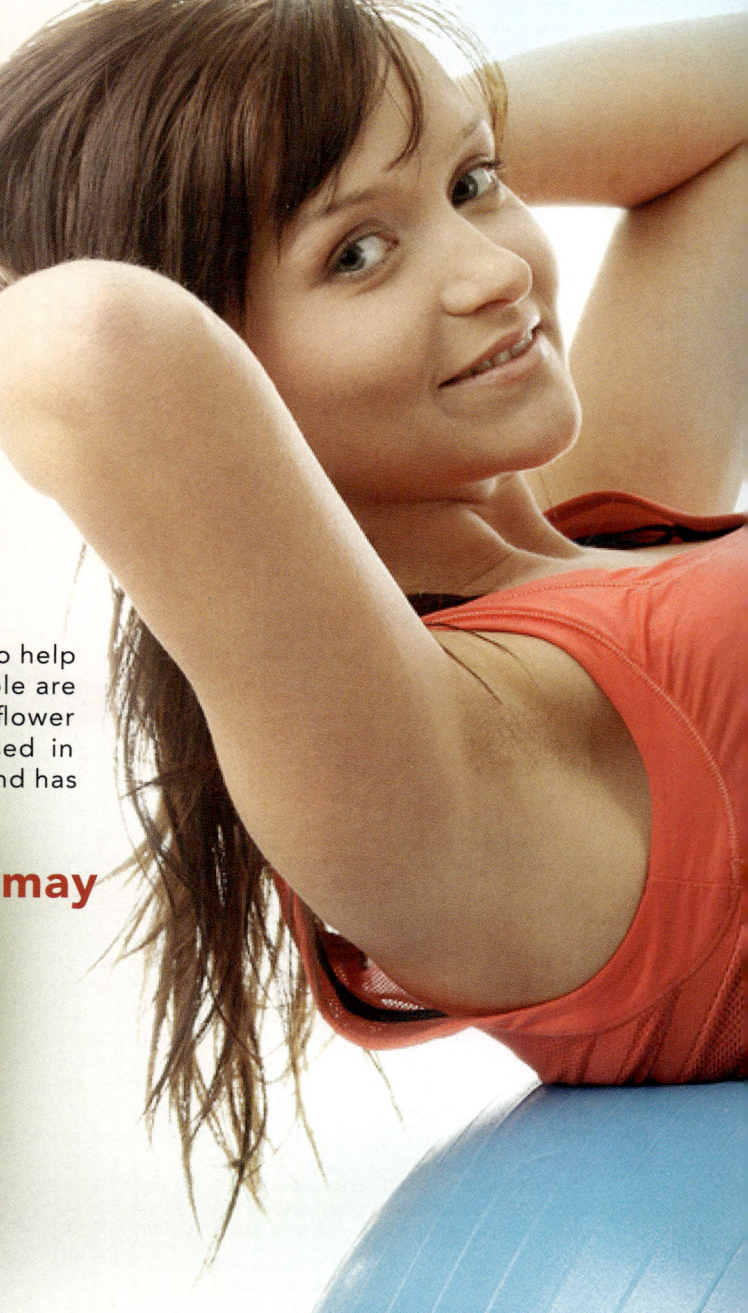

Flaxseed Oil:

Flaxseed oil comes from the seeds of the flax plant (Linum usitatissimum, L.). Flaxseed oil contains both omega-3 and omega-6 fatty acids, which are needed for health. Flaxseed oil contains the essential fatty acid alpha-linolenic acid (ALA), which the body converts into eicosapentaenoic acid (EPA) and docosahexaenoic acid (DHA), the omega-3 fatty acids found in fish oil. Some researchers think that flaxseed oil might have some of the same benefits as fish oil, EPA and DHA. Omega-3 fatty acids, usually from fish oil, have been shown to reduce inflammation and help prevent certain chronic diseases, such as heart disease and arthritis.

Getting a good balance of omega-3 and omega-6 fatty acids in the diet is important. These essential fats are both examples of polyunsaturated fatty acids, or PUFAs. Omega-3 fatty acids help reduce inflammation.

Flaxseed oil may be helpful in treating:

- High Cholesterol
- Heart Disease
- Sjogren's Syndrome
- Cancer

Coconut Oil:

Coconut oil is an edible oil that has been consumed in tropical places for thousands of years. Studies done on native diets high in coconut oil consumption show that these populations are generally in good health, and don't suffer as much from many of the modern diseases of western nations where coconut oil is seldom consumed anymore.

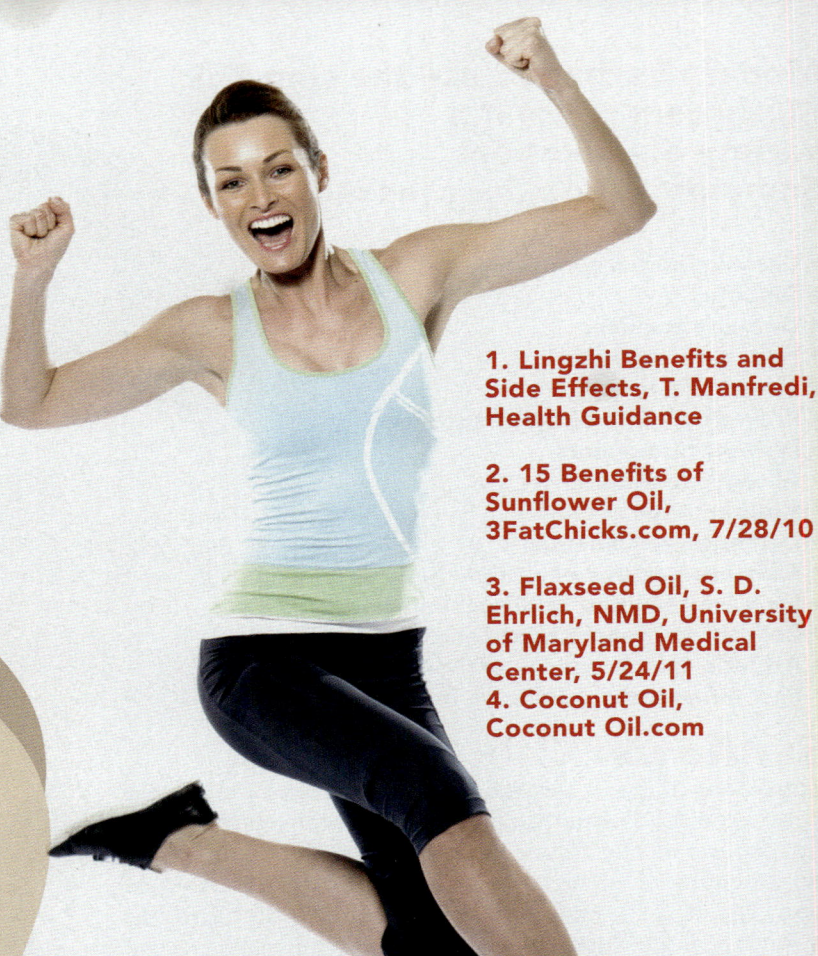

Coconut Oil Health Benefits

So, how are people using coconut oil? What are some of the health benefits of coconut oil being reported? Some of the most recent research has come from people suffering from Alzheimer's disease, with reports of people improving or even reversing the effects of Alzheimer's by using coconut oil. For years we have seen positive results from people with both type 1 and type 2 diabetes in using coconut oil. We have also seen a lot of reports of coconut oil health benefits from those suffering from hypothyroidism, as coconut oil helps boost metabolism and raise body temperature. Restricting carbohydrates and increasing coconut oil in the diet has also led many to report losing weight. Candida sufferers also report health benefits with coconut oil as research now confirms, and those suffering from various skin diseases are also seeing tremendous health benefits by applying coconut oil directly on the skin. The benefits of coconut oil for healthy hair are also well known. Other health benefits of coconut oil included fighting off bacterial infections and viruses. Coconut oil is also increasingly being seen to benefit athletes and fitness trainers giving them an advantage in sustaining energy levels longer, without drugs or stimulants.

1. Lingzhi Benefits and Side Effects, T. Manfredi, Health Guidance

2. 15 Benefits of Sunflower Oil, 3FatChicks.com, 7/28/10

3. Flaxseed Oil, S. D. Ehrlich, NMD, University of Maryland Medical Center, 5/24/11

4. Coconut Oil, Coconut Oil.com

Directions:
Shake well. Take 2 droppers full 2 times daily for excellent health and energy. For higher dosage see your health consultant.

Ingredients:
Unrefined, Organic, Cold Pressed Ling Zhi Oil, Sunflower Oil, Flax Seed Oil, Coconut Oil

These statements have not been reviewed by the FDA. This product is not intended to diagnose, treat, cure, or prevent any disease.

Dr. Tai's Pearls:

If you ever go to visit the Forbidden City at the heart of Beijing, tiny conclaves of buildings created thousands of years ago created by the grand emperors of China, you will notice that at the epicenter of the doorway there is a symbol of the Royal Ling Zhi. This fabulous mushroom has been a historical icon for Chinese medicine. My only great contribution is that trying to take Ling Zhi can be extremely frustrating. On one hand you have the promise of longevity and great benefits to your health. On the other hand, you have the difficulty of absorbing the active ingredients because it is a woodsy mushroom – so hard that you can actually drive a nail through it or kill someone by knocking them on the head – hard as a block of wood. We were able to discover the top secret of extracting the active ingredients of Royal Ling Zhi using a medium of natural organic oils that actually contribute to the essence of all the goodness that comes from this mushroom. After many years of research, we were able to discover the proper temperature, timing, and quality of this extraction. So now, the taking of the supplement is as easy as using two droppers sublingually every day. After a short 30 – 60 days, you have an absolutely marvelous transformation of your skin to a baby soft luster and healthy glow that can only come from the inside out, with the help of Royal Ling Zhi. Having beautiful skin as a marker, I can assure you that all the other tissues inside your body, including your lungs and every single organ, is also transformed and rejuvenated. Like the transformation of your skin, the inner lining of your blood vessels will slowly and methodically clean itself from the atheromas and plaques that cause problems for the heart, all the way to the carotid arteries of the brain. This is an extraordinary achievement toward a healthy cardiovascular system and for prevention of stroke, heart attack, and cancer.

Clinical Case:

Katherine, a 61-year-old executive of a supplement company taking Royal Ling Zhi for 40 days came to an extraordinary discovery of the most beautiful skin she has had her entire life. Now we can tell, just by looking at the skin on her arms, legs and face, the magnificent glow, the softness of virgin silk. She also noticed that when doing exercises, she used to have severe cramps and pain of the muscles. With a great deal of surprise, the pain is now gone and any muscle spasm is just the feeling of tightness, but with no discomfort. This was a great revelation to her of the oxygenation to her muscles increasing circulation and natural ability of the Ling Zhi to balance lactic acid in the muscle.

Side Effects: None

Contraindications:
Do not take product if you are allergic to any of its ingredients.

S.O.D. & CATALASE SPECIALIST
Extraordinarily powerful Antioxidants

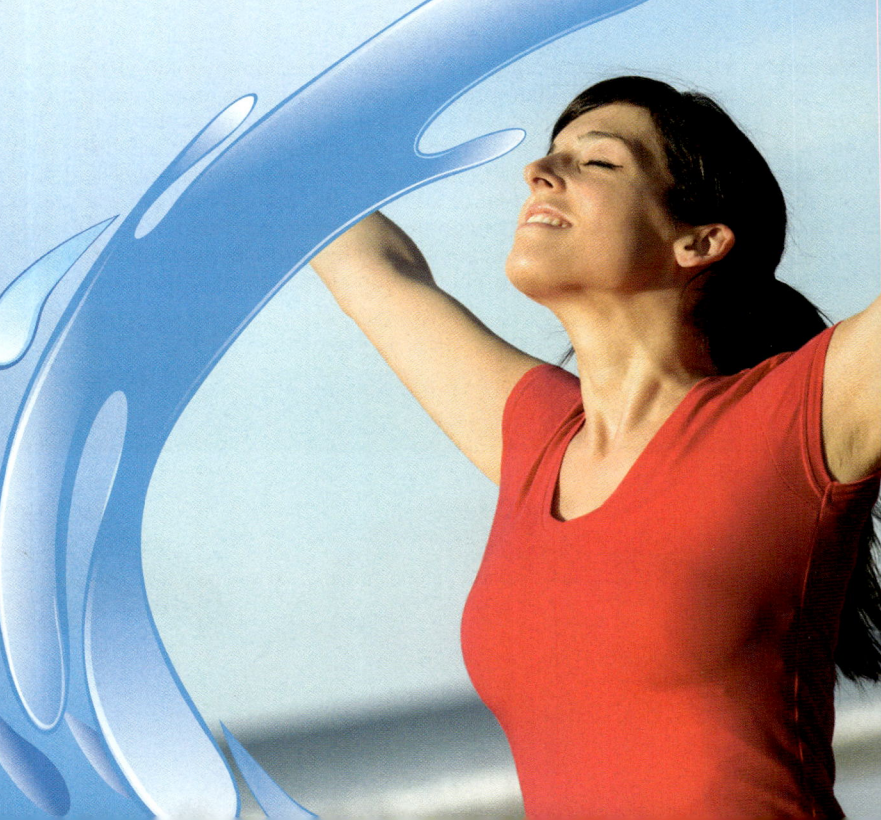

Catalase Specialist Super Oxide Dismutase (SOD) Extends Life

Anti-Aging Journals and textbooks from all over the world are scientifically documenting that viruses and living organisms, like pigeons with higher SOD levels, live up to 1200% longer. This is an incredible accomplishment.

We hear all about antioxidants protective qualities from the media and the supplement industry, making antioxidants the "darling" of the industry, and the fastest growing segment of the natural supplement market. We have antioxidants from grape seed, pine bark and even tomatoes, but these are all comparatively minor antioxidants. In the human body there are three "Super Antioxidants" known by the scientific medical community as: Glutathione, Super Oxide Dismutase (SOD) and Catalase. These three Super Antioxidants hold the secret to life itself. It is so essential to our lives that the human body actually produces them. Why? Because without the three "Super Antioxidants", you die!

When younger, we naturally produce a great deal of our body's crucial antioxidants called Super Oxide Dismutase and Catalase. As we get older, the levels of our body's production of SOD and Catalase decline with age just like hormones. This depletion leaves our bodies severely unprotected from the destructive ravages of super powerful free radicals called **Super Oxides and Reactive Oxygen Species (ROS).**

Publications by eminent scientists have warned us that Super Oxides and ROS are capable of enormous destruction to our tissues and organs. Imagine the permanent damages of these Super Free Radicals, leaving holes in our vital cells, disrupting DNA strands, leading to possible cancer, auto immune diseases and rapid, permanent aging.

Inoue M. et al, Current Medical Chemistry 12/2003, Ahsan H. et al, Exp. Imm. 3/2003, Allen, RG, Free Rad. Biol. Med. 2/2000.

We are not talking about minor antioxidants! The Super Antioxidant SOD is about 3,500 times more potent than vitamin C in stopping the destructive forces of Super Oxide Free Radicals, neutralizing the damage and preventing genetic and inflammatory diseases. Like Batman and Robin, SOD is the primary defense against the super powerful and super destructive free radicals, but it needs Catalase to mop up, clean up, and finally neutralize the left over oxidants into harmless WATER.

We are offering, for the first time, the dynamic duo of SOD and Catalase using *Pleo-Lyposome Technology,* microencapsulating the fragile antioxidants, keeping and safeguarding them fresh for enhanced instant absorption technology on sublingual or topical application. These special breakthrough technologies are proprietary and only available from Health Secrets USA.

Directions:
Shake well. Take sublingual 2 pumps in the AM & PM, hold for 1 minute before swallowing. You may apply to the skin if you choose. Adjust dosage to individual needs. Take on an empty stomach.

Ingredients:
Essential Phospholipid, Phosphotydylcholine, Super Oxide Dismutase, Catalase, Alpha Lipoic Acid

These statements have not been reviewed by the FDA. This product is not intended to diagnose, treat, cure, or prevent any disease.

Dr. Tai's Pearl

Free radical attack of these terrorists created in our bodies from the metabolism of energy and mitochondria set the stage for possible cancers and toxicity within our bodies. There are only so many antioxidants in nature that can actually deal with the severity of the most active free radicals that result in superoxides. These larger than life terrorists cause severe damage and injury to our tissues. Our body creates superoxide dismutase specifically to neutralize them, or our life would be in danger.

Clinical Case:
71-year-old New Zealand male feeling exhausted after 30 years in metal manufacturing exposed to light levels of chemical toxins. After six weeks of S.O.D. & Catalase Specialist he felt fantastic, life seems brighter, he's less tired, and to his astonishment, "even [his] hair is returning to [his] normal dark color!" It's fantastic!

Side Effects: None

Contraindications:
Do not take product if you are allergic to any of its ingredients.

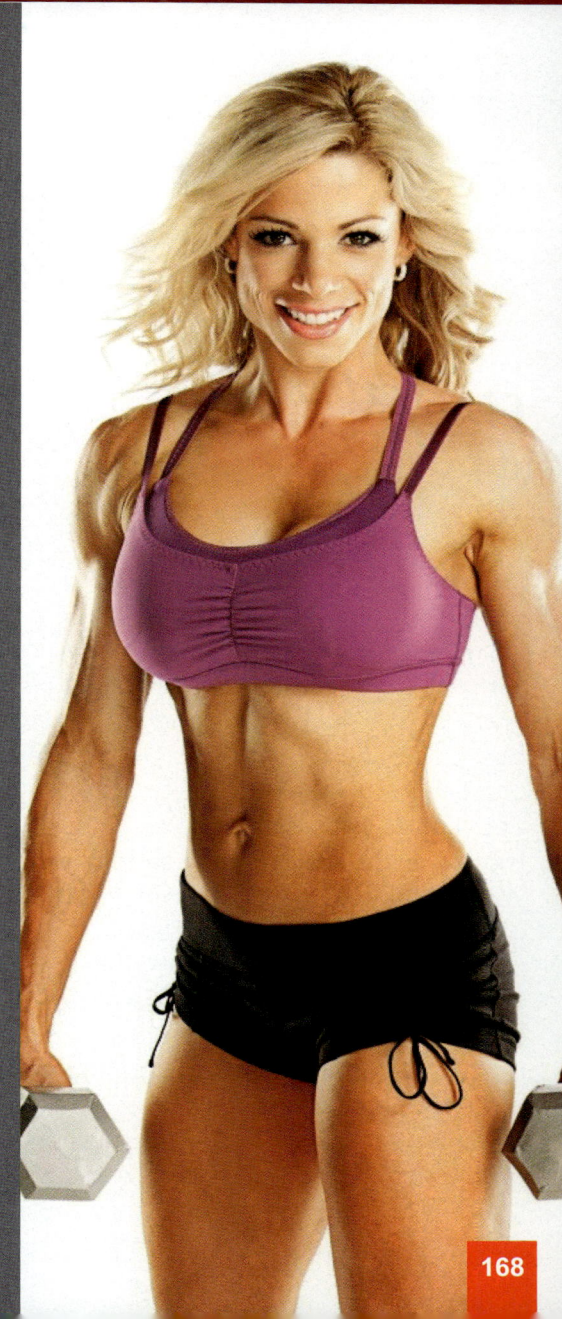

168

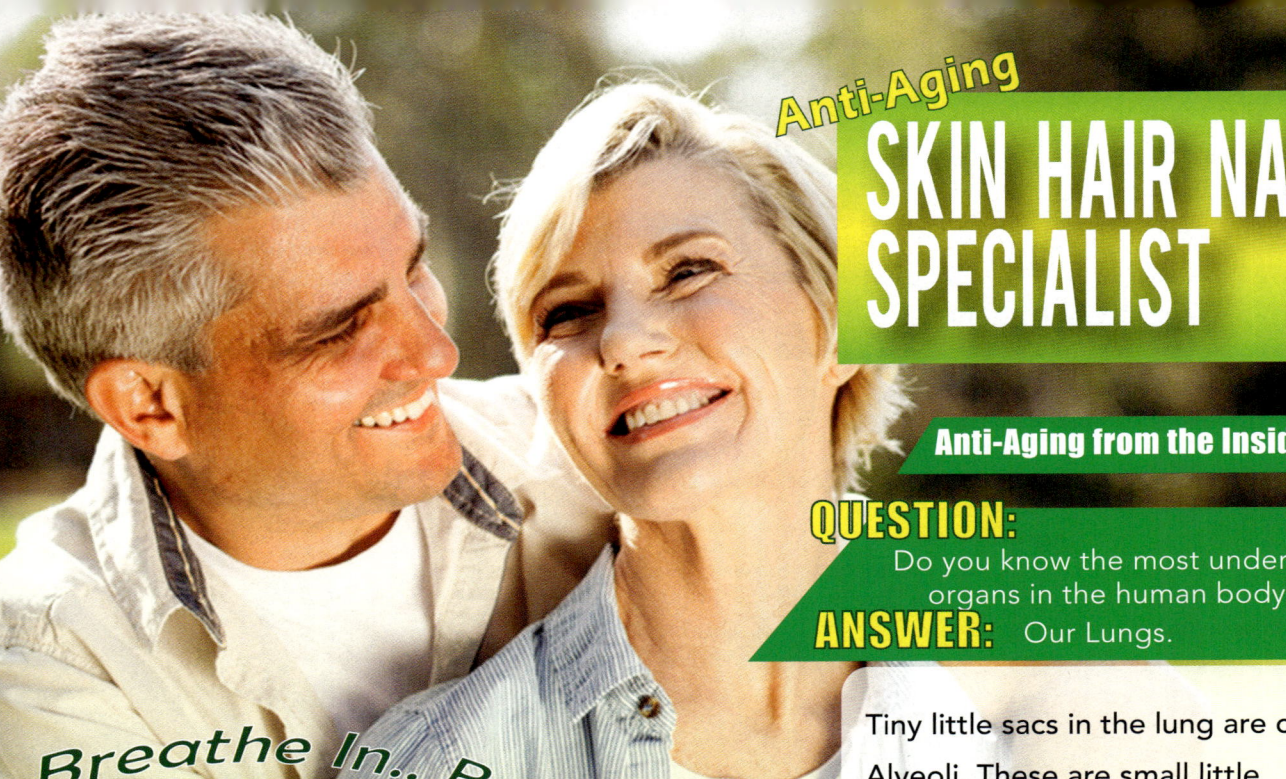

Anti-Aging
SKIN HAIR NAIL SPECIALIST

Anti-Aging from the Inside OUT

QUESTION: Do you know the most underrated organs in the human body?

ANSWER: Our Lungs.

Breathe In.. Breathe Out...

Breathing is more than just a way to pass the time, it is a vital function so important that if you stop for more than a minute, you will pass out and Death will soon follow. A few moments without oxygen? Your brain will go into a coma and in 4 to 5 minutes, your all-important heart will cease to beat, and you are DONE. Period!!

The Lungs, this rather spongy organ that fills your thorax cavity, are one of the most important organs for you to take care of. It does an extraordinary job at getting life-sustaining Oxygen while blowing off Carbon Dioxide that is left over in your body. This keeps you from going into Acidosis. These are the obvious simple jobs of a good, healthy Lung. What you don't realize is that the air you breathe is filled with dust, dirt, bacteria, fungi, viruses, chemicals, and the left-over sneeze that the guy next to you was kind enough to share! Thanks, but no thanks. This pair of lungs is doing a lot more than just filling and emptying; it's cleaning the air before delivering oxygen to your blood.

Tiny little sacs in the lung are called Alveoli. These are small little microscopic chambers that are moist, warm, and filled with blood. Walls of the Alveoli carry abundant capillary blood that are thin-walled in order to absorb the air you breathe and transfer it to your blood vessels. This is a true miracle from God. Nature has provided you with something extraordinary – the ability to cleanse dirty air and dissolve it into the Oxygen in your blood that rejuvenates tissues so that they can live, reproduce, metabolize, and create energy. Without Oxygen no energy can be created in your body.

To put it simply...

The Lungs are an entirely open organ. All the blood in your system is exposed to the dirty, filthy air and the environment we live in. The poor tissues in your lungs are subjected to constant attacks & Chronic Diseases such as Emphysema and Chronic Bronchitis. For those of you who smoke, the added Carbon Monoxide, tar and black soot coat your Lungs and plug the Aveoli. You are CONSTANTLY being ATTACKED on all fronts. If it's not infections from common Streptococcus, viruses, or fungi that is in the polluted air and grows in trees, it's allergies that batter your Lung Tissues. This causes you to develop Asthma, Pneumonia, or other major complications in your body that infect your blood, killing you as quickly as possible. We have concluded that your Lungs have to be constantly rejuvenating as they are constantly under attack. Therefore, Lungs have a great amount of scarring from the millions of battles they go through daily. If you have other diseases, such as Cardiovascular Heart Disease, Hypertension, Diabetes, or Immune Diseases, then you are DOUBLY AT RISK. While your Lungs tirelessly fight those environmental toxins, your own diseases sneak up and stab them in their unguarded back.

So you say
"BUT! DR. TAI!! My Doctor takes chest X-Rays and gives me antibiotics. I'm SURE I don't have any lung diseases!"

I want to caution you – Chest X-Rays certainly do not show any diseases until it is WAY TOO LATE! By the time it shows up on a Chest X-Ray, you are already 1-foot in the hospital or the grave.

The best protection that I can advise you is to clean and rejuvenate your lungs every second and every minute of the day. People assume that as long as they're not outside, they're not at risk. Regardless, you are still surrounded by harsh chemicals in your home, your car, and in your office that add on even more pollution for your poor body to deal with. Are you having problems breathing? Well it's NO WONDER with all the soot and smoke bellowing out of the tailpipe of your car and sneaking into your lungs. Are you having problems with fatigue? I can't say I'm surprised – pollution is treating you like an abandoned lake filled with toxic chemicals and debris. Are you having problems with a cough or experience wheezing? It's only a matter of time until you see yellow or dark colored sputum coming from your lungs.

Do you have difficulty going up and down stairs, accompanied by heavy breathing? Are you plagued with feelings of Weakness or Stress? Do you have difficulty sleeping at night or find yourself waking up in the morning with drowsiness or severe headaches? These are all the signs and symptoms of an underperforming lung. You wouldn't expect some of these symptoms, but the Lungs are key to your energy and health. When the Lungs aren't functioning properly, they take every other system in the body down with them.

I'll openly admit that I created Skin · Hair · Nail Specialist with myself in mind. I'm the one that needs this product so that I can take advantage of a healthier lung. My resume is a long and dirty one. I've worked in conditions ranging from chemical factories surrounded by toxic substances to all-natural farms with dust, fungus and animal bacteria and viruses. Between all my jobs across America and Brasil, I've inhaled more chemicals and toxins than all of you put together. It was ME that was in need of a rejuvenating herbal formula for the lungs.

I put together **Skin · Hair · Nail** Specialist starting specifically with Bamboo. Organic bamboo from Old Chinese Medicine has a very special place in modern herb technology. Bamboo is an herb that has very high Silica and Antioxidants - the key ingredients for healthy tissue and healthy functioning vital organs. Your tissues require high amounts of Silica, principally the elastic and very soft tissues of your lung. Silica is a key component in protein and what Panda Bears and all other animals live off of. Humans need silica. We need Silica for all the tissues of our skin and hair, and to help build the collagen in our nails. Collagen and elastins make the connective tissues (bones, joints, and ligaments) to your body that give you beauty as well as strength and allows for the healing of your skin. Your teeth and gums are also very special tissues that require high amounts of silica.

When we were young we used to have a lot of silica that our bodies were able to absorb. Our young and healthy bodies could retain silica for the rapid growth of our hair, skin, and abundant tissues. By the time we get to be 20 years-old, we have done all of our essential growing and now move on to cultivating our strength and flexibility in order to withstand the rigors of daily activity. Past the age of 30, our bodies start to lose the ability to absorb and retain silica therefore you can see that as you grow old that you lose the strength of your follicles and hair begins to fall out, you lose the strength of your nails and you start to lose the density of your bones. Your once wonderful skin no longer has the same beauty it did when it had adequate amounts of collagen and elastin. Instead it starts to show small and the large wrinkles and folds around your mouth, and they create those deep ridges that makes you look old.

It is the Bamboo that can give you large amounts of Organic Silica that goes to work immediately. Beyond the silica, Bamboo even provides antioxidants that protect you from breaking down due to allergies, the attacks of bacteria and viruses, and potential Cancer formations from abnormal growth of cell tissues . Numbers of different published Medical Research reveal that silica is the key ingredient for protection from the damage of occasional inflammation, the ravages of Overweight and Obesity, the complications of Diabetes, the devastation that comes and attacks your body due to Chronic Inflammation

It is undeniable that your whole entire body needs silica, and therefore it needs Bamboo. Even though many companies have used Bamboo parts and extracts in their haircare and facial scrubs, it isn't until you can actually build up a reservoir of silica in your own body that you will be able to enjoy adequate protection. Silica is the most important ingredient in regards to total anti-aging and restoration of beautiful tissues. In order for your body to continue to be young, healthy and strong **YOU NEED SILICA.**

Medical Herbal Journals have written about the silica in Bamboo extracts for decades as a powerful anti-inflammatory, anti-tumor, anti-microbial, and anti-ulcer ingredient. From this product, not only will your lungs be rejuvenated, but the research from Columbia University has shown that the average human being needs a minimum of 7grams of silica in the body. Without this minimum, we see a major imbalance of Calcium and Magnesium, as well as all the other Hormonal disturbances that come from this imbalance. Silica is very important in the natural assimilation of Phosphorus, which is the key element in bones. It is medically proven that with silica and the collagen it creates, you can stay younger and healthier. Your hair will grow abundantly due to the strengthened hair roots, your teeth will be reinforced with harder enamels and enjoy the prevention of cavities, and your gums will be protected from inflammation and attacks from the bacteria in your mouth.

If you have fragile, brittle and flaking nails, you should pay closer attention to your tissue's needs. Fragile nails are a clear indicator that you are going to have fragile bones. When you neglect your nails they demineralize, and you can bet money that you are also demineralizing and decalcifying your bones. With the Bamboo Extract in Anti-Aging Skin · Hair · Nail Specialist, your nails will be strong and grow from the nail plates thanks to the complex protein structures that requires the silica.

Ancient Chinese Herbalists offer Bamboo as a strong and abundant source of silica for higher antioxidants, prevention of premature aging and the preservation of youth as Earth's ultimate source of anti-aging. If you are a smoker or live in the city where you're exposed to great amounts of environmental toxins, if you work in a factory, if you work many hours with lots of human contact and other humans as a source of toxins, then Skin · Hair · Nail Specialist is made especially for you to strengthen the lungs and provide silica to inhibit all of those chemicals, nitrosamines, and toxins that surrounds us daily.

I was able to utilize Bamboo together with an ancient Chinese Herb called **Snake Gourd**, or Trichosanthes. Trichosanthes is a powerful ancient Chinese All-Natural Antibiotic. It's an expectorant that helps to eliminate infections and pus, it is cleanser of the phlegm in your lungs, and expels a wide array of toxins and poisons from your system while being a powerful anti-inflammatory. , Snake Gourd is used in China to help to tone the heart and to also normalize all physiological systems and rejuvenate your lungs by stopping serious illnesses such as pneumonia. Snake Gourd was even used in Ancient China for treatment of Tuberculosis. The Chinese have used this concoction of herbs for the successful treatment of fevers and erasing diabetes, stopping toxins of heart disorders and helping to remove Jaundice from the liver.

Snake Gourd is an excellent source of Vitamin A, Vitamin B, Vitamin C, and many of the minerals such as Manganese, Potassium and Iodine that are SUPER CHARGED to reduce the harmful toxins hidden in air particles and inside the food that we eat. Snake Gourd starts by calming the inflamed Nervous System before cleansing the body from bacteria and viruses. Its abundant minerals and vitamins, including the COMPLETE Vitamin B Complex with Riboflavin, Keratin, Niocin, and Thiamine, are all important to balance bodily fluids, decrease heart palpitations, treat night fevers, and has the ability to neutralize toxins in the lungs and body.

Clinical Cases:

43 year-old female waitress Suzanne T was a smoker for many years and quit in the last ten years. Despite quitting, Suzanne continued to have a raspy voice and suffered from a harsh smoker's cough complete with phlegm every morning, and difficulty breathing while working, which put her at risk of losing her job. Although she wanted to turn her life around for the better, Suzanne discovered she couldn't even exercise because she didn't have the strength, energy, or the breath to keep up with even the shortest workout DVD. You could immediately notice dark, black circles around her eyes with just a passing glance, and thick, large wrinkles aged her beyond her years. Suzanne used Skin · Hair · Nail Specialist to help to rejuvenate the lungs, the liver and the kidney as well as giving her the health that she needed to improve the appearance of her hair and skin. Her complete protocol was using Skin · Hair · Nail Specialist together with Super B12, Max Performance, Ionic Micro Mineral and Total Circulation in order to increase the circulation. Within 3 months she showed drastic improvement. Now, 6 months after beginning her Anti-Aging Protocol, she works out 45 minutes twice a week, has been marked as a "hard-working and reliable worker" at the same job that threatened to fire her, and her demeanor and outlook is at least ten years younger than before.

Lu B, Wu X, Tie X, et al. Toxicology and safety of anti-oxidant of bamboo leaves. Part 1: Acute and subchronic toxicity studies on anti-oxidant of bamboo leaves. Food Chem Toxicol 2005;43(5):783-792.

Hu C, Zhang Y, Kitts DD. Evaluation of antioxidant and prooxidant activities of bamboo Phyllostachys nigra var. Henonis leaf extract in vitro. J Food Chem 2000;48(8):3170-3176.

Kim KK, Kawano Y, Yamazaki Y. A novel porphyrin photosensitizer from bamboo leaves that induces apoptosis in cancer cell lines. Anticancer 2003;23(3B):2355-2361.

Clinical Cases:

Executive in the I.T. Industry, 58 Year Old female Jo C noted that she was losing hair, her skin was dramatically dry with a lack of elasticity and she was having tremendous outbursts of wrinkles and big pores. Jo's nails were constantly fragile and breaking and even though she went to have her manicure maintained on a weekly basis, they didn't seem to help the quality and strength of her nails. She started taking Super B12, Skin · Hair · Nail Specialist, Glutathione, Royal Ling Zhi and applying Melatonin at night. This protocol helped her to reestablish the foundation for wonderful new skin. The texture, strength and thickness of her hair slowly came back. Slowly, the nails that flaked and broke grew back stronger and healthier than they'd ever been in her adult life. Jo C followed up this protocol and upon realizing her health could be even GREATER, decided to implement a protocol for hormonal balancing. After receiving the Results & Recommendations of her Salivary Hormone Testing, Jo discovered Vitamin D3-K2 and Ionic Micro Minerals, which helped tremendously to strengthen her bones as well as increase the quality and beauty of the skin. To care for her new, glowing skin, Jo began using the skin care that I designed and slowly replaced her old harsh products that did NOTHING besides clogging her pores. With the help of Nano-Technology and natural cucumber extract, Smart Skin rejuvenated her skin and gave her a beautiful shine and healthy glow. Pretty soon she became well known by her colleagues for having a fantastic, baby-soft face! This is a truly successful case in which Silica and a proper protocol can revitalize your skin, your hair, your nails and stomp out Osteoporosis. This is anti-aging at its absolute best.

Dr. Tai's Pearl

I am a REAL Momma's Boy. My mother had a wonderful influence on me starting from a very young age. I can still hear my mother telling me to eat bamboo salads with shoots simmered in broth until very soft. Of course, she used to tell me to eat it because it's good for my skin, hair, and nails. Now this is an everyday conversation on the table because I hated celery as a child and she would say that I had to eat it because it's good for my circulation.

You can just imagine folks, every meal of everyday being bombarded by mother to eat the right vegetable for improving certain aspects of your organs and body parts.

God bless my mother!

Side Effects: None

Contraindications:
Do not use this product if you are allergic to any of its ingredients

Directions:
Take 1 Capsule twice Daily A.M. & P.M.

Ingredients:
Bamboo Extract, Green Tea Extract, Snake Gourd Extract

These statements have not been reviewed by the FDA. This product is not intended to diagnose, treat, cure, or prevent any disease.

SKIN SPECIALIST
Prevention & Treatment of Skin Diseases

Have you ever been criticized for having rough hands and rough feet? Is your skin very dry and cracked? Do your hands and feet feel like a "cactus"?

Don't despair Help is here!

This new technology was created specifically for people with very dry, very cracked, very rough skin of their hands and feet, and also for those suffering from dermatitis, including rosacea and eczema of the face.

Skin Specialist contains natural essential phospholipids in combination with powerful anti-inflammatory extracts from natural Asian herbs. These special active ingredients have been preserved with new water extraction technology that is delivered through a liposome transdermal transport into your skin that may result in invigorating repair of damaged skin.

Diabetics know that dried, cracked skin is the leading cause of potential ulceration and infection that can result in amputation. This special formulation used daily and consistently may rejuvenate your skin, giving you smooth and soft skin, healing even the worst areas such as around your finger nails and on your heels. It is simply awesome!!!

- May Repair Damaged Skin
- Cracked and very Dried Skin
- May Penetrate Eczema
- Rough Skin of Hands and Feet
- Facial Rosacea
- May Smooth & Rejuvenate skin
- The most beautiful skin of your life

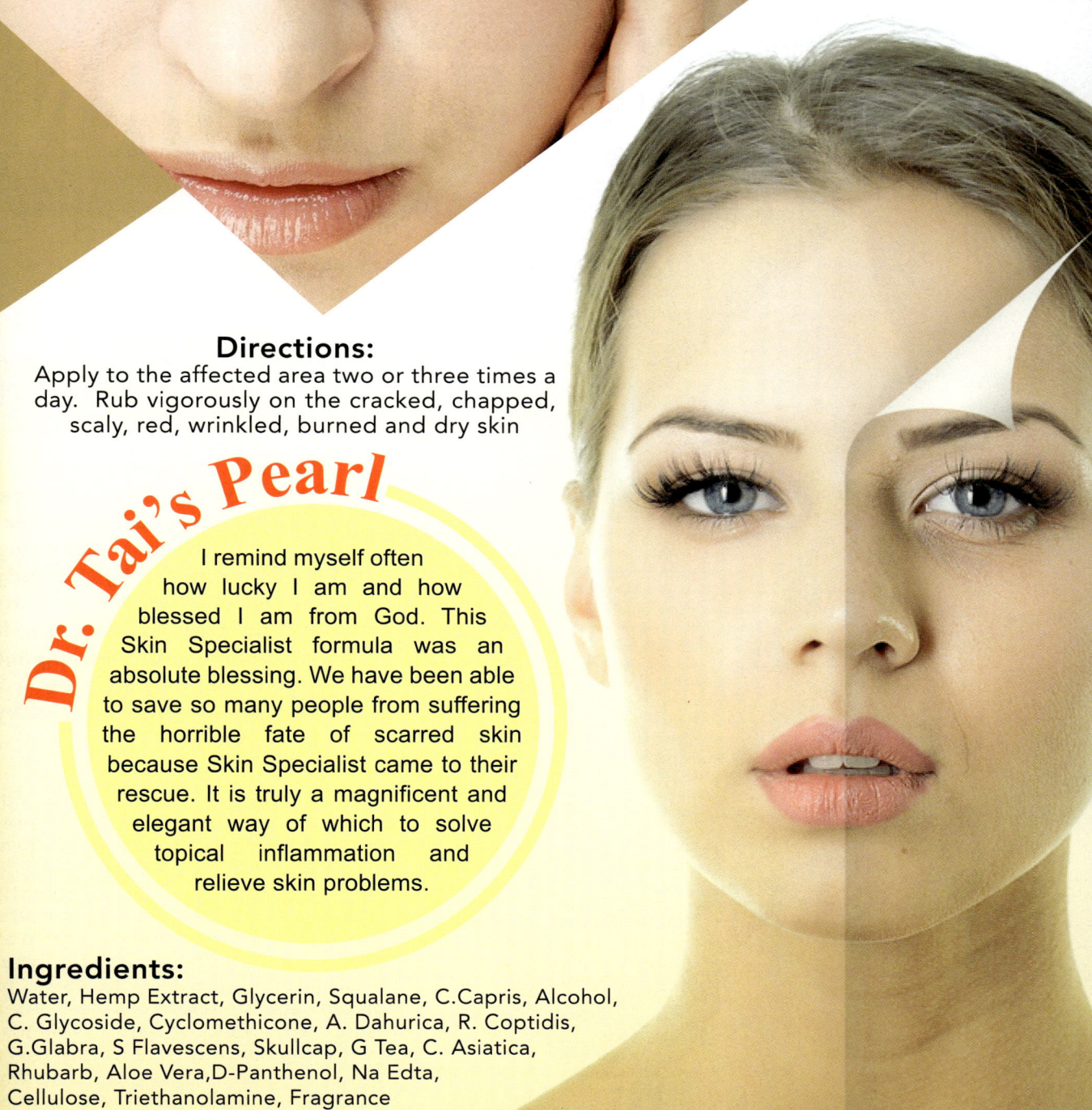

Directions:
Apply to the affected area two or three times a day. Rub vigorously on the cracked, chapped, scaly, red, wrinkled, burned and dry skin

Dr. Tai's Pearl

I remind myself often how lucky I am and how blessed I am from God. This Skin Specialist formula was an absolute blessing. We have been able to save so many people from suffering the horrible fate of scarred skin because Skin Specialist came to their rescue. It is truly a magnificent and elegant way of which to solve topical inflammation and relieve skin problems.

Ingredients:
Water, Hemp Extract, Glycerin, Squalane, C.Capris, Alcohol, C. Glycoside, Cyclomethicone, A. Dahurica, R. Coptidis, G.Glabra, S Flavescens, Skullcap, G Tea, C. Asiatica, Rhubarb, Aloe Vera, D-Panthenol, Na Edta, Cellulose, Triethanolamine, Fragrance

These statements have not been reviewed by the FDA. This products is not intended to diagnose, treat, cure, or prevent any disease

Side Effects: None

Contraindications:
Do not use this product if you are allergic to any of its ingredients.

SLIMMING FAT BURN
Localized Fat Melting

Diet drugs just not working?
Feeling sluggish and unattractive?
Want to lose inches in just a week?
Health Secrets has created a new product just for you!!!

Slimming Fat Burn (7-Keto) liposome transdermal topical cream may help you lose inches! 7-Keto is a naturally occurring substance produced by the body in the adrenal glands and its production declines with age. It is a non-stimulant, thermogenic agent that may increase metabolism and promote healthy weight loss.

Supplementing with Slimming Fat Burn Liposome cream (7-Keto) may create a more youthful metabolism and when used with a healthy diet and exercise program, may greatly accelerate your weight loss results. Unfortunately, when you reduce food intake with diet drugs, your metabolism slows down to compensate for fewer calories. As a result, any weight lost is almost always regained with a return to a normal diet. It's a no-win situation. And it just gets worse.

Clinical trials were done over an 8 week period using 30 overweight healthy volunteers consuming an 1800 calorie diet with light circuit training. With 7-keto, the results were 300% more weight loss vs the placebo! Slimming Fat Burn Liposome cream produced no adverse effects and hormone levels remained in normal clinical ranges.

Scientifically Backed Active Ingredient – 7-Keto

- May result in 300% more weight loss than diet and exercise alone
- May result in majority of weight loss being fat loss
- May promote weight loss without use of stimulants
- Active ingredient awarded a patent for weight loss

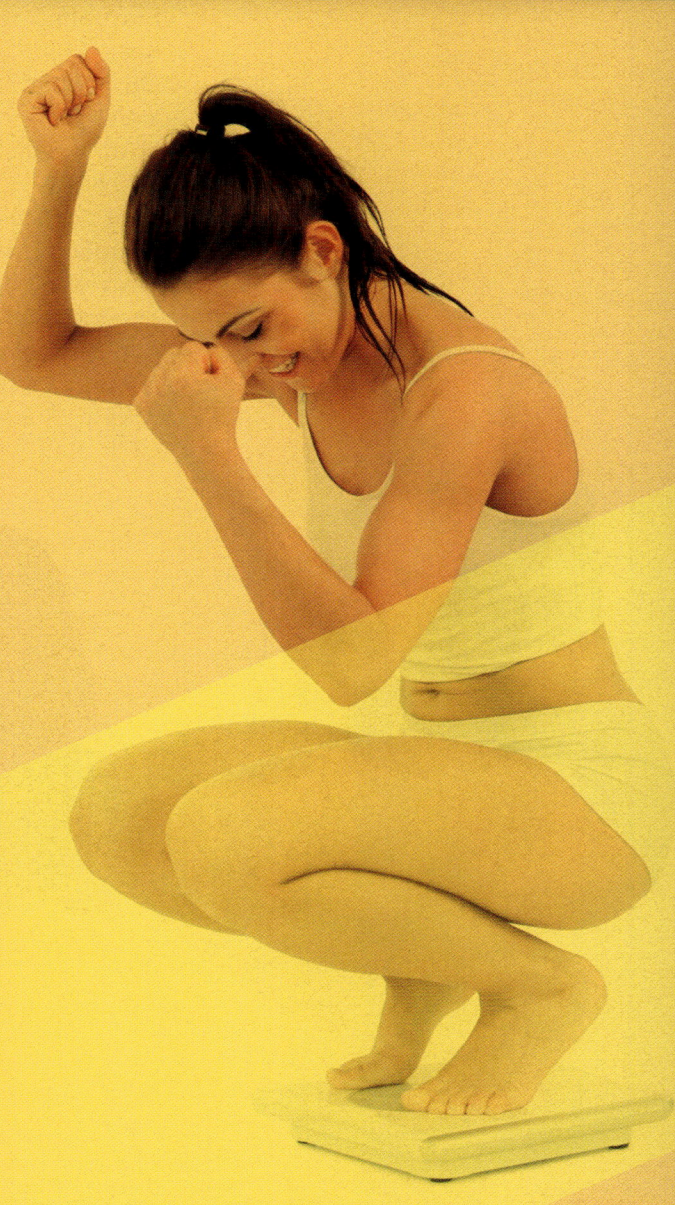

Dr. Tai's Pearl

When I was losing weight in my quest for getting myself healthy, I had severe problems with loose skin under my chin and arms. Flabby skin and excess fat nearly drove me crazy!! *Slimming Fat Burn* was a creation to save my own skin. Extensive research showed how well these ingredients worked in tightening the skin and burning the fat subcutaneously.

Side Effects: None

Contraindications:
Do not use this product if you are allergic to any of its ingredients

Directions:
Apply to soft parts of skin, 3 pumps AM & PM. Rub vigorously into your skin until dry.

Ingredients:
Fulvic Ext., Essential Phospholipids, Evening Primrose Oil, Shea Butter, 7 Keto-DHEA, Aloe Vera, Vitamin A, Vitamin E, Allantoin

These statements have not been reviewed by the FDA. This product is not intended to diagnose, treat, cure, or prevent any disease.

Stress Specialist

Help with Stress that leads to Fatigue!

Doctors have seen stress's tired face, and their patients have felt it. Doctors know what stress looks like while their patients know how terrible it feels. Over 80 percent of the medical conditions seen in medical practices have an underlying cause of stress. And everyone has a story- Even stress does.

And Stress is born…

Once-upon-a-time in a faraway land where the "Emotions" lived there was a frantic Emotion named "Overwhelm" who unwillingly married an Emotion she was always too busy to feel. This was fine for Overwhelm because her biological clock was ticking and needed to bear a child as soon as possible. She found a perfect match named " Frustrate." He was crazy about her.

Oh… what a tense couple they were.

With the help of the Tantrum Witch the two immortal Emotions conceived a child they decided to name "Stress." The Emotions of the land had enough of the couple and would not be able to tolerate their offspring, so they closed the gates of feelings and forbade the family from ever going back. The Emotions weren't sure their locked gates would keep them out so they asked Dr. Tai to help cast the three into oblivion. Since Stress's birth,

Dr Tai has tried to stop the wandering family from visiting people across the world with an elixir he calls "Stress Specialist" a potent formula specially concocted to kick nasty sensations out of the body. Will Dr. Tai be able to keep the troublesome trio out of everyone's lives? It all depends on who decides to try his Stress Specialist formula.

To be continued…

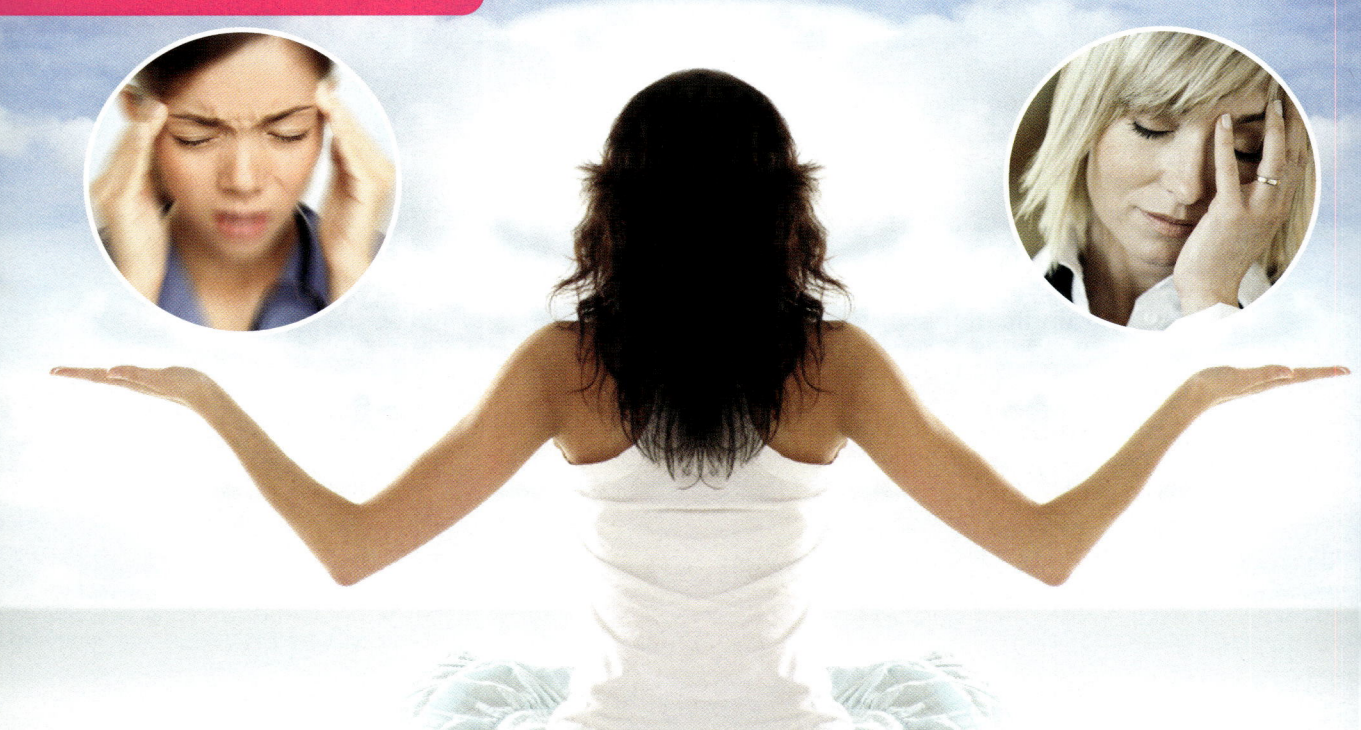

Stress Specialist is an all-natural formula made from Passion Flower, Valerian and Rhodiola Rosea. It is a superb blend of herbs that may strengthen the nervous system and fill you with more positive energy than you thought you had.

Stress is pressure, strain and anxiety. It is exhausting, nerve wrecking and hectic. To be free of these negative sensations would make you unstoppable, free to achieve your goals, and be the person you know you really are. On a sunny day, stress is the gray cloud that spoils the picnic. Don't let the darkness of stress dim your day or spoil your plans.

We flock together like birds of a feather

- **Passion Flower,** the Native American flower of passion will do what it promises. Powerful in Flavanoids, it exhibits anti-anxiety effects so you can rekindle the passion you have for all the things you love to do, but no longer have the energy for. As a mild aphrodisiac it decreases the strain in your lungs to bring more oxygen into your system, allowing you to go that extra mile with pleasure (Kelly, G.S. Alternative Medicine Review—2001).

- Used for thousands of years in ancient Greece and China, **Valerian** helps provide calming and sedative affects. It provides relief from tension, headaches and gastrointestinal spasms. Packed with amino acids GABA, Tyrosine and Arginine Valerian has all the active ingredients for relief that's nothing short of powerful (Dr. Weiss R.F. Herbal Medicine.2nd edition Stuttgart Germany--2000).

- **Rhodiola Rosea,** the Russian resistance builder helps provide cardio-pulmonary protection as it works as a stress fighting hormone that balances the adrenal glands. It may provide relief from chronic fatigue syndromes as it secures and fastens the Stress Specialist formula together turning it into a complete system for your body (Kelly, G.S. Alternative Medicine Review—2001).

Summary

Stress Specialist is made up of: Passion Flower which may help you to relax, Valerian which may remedy and Rhodiola Rosea which may create resistance.

You're not the only one. In a 2002 clinical study conducted by Andrea Tini et al. tested the effects of Valerian extracts on 48 adults and split the group in half. Three times a day, one group was given 2.5 mg Valium (a sedative pharmaceutical drug) while the other group was given 15 mg of Valerian. The group that took Valerian showed significant improvement in their moods. Their scans showed that their anxiety sensations reduced dramatically.

Directions:
Take one capsule twice a day

Ingredients:
5-Htp, Valerian, Ashwaganda, Passion Flower, Rhodiola Rosea, Citric Acid, L-Theanine

These statements have not been reviewed by the FDA. This product is not intended to diagnose, treat, cure, or prevent any disease.

Dr. Tai's Pearl

During a very difficult phase in one of my Best Friend's life, he was ready to hang himself from the stress that overwhelmed him from personal and family problems. My only useful act in him sharing this pain was finding someway to relieve this over-stressed situation. I gave him Stress Specialist as a way to reach out and be with him, day and night, through these capsules. Years later he told me that the Stress Specialist actually saved his life. Unable to sleep from the over-stress, Stress Specialist was able to lower his stress and instill a sense of peace and calm in him and restore the rest that had been robbed.

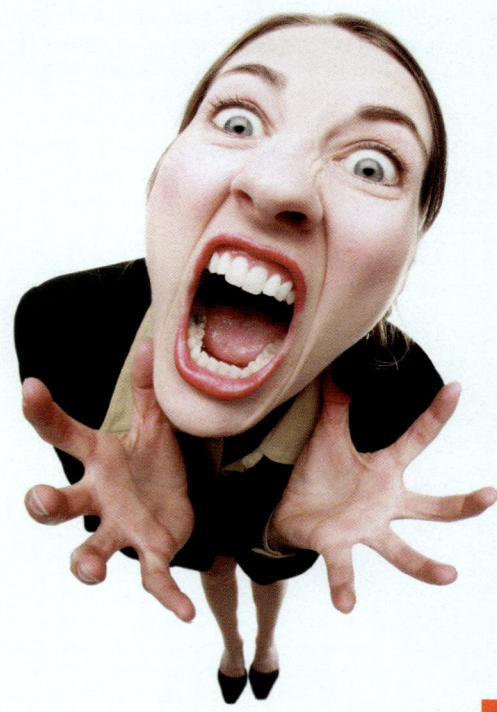

Side Effects: None

Contraindications:
Do not use this product if you are allergic to any of its ingredients

Stress & Anxiety Specialist
Serotonin to Stabilize Stress Centers in the Brain!

Stress
is a serious illness involving imbalances of neurotransmitters in the brain. A neurotransmitter is classified as a chemical messenger, traveling through the brain, sending messages from one neuron nerve cell to another. Different neurotransmitters produce different functions, ranging from feelings of pleasure to the ability to manage stress. An imbalance in chemical neurotransmitters leads to, but is not limited to anxiety, anger, impulsive actions, and stress.[1]

List of some Neurotransmitters and their Functions:
- Dopamine – pleasure, attachment/love and altruism.
- Norepinephrine – Arousal, energy, drive, stimulation and fight or flight.
- Serotonin – Emotional stability, reduces aggression, sensory input, sleep cycle and appetite control.
- GABA – Controls anxiety, arousal, convulsions and keeps brain activity balanced.

Depleted serotonin has been viewed as a major cause of Stress.[2] When levels are low, symptoms may include troubled sleep, anxiety, headaches and irritability. The ratios of dopamine and serotonin activity are very important. Keeping them balanced is the key to relieving symptoms of stress.[2]

Serotonin modulates stabilizing actions in the brain, creating a balance in chemical activity allowing those suffering from stress to be cool, calm and collected. With sufficient amounts of serotonin in balance with other neurotransmitters, our brain may approach intellectual challenges and accomplish accurate conclusions successfully and with ease.

Natural extracts of very young grass leaves are precursors to serotonin, have varying benefits, which are highly effective and natural. **Dosage is the key!** Dosage may need to be adjusted to individual needs. In the beginning, dosage may be increased given individual circumstances.

Products promising to balance serotonin in the brain do not work! The reason is that Blood Brain Barrier does not allow transport of serotonin into the brain. The Blood Brain Barrier is like The Great Wall of China. It keeps every unknown compound out. Stress & Anxiety Specialist possesses the ability to cross the Blood Brain Barrier because the carriers are recognized by the brain cells itself as friendly natural compounds. Stress & Anxiety Specialist may be very effective in balancing stress, and even coping with depression. It is a special proprietary formula created by Dr. Tai. It not only contains the proper ingredients but also the proper ratios, which is crucial to relieving the symptoms and causes of stress.

Serotonin Adaptogens Report the Following Benefits:

- Positive mood
- More constant mood
- More balanced mood
- Lessened anxiety
- Lessened anger
- Less erratic and irritable
- Better social skills
- Heightened self confidence
- Enhanced energy
- Improved sleeping patterns
- Heightened learning ability
- Heighted capacity for learning
- More attentive behavior
- Better mental focus

Dosage:
Take 1-2 full droppers twice daily.
Dosage **must** be adjusted for individual needs.

Ingredients:
Grass 10 Leaf Extract, Virgin Coconut Oil, Mint Flavors, Stevia

These statements have not been reviewed by the FDA. This product is not intended to diagnose, treat, cure, or prevent any disease.

1. Gainetdinov, R.R., Wetsel, W.C., Jones, S.R., Levin, E.D., Jaber, M. and Caron, M.G. (1999) Role of serotonin in the paradoxical calming effect of psychostimulants on hyperactivity. Science 283:397-401.

2. H. Soderstrom, K. Blennow, A-K Sjodin, and A. Forsman. New evidence for an association between the CSF HVA: 5-HIAA ratio and psychopathic traits. Journal of Neurology, Neurosurgery and Psychiatry, Vol. 74, 2003, 918-21.

Dr. Tai's Pearl

My life is not a bowl of cherries- that is for sure. I live a very stressful life, traveling through many time-zones and crisscrossing the skies from one city to another, and one country to another, speaking on behalf of natural health solutions. The stress level that we live under is tremendous. Having the weight of many sick individuals on my shoulders and the obligation to bring natural solutions to all corners of the world is a major responsibility. I personally use Stress & Anxiety Specialist to bring serenity, calmness, and a more positive outlook towards my work and my life. I can honestly say it has been one of the most important additions to my own personal treatments. I will be forever grateful to Stress & Anxiety Specialist and I never leave home without it.

Side Effects: None

Contraindications:
Do not use this product if you are allergic to any of its ingredients

SUPER B12 SUBLINGUAL

Maximum Energy, Brain Power & Vigor RIGHT NOW!

The whole B complex and individual components of Vitamin B are most important to maintain healthy human metabolism by neutralization of toxic amino acids naturally formed in our body, like Homocysteine. Homocysteine is known for creating destructive metabolism contributing to Cardio vascular diseases. Folic acid and other B vitamins are also very important in the fight against elevated homocysteine.

Another vital function of Vitamin B12 is in the healthy physiology neural transmission and neural pathway. It plays an important role in the regeneration of the perineural sheath, the very site of biochemical exchange and conduction of our nervous system. Unfortunately, there is a gastrointestinal barrier that often limits the absorption of B12 taken in capsule or pill form - you will often lose over 95% of vitamin B12 through excretion without absorption. As our body ages, we see a greater deficiency of vitamin B complex, especially vitamin B12 and concurrently, a higher and higher demand of B12 as part of our energy metabolic pathway and for rebuilding of neurological tissues.

Super B12 Lipo Spray is specially designed with a New Delivery Technology using the micronized liposomes, only a few hundred nanometers in size. This new technological breakthrough utilizes natural essential phospholipid microspheres. The center hollow vesicle carries the B complex, especially B12, allowing it to bypass the "gastrointestinal barrier", increasing the effectiveness of absorption in the sublingual and the bucal mucosa of our mouth. This ultra-fast absorption from the oral cavity takes the B complex and B12 directly into the blood vessels that are located anatomically beneath the tongue. There are abundant capillaries throughout the mouth mucosa. It is a unique and very efficient delivery process without the painful utilization of injection. This oral liposome is a major improvement in providing a delivery of uniform dosing on a daily basis, preventing the high and low peaks of B12 and B complex in the human body.

B12 and B complex is well regarded as the best way to achieve high energy and an incredible sense of well-being. Enjoy it!

Super B12 Sublingual may:

- Provide energy and vitality
- Provide homocysteine balance
- Improve memory sharpness
- Improve neuro conduction
- Support vascular health

Directions:
Shake well before use.
Place 10 drops in mouth under tongue.
Hold for 1 minute before

Ingredients:
Vitamin B12, Methylcobalamine, Folic Acid, Vitamin B2, Vitamin B6, Essential Phospholipids

These statements have not been reviewed by the FDA. This product is not intended to diagnose, treat, cure, or prevent any disease.

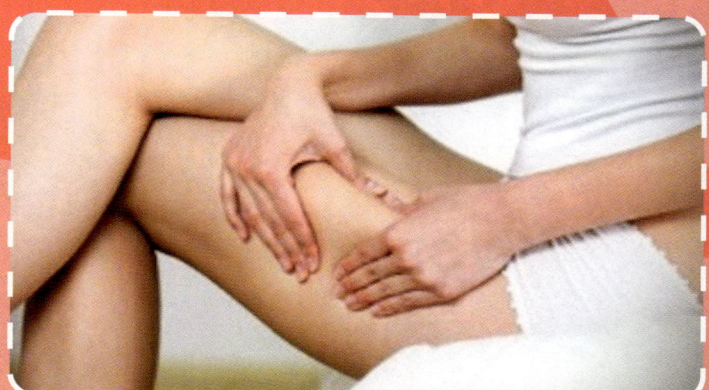

Dr. Tai's Pearl

All of our lectures require me to be dynamic and put out a maximum 150% of my energy. I depend on Super B12 as my starboard and go-to supplement to carry me through the low points of my presentations. I sometimes have to stand and lecture for 8 to 10 hours (such as many of the workshops that I do all over the world). I depend on Super B12 to give me the consistent energy and passion that I put into every single lecture. You can depend on Super B12 Specialist to deliver over, and over, and over again.

Side Effects: None

Contraindications:
Do not use this product if you are allergic to any of its ingredients

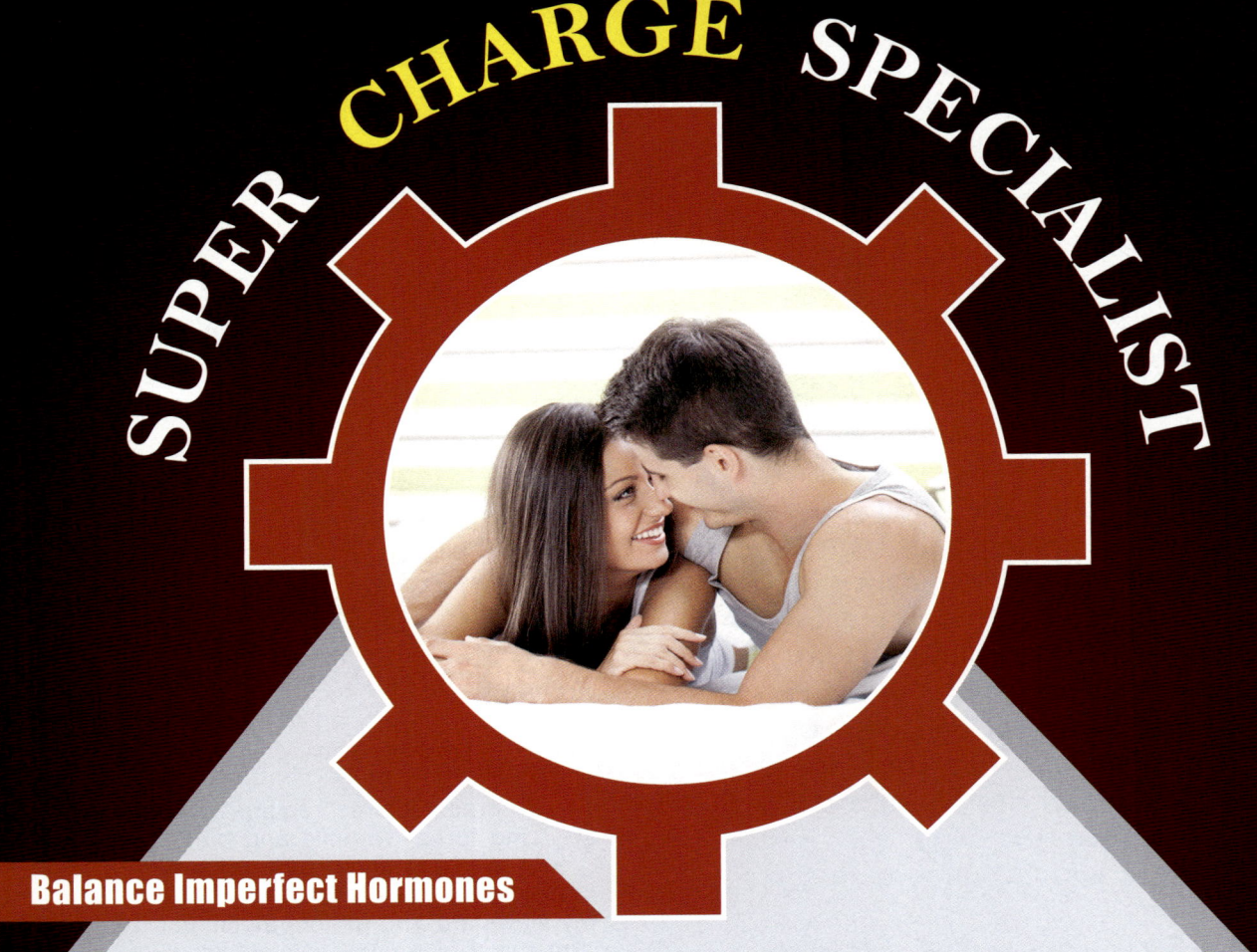

SUPER CHARGE SPECIALIST

Balance Imperfect Hormones

What is the Importance of Testosterone?

Testosterone is a male and female sex hormone essential for sexual stimulation. In addition, testosterone stimulates metabolism, helps build muscle, increases energy and enhances mood. As a man ages his testosterone levels decline as well as all the beneficial effects of the hormone. With its decline, comes emotional instability, loss of muscle mass and decreased or no libido. Erectile Dysfunction, or ED, affects about 30 million men in the United States and is a common health problem.

What can be used to Treat Andropause and Testosterone Deficiency?

In a recent study in the **British Journal of Sports Medicine by Hamzah, S., and Yusof, A., in 2003**, the beneficial effects of eurycoma are impressive. This exceptional ingredient has resulted in increased levels of testosterone in the blood, improved sexual function and increased psychological parameters including mood, energy and a sense of well-being. One of the most significant improvements was the increase in the libido of men and it had given fertility to men that had seemed infertile. Calcium fructoborate, present in fruits, gives an **increase of 12% in testosterone levels**[1] and works alongside eurycoma to quickly pack an even more favorable outcome for your body's health, vitality, increased muscle strength and endurance.[2] After treatment with Eurycoma, an increase in testosterone has ranged from **49% in a 50 year old male to 133% in a 24 year old male.**[3]

Additional Synergistic & Substantial Benefits of Eurycoma and Calcium Fructoborate

Treatment of andropause using eurycoma and calcium fructoborate raises testosterone naturally with no outsource of the hormone, therefore helping your own body produce testosterone. Eurycoma also increases the levels of DHEA and lowers SHBG leaving you with more "free testosterone" to work in your body. Eurycoma has also been proven to raise DHEA, a hormone essential for energy, vitality and youth and considered the grandfather hormone, raising levels by 47% in only a matter of three weeks.[3] Of 49 men who had been infertile for[5] years, 11 spontaneous pregnancies had occurred during the first 6 months of a trial.[4]

Epimedium Grandiflorum, or **"Horny Goat"**, is known throughout China & Asia as a supplement for improving performance. Aptly named "Yin Yang Huo," Epimedium Grandiflorum balances the energy meridians & channels of the Human Body. Epimedium Grandiflorum is used most often to combat weakness & fatigue for mental as well as physical lows. It also excels at improving heart & blood vessels with superior lung functions & supplying better memory for the brain.

Most important for women in Menopause or men in Andropause, helping with sexual activity & desire as well as improved circulation to the sexual organs.

The Polyphenols in this herb increase the blood flow & performance of sexual organs. The magic of this ingredient doesn't stop there, but also works to balance Women's Estrogen & Men's Testosterone. Epimedium Grandiflorum is also excellent as a tonic.

- **Increases blood flow**
- **Increases testosterone**
- **Increases DHEA**
- **Increases libido**
- **Increases sperm count**
- **Increases sexual desire**
- **Increases lean muscle mass**
- **Increases energy and vitality**

Directions:
Take 1 to 2 capsules daily for men and women. May increase the dose if needed or recommended by your health practitioner.

Ingredients:
Maca Root Powder, Epimedium 10%, Epazote, Eurycoma, Calcium Fructoborate, Panax Ginseng, Lepidium Meyenii

These statements have not been reviewed by the FDA. This product is not intended to diagnose, treat, cure, or prevent any disease.

1. Traish, A.M., et al. "The Dark Side of Testosterone Deficiency: II. Type 2 Diabetes and Insulin Resistance." Journal of Andronology. Vol. 30, No. 1, Jan/Feb 009: 23-32

2. Talbott S, Talbott J, Negrete J, Jones M, Nichols M, and Roza J. Effect of Eurycoma longifolia Extract on Anabolic Balance During Endurance Exercise. Journal of the International Society of Sports Nutrition. 3 (1)S1-S29, 2006.

3. Hamzah, S., and Yusof, A (2003) The ergogenic effects of eurycoma longifolia jack: A pilot study. British Journal of Sports Medicine. 37:464-470.

4. M.I. Tambi, M. Kamarul Imran. Wellmen Clinic, Damai Service Hospital, Kuala Lumpur, Malaysia. Dept of Community Medicine, School of Medical Sciences, Universiti Sains Malaysia, Kbg Kerian, Kelantan. Efficacy of the 'Malaysian Ginseng',US Patented, Standardised Water Soluble Extract of Eurycoma longifolia jack in Managing Idiopathic Male Infertility

5. Gri Glianur MD. et all. Alt. Med. Alert 2001, 4:10-22

Dr. Tai's Pearls:

The problem with Bio Identical Hormones has always been the "Negative Feedback" loop of side effects, the "White Elephant" in the room that no one wants to talk about. Having negative signs & symptoms of shrinking, small, soft testicles has never pleased me much, so I have always found that taking SUPER CHARGE Specialist alone or together with Transdermal Bio Identical Testosterone makes a wonderful & great combination in minimizing & bypassing the negative feedback loop by stimulating your own Testicular production of Testosterone.

Another Clinical Pearl for a Bonus is that maybe you can use less Bio Identical Testosterone for your body's needs & thereby further reduce excess Testosterone your body cannot use & thereby reducing Aromatization of too much Testosterone that can occur in injectable, oral, or too much BioIdentical Testosterone given by careless Doctors.

Remember the negative – too much Estrone & Estradiol from the excess Testosterone Aromatization can actually make you more feminizing, which is exactly the opposite effect of what you are trying to achieve. In addition, too much Estrone will have a negative effect on the Prostate.

Side Effects: None

Contraindications:
Do not use this product if you are allergic to any of its ingredients.

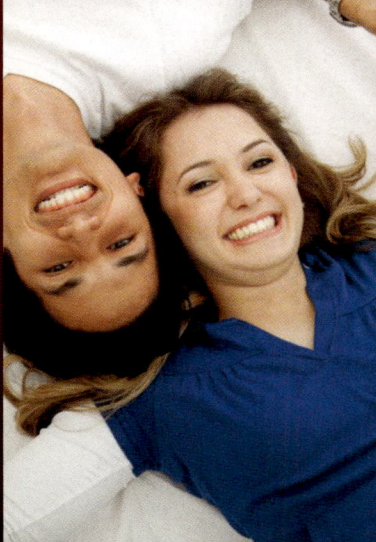

Thin Factors & Thin Factor Liquid (Homeopathic)

Stop Leptin Abnormalities that cause Obesity!

From the leaves

of the bauhinia forficata, indigenous tribes of Brazil make teas and broths, which they drink as a tonic to soothe upset stomachs or, in the case of graying elders, to simply feel younger. It's regarded as a diuretic with antibacterial, antifungal and anti-Candida properties. Its bark is prepared and consumed as an anti-diarrheal agent. The locals use extracts for snakebites and even bathe their babies in it. Significantly, they also employ Bauhinia forficata to fight diabetes. A teabag's worth consumed after a meal purportedly helps regulate blood sugar levels. Since 1929, several Brazilian studies have affirmed the leaf's reputation as a sort of "vegetable insulin."

About one-quarter of Western pharmaceuticals are derived from rain forest ingredients, but less than 1 percent of tropical trees and plants have been tested by scientists. Could bauhinia, long revered as a rich source of salutary phytochemicals, offer other life-changing gifts? Given its apparent effects on blood sugar, would it also function as a powerful tool in weight loss?

Mechanism of Leptin

Laboratory tests revealed that bauhinia contains compounds that appear to enhance satiety after a meal. Too often, we overeat because the hypothalamus—the appetite center of the brain--is slow to receive those "stop right there!" signals from hormones such as leptin. This hormone acts like a biochemical traffic cop, helping regulate metabolism and energy intake.

Leptin originates in fat cells and circulates at levels proportionate to body fat. Leptin talks directly to the hypothalamus gland in the brain. When leptin levels are high in normal function, it tells the brain to decrease food intake and increase sympathetic nerve activity, thus increasing metabolic rate. Leptin is a hormone that is secreted in white adipose tissue. Leptin regulation signals the brain, having a primary influence on body weight, insulin, cardiovascular health, reproductive function, sex hormones, immune function, adrenal function, stress, thyroid function, bone health, cancer and inflammation.

Because its receptors respond to sweetness, it affects sugar cravings in a way that, when rewarded, fosters a "learned addiction." Excess eating of sugar and calories in turn, raises the blood's level of triglycerides, which can impede leptin from reaching the brain. So the body is tricked into thinking its starving. The overeating that typically ensues then clogs the fat cells even more, signaling the liver to create extra cholesterol. The result is that with overeating, the hormone's receptors become less sensitive--a syndrome known as "leptin resistance." The hypothalamus, functioning much like thermostat, gets continually dialed up in a way that further increases appetite. Overeating begets more overeating.

Leptin miscues are one reason we can gorge on a heavy meal, capped off with dessert and not feel uncomfortably full until the regretful ride home, half an hour later. Like a crackerjack cleaning crew, bauhinia essentially scrubs and cleans up the leptin receptors, enabling them to work with brisk efficiency again, fostering a sense of satisfaction to stop hunger pangs. The hormonal signals reach the brain with greater effectiveness so metabolism, regulated by the hypothalamus, returns to a healthy function. Suddenly, that second slice of pizza doesn't beckon so irresistibly.

Further research confirmed this response. Recently, we conducted a placebo-controlled, double-blind study. It started as a four-week program, involving 31 patients (18 male, 13 female) and was extended to an eight-week study of eight subjects (three male, five female) from the treatment group. In the initial pilot program, subjects were randomly divided into two groups and instructed to take five milliliters of the test material--either bauhinia leaf extract or a placebo solution--half an hour before each meal. In addition to noting their weight, we measured the circumference of the chest, waist and hips, as well as body mass index and waist-to-hip ratio. The subjects were ordered not to alter their diet and exercise regimens in any way.

Dr. Tai's Pearl

Once in a while in the life of a researcher we stumble across something so extraordinary that it defines who we are. Thin Factors with Bauhinia is one of those discoveries. My professional life and research have all been impacted and changed by my participation in a double-blind study that was followed by multiple publications in major medical journals. I used the Thin Factors personally for the 50 pounds I had to shed to get my health back. Without it I would have never succeeded, and I could never perform to the level that I do today. The Thin Factors is a true gift to all of human kind to not only cleanse the Leptin Receptors, but also lower inflammation and normalize our satiety factor so that we can go back to being healthy individuals with healthy eating habits.

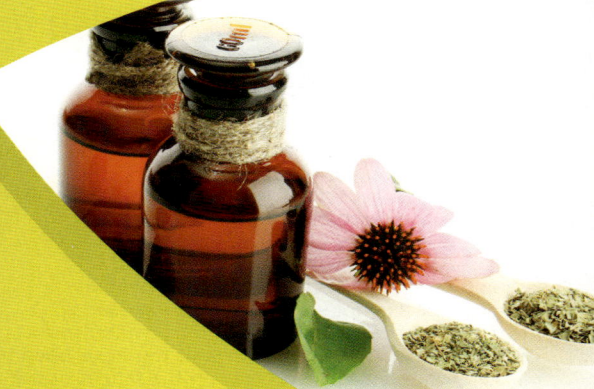

Directions for Gel Caps:
Take 1 or 2 gel caps (3) times daily, preferably (1) hour before each meal. For higher dosage, consult your health care practitioner.

Ingredients:
Extract Of Bauhinia, Essential Oils

Directions for Liquid:
Take 1/2 dropper (3) times daily 10 minutes before eating.

Ingredients:
Aloe Water, Homeopathic Bauhinia 3C, Homeopathic HCG 3C, Grapefruit Seed Extract

Side Effects: None

Contraindications:
Do not use this product if you are allergic to any of its ingredients

These statements have not been reviewed by the FDA. This product is not intended to diagnose, treat, cure, or prevent any disease.

TOTAL CIRCULATION

Improvement of Circulation for Sexual Wellness & Body

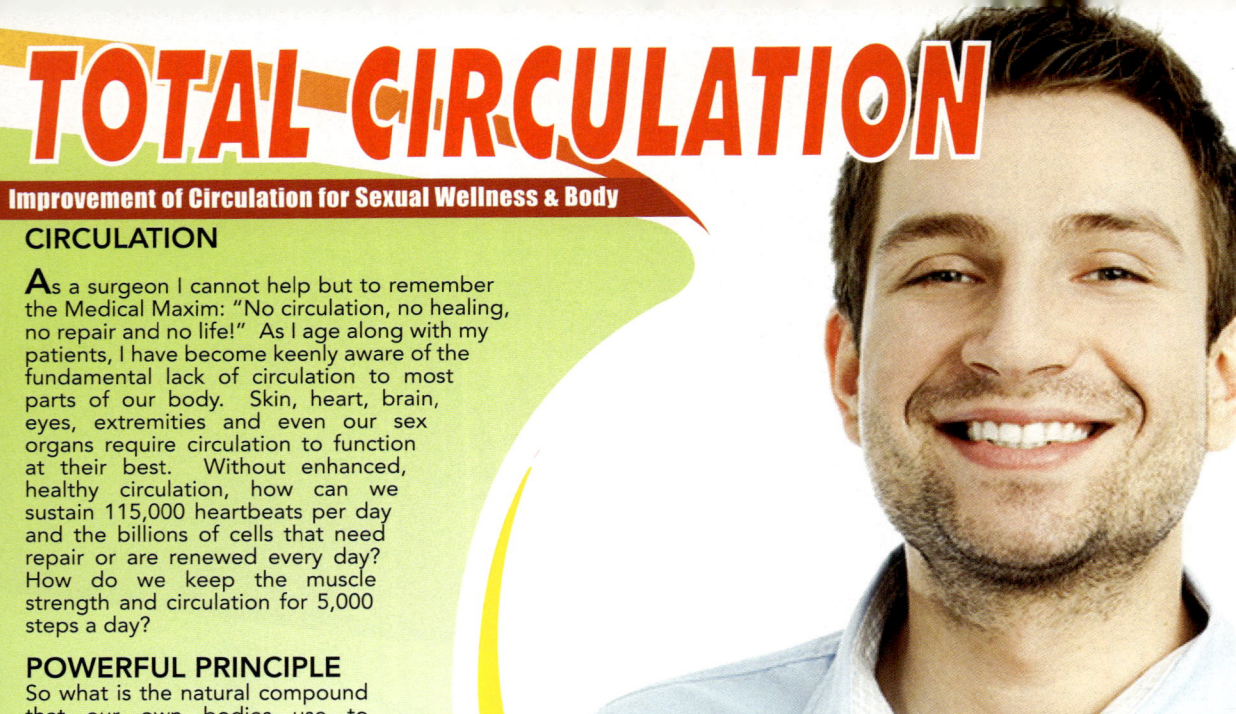

CIRCULATION

As a surgeon I cannot help but to remember the Medical Maxim: "No circulation, no healing, no repair and no life!" As I age along with my patients, I have become keenly aware of the fundamental lack of circulation to most parts of our body. Skin, heart, brain, eyes, extremities and even our sex organs require circulation to function at their best. Without enhanced, healthy circulation, how can we sustain 115,000 heartbeats per day and the billions of cells that need repair or are renewed every day? How do we keep the muscle strength and circulation for 5,000 steps a day?

POWERFUL PRINCIPLE

So what is the natural compound that our own bodies use to maintain healthy circulation? The simple answer is NITRIC OXIDE. This is a natural compound that our bodies make to keep the blood circulating throughout the heart, the brain and the major organs. Nitric Oxide contributes to the elasticity of the blood vessel walls that allow for the accommodation of our heartbeat as the wave of pressure circulates throughout the entire body keeping the blood vessels elastic and pliable. Imagine, for example, a water hose exposed to the drying elements of the sun and the winter snow. As time passes, the rubber walls of the hose become cracked, hard and dry. Turning on the faucet of the water hose, even just a little bit, will cause the sudden higher pressure to burst the hose and send water all over the place. This is the deadly scenario of heart disease, stroke and gangrene.

All the different major illnesses of immune disease, diabetes and even natural aging, are associated with lower production of Nitric Oxide, which protects the blood vessels throughout our body.

Think of a diabetic losing their eyesight, suffering from kidney shut down and staring at a below-the-knee amputation. Or maybe it is the libido for both the man and the woman, not working like it used to because of the falling level of Nitric Oxide.

Yes, the mind is willing! But the body is unable. Sexual activity is the powerful result of our ability to have good circulation in our genital areas. For a man, an erection is an increase circulation to the penis. For a woman, the attainment of orgasm is facilitated by increased circulation in the clitoral area.

The market for natural supplements of Nitric Oxide precursors is primarily a result of increased products with massive dosages of Arginine (1 gram or more) in order to stimulate healthy circulation and higher levels of Nitric Oxide. However, research has shown reliably and very negatively that high doses of Arginine (greater than 1 gram) daily results in the activation of viral infection such as herpes outbreak to the lips and increased viral lodes production throughout the human body.
Total Circulation is the first unique and proprietary formulation that delivers powerful levels of Nitric Oxide for immediate availability, increasing circulation to the brain, heart and extremities where the vessel dilation to our head and face, extremities and large organs is noticeable within an hour of taking Total Circulation! You can actually feel the warmth of the skin and slight flushing from the healthy abundance of circulation to the tissues!

As a result, an increase in libido and circulation throughout the body is accomplished without the large dose of Arginine.

Breakthrough technology in the combination of Arginine, Ornithine and Citruline at the prescribed ratio and the microencapsulation of the power of liposome allows for delivery and absorption intra-cellular availability of these essential ingredients to the immediate formation of Nitric Oxide in our circulation.

Total Circulation will last for 24 hours afterwards. Minor transient, flushing or warmth to the skin is expected and desirable to show the increase circulation from the Nitric Oxide being present in our body within the hour. This is only temporary. The feeling passes away without any side effects.

Total Circulation Indications: Improved libido for males and females, improved circulation of the extremities, to the brain and to the heart, improved blood pressure, as well as, diabetics, glaucoma, Raynaud's disease and cold hands and feet.

Directions:
Max Nox can be taken daily. (1) Dropper full on an empty stomach at least one (1) hour before eating and do not eat for at least one (1) hour afterwards. Drink only clear water for maximum absorption.

Ingredients:
Eurycoma, Andrographis, Butea, Watermelon Extract, Citrulline, L-Arginine, L-Ornithine These statements have not been reviewed by the FDA. This product is not intended to diagnose, treat, cure, or prevent any disease.

Dr. Tai's Pearl

It is very difficult to increase circulation to the brain and the heart with supplementation. Many have tried without success. Using citrulline and the extraordinary ingredients of Total Circulation, we have been able to demonstrate by thermography, an increase of the circulation to the brain by over 37% within 30 – 40 minutes. This is a spectacular result. Just consider what you can do to help those patients and individuals who have 70 – 80% blockage to the carotid or arteries to the brain or extremities, which create extreme impairments of function and performance. Having collateral circulation increase in tissue perfusion to those areas with the help of Total Circulation, can achieve potential improvements and progress, increasing circulating without surgical intervention. This is not a small clinical pearl; this is a large discovery for mankind.

Side Effects:
The side effects are definitely relative to the dosage. If you take higher dosage, the higher the side effects lower dosage, the lower the side effects. Because of the higher dosage, the large amount of vassal dilation causing problems such as stuffy nose and heavy head, related to increases circulation to the brain and flushing of the skin of the face. You may actually feel the warmth because of the increased circulation.

Contraindications:
Mostly with other medications that are vassal dilators which compounds the increased circulation due to Total Circulation. Sublingual nitro glycerin is contraindicated and other prescriptions which are Vasodilators through the coronary artery for the treatment of angina pectoris. Do not take product if you are allergic to any of its ingredients.

Clinical Cases:
Diabetic lady of 67-years. Suffered from previous ovarian cancer and was treated with chemotherapy and radiation. She has successfully been in remission for seven years; however the consequences of diabetes and circulation combined have created a large ulceration on the medial aspect of her left ankle. This has created very large discoloration and alteration with severe pain and doctors from all over the area have attempted to close the open ulcer without any success. One surgeon decided to amputate because of the infection that has now progressed to the deeper tissues, exposing medial blood vessels, superficial veins, and tendons and ligaments. When we saw this patient, she was in severe discomfort, barely able to walk with the assistance of crutches, her foot and ankle was extremely swollen with large ulceration, approximately 5 – 8 cm in diameter. Treatment of increasing circulation was begun, using a few drops of Total Circulation three times a day, multiple vitamin B, support for the immune system, as well as diabetes. We changed her diet; we worked on the topical antibiotic with compression in order to relieve the edema and swelling. Patient was supplemented with microminerals and Royal Ling Zhi. Upon control of the infection, granulation base started to be deposited with the help of the collateral circulation from Total Circulation and improving of microcirculation using Clot Buster. Debridment of the necrotic tissues on a weekly basis and after several months, the ulcer was successfully closed and patient able to walk without the use of crutches, as well as wear shoes with compression support stockings to control edema.

ULTRA CHARGE

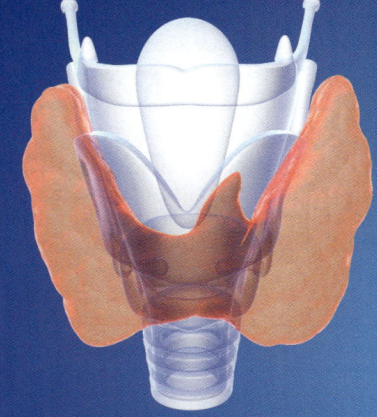

Some Thyroid-Specific Disorders Include:

Hypothyroidism
Goiter
Thyroid nodules
Thyroid cancer

As a physician entering my fifth decade of practice, I have come to find through others and my own experience, that the Thyroid is the gate keeper to all health. When taking the whole body into consideration, the Thyroid is relatively small, however it is the conductor to all of the most important organs. We're talking the heart, brain, liver, kidneys AND skin! Now what do you call the one at the top, controlling all the big movers? The Boss.

Behind every Boss, there's a corporate entity monitoring each process that a business is set up to do. In thyroid's case, that would be the Brain's Hypothalamus. The Hypothalamus produces a hormone called Thyrotropin Releasing Hormone (TRH) that causes the pituitary gland at the base of the brain to release Thyroid Stimulating Hormone, or TSH. This hormone is vital to thyroid function because it goes on to stimulate the Thyroid Gland to release its primary hormone Thyroxine, also commonly labeled T4.

This feedback mechanism in the brain makes it so when Thyroid Hormones are low, the Hypothalamus gets to work, producing the TRH, triggering TSH that releases T4, thusly keeping your whole body in balance.

Disorders of the Hypothalamus Gland or Pituitary Gland can cause severe Thyroid problems that could permanently compromise Thyroid Function.

I know that I have brought something truly special to the realm of supplements by integrating Eastern Herbals with Western knowledge. I strongly depend on my knowledge of Chinese Herbal Medicine when formulating new supplements and Ultra Charge Specialist is no exception. As far back as 400 A.D., the Epimedium used in Ultra Charge Specialist has been used to treat health issues such as Hypertension, Coronary Heart Disease, Memory Loss and Joint Pain.

191

Trials with **Epimedium** have shown that the herb has the ability of reducing cortisol levels. What does THE Stress-Hormone have to do with your Thyroid? Well, it's a simple truth that frenzied, HIGH Cortisol Levels will adversely affect Thyroid Hormones by lowering them to abysmal levels. When you are stressed, your Adrenal is triggered to chug out Cortisol by the boatload – meanwhile this fresh Cortisol is causing severe resistance to not only your Thyroid Hormones, but every single Hormone in your body!!

Sure, you think Cortisol may cause just a 'little' mischief, making body's tissues to resist against the thyroid hormones, but excess Cortisol actually goes as far as suppressing TSH secretion. If you remember, TSH is the controller hormone which is produced by the brain and tells the Thyroid when to show up to work. By suppressing TSH you are literally disabling the Thyroid from making ANY THYROID HORMONES! You are DISABLING the BOSS from directing a WHOLE BODY OF WORKERS – YOUR ORGANS!!

Low Cortisol can also cause complications with TSH levels, causing an unnatural increase. T3 function also suffers as T3 receptors find it harder and harder to react in the presence of T3 – regardless of the amount. This throws thyroid function completely down the drain!! Remember that we want for the levels of the body to be in Balance. If things are not balanced, your biochemical foundation is slanted and left with severe dysfunction. Deficiency or Excesses are NEVER good things.

"Alright, Dr. Tai, I understand the severity of Thyroid Dysfunction & Disease, but MY Thyroid is FINE!"

"Are you Sure About That?"

This is why I thank Epimedium for FIGHTING TIRELESSLY against receptor resistance, and all excesses, and deficiencies that affect the Thyroid and its related hormones.

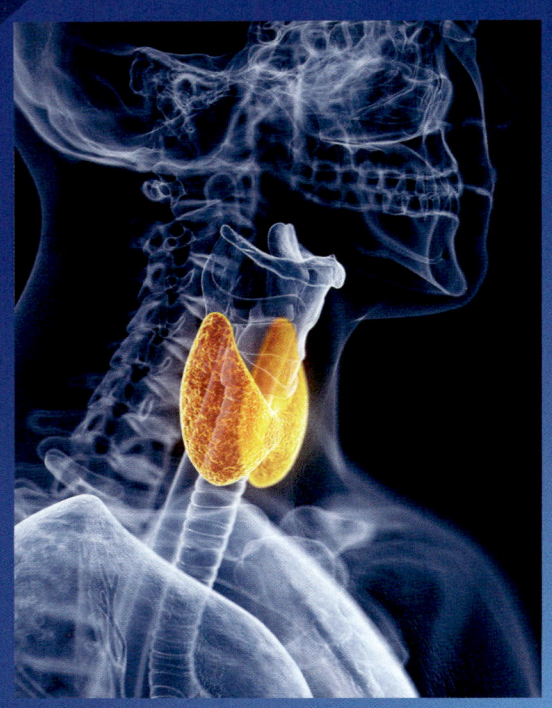

The Symptoms of Hypothyroidism can be surprising, covering a large spectrum of body parts and systems. You would probably expect a sign, like enlargement of your Thyroid, and you wouldn't be incorrect. Many people are aware of the Goiter that can form due to Hypothyroidism and the subsequent Adrenal Fatigue. However… are your nails brittle? It's a common enough problem that at least a handful of your friends would admit to it. Is your hair dry, unable to ever get enough moisture? What about your skin? Do you scratch and scratch and scratch, exfoliating all over your keyboard and desk, leaving behind a fine layer of skin-dust because you're just so dry and itchy!?

You may say coincidence, but thousands of Physicians, Medical Publications and the ENTIRETY of Modern Medical Science say something else: **Hypothyroidism!!!**

Hypothyroidism can present itself in the form of very subtle symptoms that don't cause alarm until it's TOO LATE.

COMMONLY IGNORED SYMPTOMS OF HYPOTHYROID:

Tiredness & Fatigue	Weight Gain (Due To Fluid)
Low Energy	Increased Sensitivity to Cold
Brittle Fingernails & Hair	Hair Loss
Dry, Rough, Pale Skin	Constipation
Muscle & Joint Pain	Heavy & Irregular Period
Muscle Weakness	Hoarse Voice
Puffy Face	Swollen Legs, Ankles & Feet
Difficulty Thinking & Focusing	Feeling Down or Depressed
Memory Trouble	Slower Speech or Movement
Swollen Thyroid Gland	All Over Inflammation

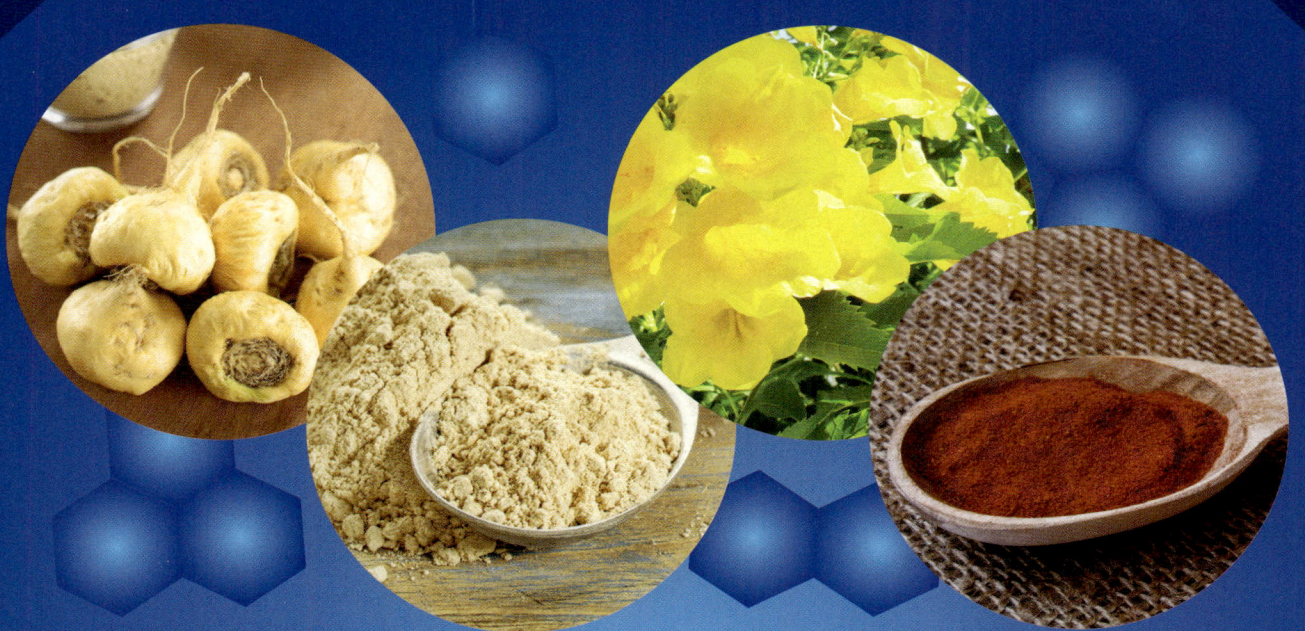

These symptoms are detrimental and can be highly devastating to a person's quality of life. This is why I worked passionately to develop the formulation for Ultra Charge Specialist. My heart swells with pride when I think of all the members and subjects that have been helped by this specific combination.

Helping Epimedium to keep control is **Una De Gato (Cat's Claw)** and **Maca Root Powder**. I have worked with both of these ingredients at length and have reviewed countless studies and spoke with authorities on their benefits

A large part of the debilitating physical effects of Hypothyroidism is the constant pain caused by the inflammation of joints and tissues. There is no living with a body that constantly feels as if it's being roasted over hot coals. Una De Gato helps directly by suppressing TNF-alpha synthesis, TNF being a cytokine that is involved in systemic inflammation.

Maca Root Powder contains a high iodine content, which is CRITICAL in supporting Thyroid Function.

Iodine is a major component of Thyroid Hormones, so it takes a pure, natural, unmodified source to properly regulate the Thyroid. Maca Root Powder has the ability to also balance all of the body's hormones without negatively affecting them. This ability to balance hormones in turn helps to boost iodine levels, making it possible to passively support the thyroid. By providing your body with an herb that can do these things, balancing hormones and naturally increasing iodine levels, you can reach a level of healthy Thyroid function and then continue to maintain that level of Optimum Thyroid Health.

It is important to also address the tissues that have been badly abused and damaged in the time that your Thyroid was run into the ground. The formulation of Ultra Charge Specialist utilizes a generous amount of Aloe Water, the most moisturizing form of hydration known to man, to help repair your hair, skin and nails by penetrating these dry and near-impenetrable tissues to break down and digest dead skin cells!! Aloe Water then wraps its job up in a neat package, helping to further reduce inflammation, working alongside the Una De Gato to eradicate surface pain and deep tissue inflammation.

These statements have not been reviewed by the FDA. This product is not intended to diagnose, treat, cure, or prevent any disease.

Dr. Tai's Pearl

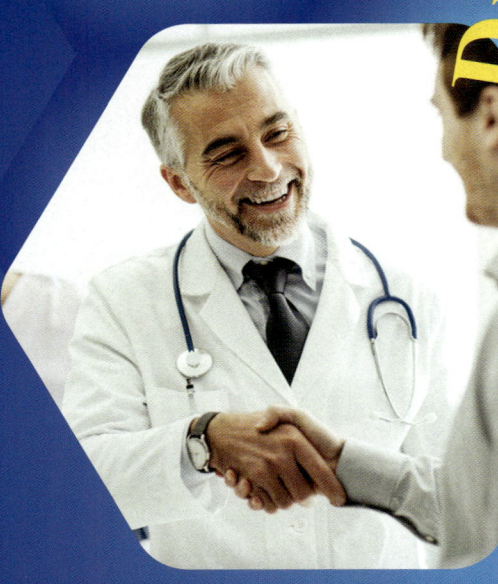

Like High Blood Pressure, you don't know the extent of your thyroid health until you measure it! Yes... you can measure the severity of Hypothyroid! It's painless and fast while still remaining affordable, accurate and simple enough that it can be done in your office. It's called **ThyroFlex.**

Directions: 1 Dropper AM on an Empty Stomach. May increase to 1 dropper full AM & PM on an Empty Stomach.

Ingredients: Aloe Water, Epimedium, Epazote, Una De Gato, Maca Root Powder, Mozuko Extract, Brown Algae Extract, Iodine, Potassium Iodide, Fulvic and Humate, Thyroidium 3C

This Product Is Not Intended for HYPERTHYROIDISM!

Side Effects: None

Contraindications: Do not take if you are allergic to any of the ingredients.

Clinical Cases:

Suzanne P. was just celebrating her 36th birthday when the Family Doctor told her that she had Hashimoto's Thyroiditis. Worry hadn't even registered in her mind before her Doctor was handing her a prescription for Synthroid. Just like that, as soon as it happened it was swept away under the rug. With Synthroid, all would be GOOD! There was nothing to worry about!

I don't believe "Good" knew her mailing address – 12 years later and she was still waiting. While she sat patiently for over a decade (the nail biting and sleepless nights don't count, of course), her symptoms had completely seized control of her life. Tiredness, Fatigue and Brain Fog were just the tip of the ice-berg, making her constantly late to meetings, perpetually stuck behind schedule and unable to follow along in simple conversation!! Just trying to comprehend what was in front of her was like attempting to open a Chinese Puzzle Box!

Hashimoto's had also robbed her of her confidence and good looks. Although those around her tried to console her, the 62lbs she had gained served as a deadly reminder of what this disease had done to her, pushing her into obesity and putting her at risk for even MORE health complications. Suzanne was so emotional that she avoided looking at herself, but shielding her eyes from the mirror on her way to the bathroom couldn't change the clumps of hair that clung to her fingers when she showered. Desperate & crying, she came to me looking for relief…

I was passionate about helping Suzanne. When I met her, I took her hands, intending to comfort her and tell her just how devoted I was…but instead I had to recoil!! Her hands were ICE COLD! As I rubbed my own hands together, trying to fight off her freezer burn, she laughed and told me that her feet are even worse!!! I had seen thousands of patients just like Suzanne P., treated by their doctors with Synthroid & other prescriptions similarly. These drugs have markers for thyroid, so that after ingestion, test results read A-OK! The Doctors may think you are fine, but the patient, like Suzanne, is miserable!

ThyroFlex best shows her Real-Life physiology hypothyroid at moderate severe level.

In my lectures all over the world, you'd be surprised how many physicians are CONVINCED that there is NO ROOM for improvement in their practice. Meanwhile, their patients aren't getting better, some get WORSE and ALL OF THEM show up to their appointments filled with dread only to leave near tears when they're still suffering despite "alright" test results. Uhmm… Excuse Me!? You may be drawing the samples and reading off charts and reports, but you are NOT CARING FOR YOUR PATIENTS!

I remind doctors in the audience of these lectures that we don't treat lab results, We Treat People! People with feelings, who are vulnerable, emotional and in pain - constantly suffering from symptoms of Hypothyroid in spite of improved blood markers in lab results!! We are People Doctors!

**Ultra Charge was conceived and born out of the desperate need of patients like Suzanne P.
It has been a Life Saver and A Game Changer.**

In most cases of Hypothyroid, I don't have to change their prescriptions, and only add several droppers of Ultra Charge Specialist in the early mornings & late at night on an Empty Stomach. WARNING! Ultra Charge will not work if you take with food – it is very sensitive! Must be taken on an empty stomach & do NOT eat for 1 hour afterwards.

At our first meeting, we gave Suzanne a fast and non-invasive ThyroFlex test. Thanks to the Instantaneous results, she was able to leave the same day with an all-natural protocol circulating around Ultra Charge Specialist and her three most concerning symptoms. When I saw Suzanne only 2 weeks later, she was beaming with a smile from ear to ear. "I am Good," she said, "As a matter of fact, I'm GRRRREAT!!"

Her ThyroFlex level in only 2 weeks showed a 72% improvement in her biologic Energy.

You feel better when the Battery of your Body gets recharged! The first thing I noticed about Suzanne at this second meeting was the light in her eyes, and her ability to follow along effortlessly with everything we talked about. Before, I had to stop just short of snapping my fingers in her face to keep her attention and understanding. The Fatigue & Tiredness were gone and now that her Brain Fog had lifted, she was thinking clearly. Even her husband noticed! I'm sure he missed her ice-cold feet scooting under the covers to find him, but ultimately it was a welcome change.

Suzanne P. continued to improve. We continued to test and monitor her recovering Thyroid Reflex level and adjusted her dosage of Ultra Charge. Suzanne P. was abuzz with excitement as her hair regrew! I had never seen her look so magnificent with all her energy & radiance.

Thank you, Ultra Charge!

References

1. Samuels, MH. Effects of variations in physiological cortisol levels on thyrotropin secretion in subjects with adrenal insufficiency: a clinical research center study. J Clin Endocrinol Metab. 2000;85(4):1388-1393.
2. Hangaard J, et al. Pulsatile thyrotropin secretion in patients with Addison's disease during variable glucocorticoid therapy. J Clin Endocrinol Metab. 1996;81:2502–2507.
3. Hangaard J, et al. The effects of endogenous opioids and cortisol on thyrotropin and prolactin secretion in patients with Addison's disease. J Clin Endocrinol Metab. 1999;84:1595–1601.
4. De Nayer, P et al. Altered interaction between triiodothyronine and its nuclear receptors in absence of cortisol: a proposed mechanism for increased thyrotropin secretion in corticosteroid deficiency states. 1987;17(2):106-10.
5. Abdullatif, HD, Ashraf, AP. Reversible subclinical hypothyroidism in the presence of adrenal insufficiency. Endocr Pract. 2006;12(5):572-575.
6. J Oral Sci. 2010 Sep;52(3):473-6. In vitro antimicrobial activity of phytotherapic Uncaria tomentosa against endodontic pathogens. Herrera DR1, Tay LY, Rezende EC, Kozlowski VA Jr, Santos EB.
7. Int Immunopharmacol. 2008 Mar;8(3):468-76. doi: 10.1016/j.intimp.2007.11.010. Epub 2007 Dec 26. Immunomodulating and antiviral activities of Uncaria tomentosa on human monocytes infected with Dengue Virus-2. Reis SR1, Valente LM, Sampaio AL, Siani AC, Gandini M, Azeredo EL, D'Avila LA, Mazzei JL, Henriques Md, Kubelka CF.

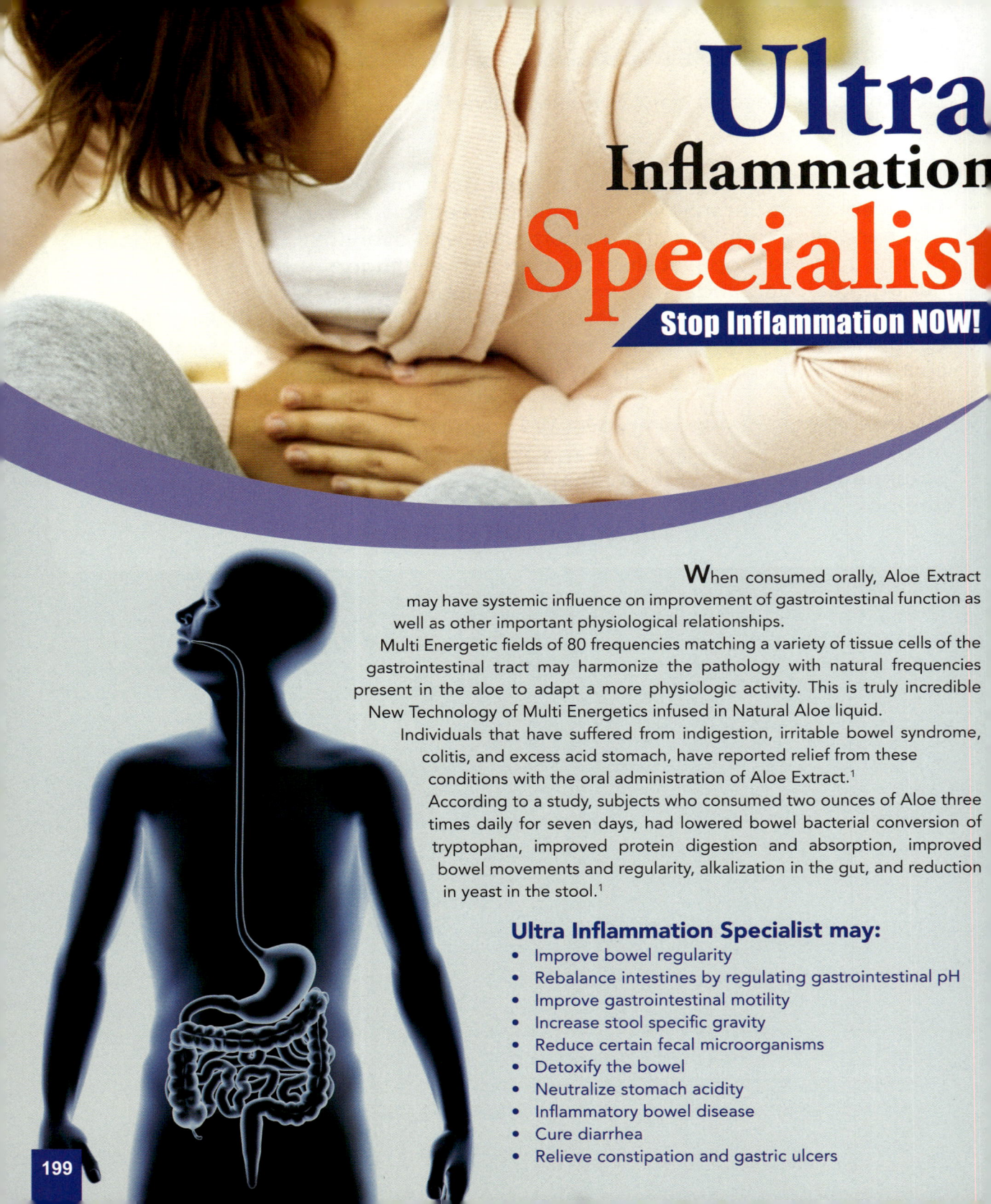

Ultra Inflammation Specialist

Stop Inflammation NOW!

When consumed orally, Aloe Extract may have systemic influence on improvement of gastrointestinal function as well as other important physiological relationships.

Multi Energetic fields of 80 frequencies matching a variety of tissue cells of the gastrointestinal tract may harmonize the pathology with natural frequencies present in the aloe to adapt a more physiologic activity. This is truly incredible New Technology of Multi Energetics infused in Natural Aloe liquid.

Individuals that have suffered from indigestion, irritable bowel syndrome, colitis, and excess acid stomach, have reported relief from these conditions with the oral administration of Aloe Extract.[1]

According to a study, subjects who consumed two ounces of Aloe three times daily for seven days, had lowered bowel bacterial conversion of tryptophan, improved protein digestion and absorption, improved bowel movements and regularity, alkalization in the gut, and reduction in yeast in the stool.[1]

Ultra Inflammation Specialist may:

- Improve bowel regularity
- Rebalance intestines by regulating gastrointestinal pH
- Improve gastrointestinal motility
- Increase stool specific gravity
- Reduce certain fecal microorganisms
- Detoxify the bowel
- Neutralize stomach acidity
- Inflammatory bowel disease
- Cure diarrhea
- Relieve constipation and gastric ulcers

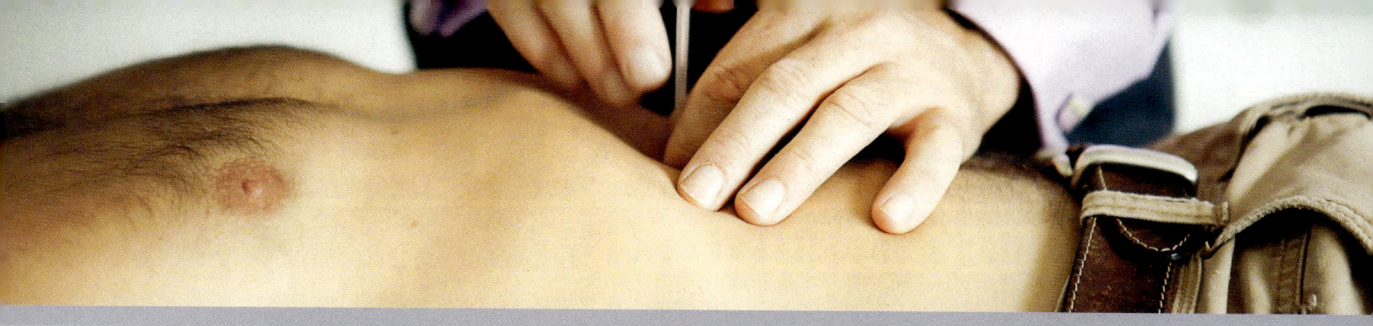

Directions:
Drink 2 ounces 3 times daily – morning, noon, and night, on an empty stomach

Ingredients:
Multi-Energetic Aloe Water

These statements have not been reviewed by the FDA. This product is not intended to diagnose, treat, cure, or prevent any disease.

1. Bland, Ph.D., Jeffrey. "Effect Of Orally Consumed Aloe Vera Juice: On Gastrointestinal Function In Normal Humans." Preventive Medicine. (19_85_)

Dr. Tai's Pearl

Now we are talking about a supplement that nears miracle. Yes, Miracle, as in removing all inflammation from your mouth and the GI Tract upon contact. There are literally millions of people all over the world suffering from inflammation of the GI Tract causing untold deficiencies in absorption, and nutrition as well as severe pain and suffering from swelling and other abnormalities. Nothing that you have ever experienced will come close to the magnificent results we have obtained using Ultra Inflammation. The only word that comes to mind when I think of it is MIRACULOUS!

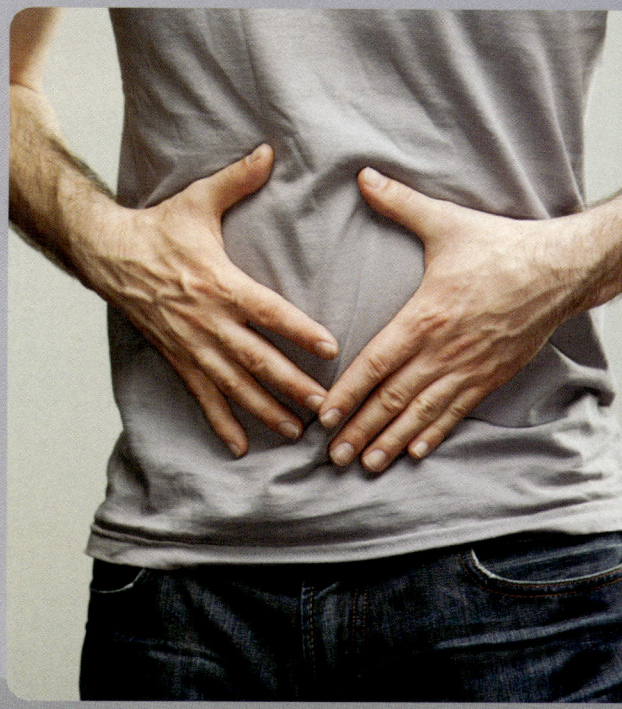

Side Effects: None

Contraindications:
Do not use this product if you are allergic to any of its ingredients

ULTRA INTENSE
Powerful Circulation & Sexual Function

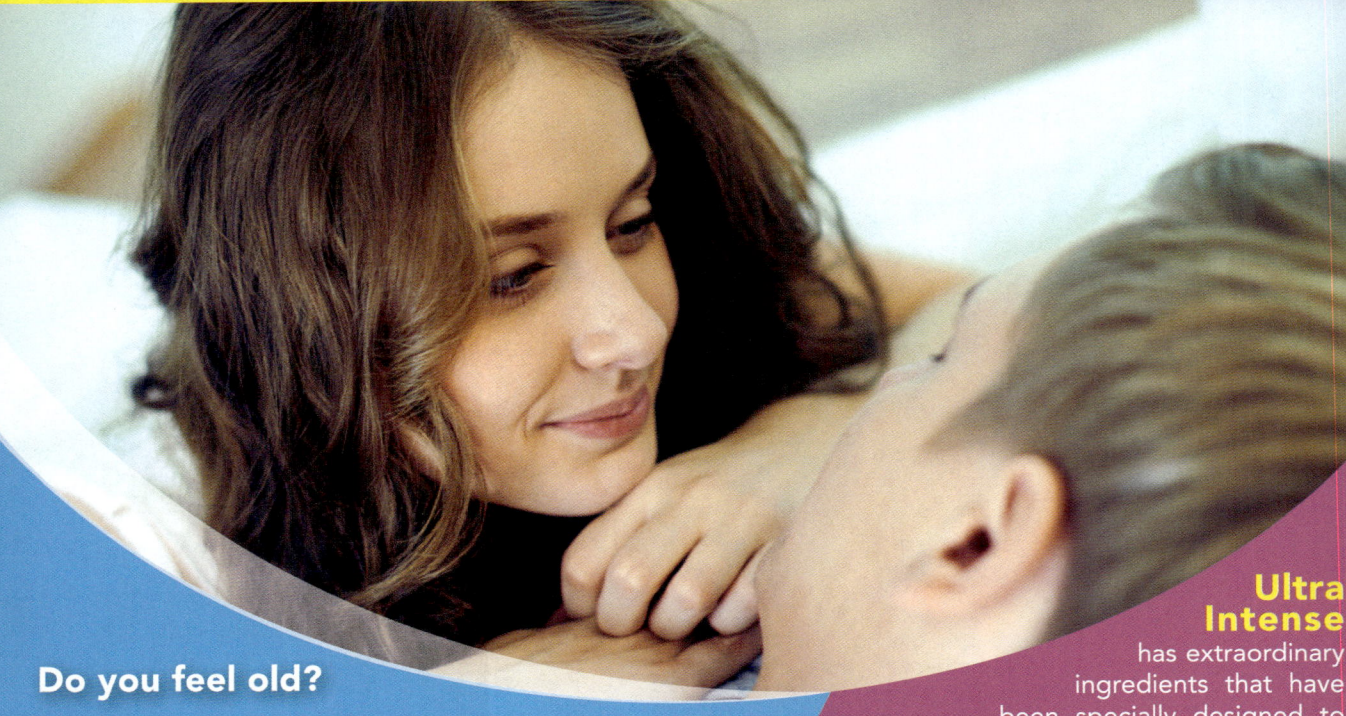

Do you feel old?

Are you lacking vitality?

Do you feel your libido is much lower than it used to be?

Ultra Intense's Special proprietary Formulation may be just what you need!!!

Ultra Intense has extraordinary ingredients that have been specially designed to Turbo Charge the sexual energy in your life. We have taken the latest research and made some wonderful extracts! Very special, very refined and very potent! In fact, the essential Bio-Extract used in this special formulation is 100:1 standardized for maximum potency. We have combined careful technology to enhance absorption and deliver the full potency exactly where it is needed. This technology is unique and has been developed especially for this formula. For maximum effect, you may take once daily on an empty stomach, with no alcoholic beverages. You may take an extra dose one hour before powerful sexual activity. The chosen ingredients such as Eurycoma and Butea are Nitric Oxide producers which may increase libido and improve sexual energy and power.

The Arginine combined with Watermelon Skin Extract may significantly increase blood vessel dilation and improvement of blood flow to the Vascular Cavernosa, increasing libido and a long lasting erection.

Cautions: DO NOT TAKE if you are suffering from Heart Diseases, Hypertension or taking medications for these conditions. DO NOT TAKE this if your physical condition, circulation or blood pressure and health cannot withstand vigorous sexual exercises.

Directions:

Take 1 capsule on empty stomach 1 hour before activity or you may take 1 capsule daily for excellent results. Do not consume food or alcohol for at least one hour. Do not exceed 2 capsules per 24 hour period. Keep out of reach of children.

Ingredients:

L-Arginine, L-Orinthine, L-Citruline, Watermellon Skin Ext, Eurycoma, Cistanche, Butea Superba

These statements have not been reviewed by the FDA. This product is not intended to diagnose, treat, cure, or prevent any disease.

Dr. Tai's Pearl

Nitric Oxide is synonymous to life itself. Ultra Intense brings you Nitric Oxide and an increase in vascular tissue perfusion that I have seen in no other product. Diabetics as well as individuals with low-circulation will be absolutely thrilled by the results that occur within thirty-minutes of taking Ultra Intense. We have literally saved life and limb because of the health giving properties of the L-Citruline in Ultra Intense.

Side Effects: None

Contraindications:
Do not use this product if you are allergic to any of its ingredients

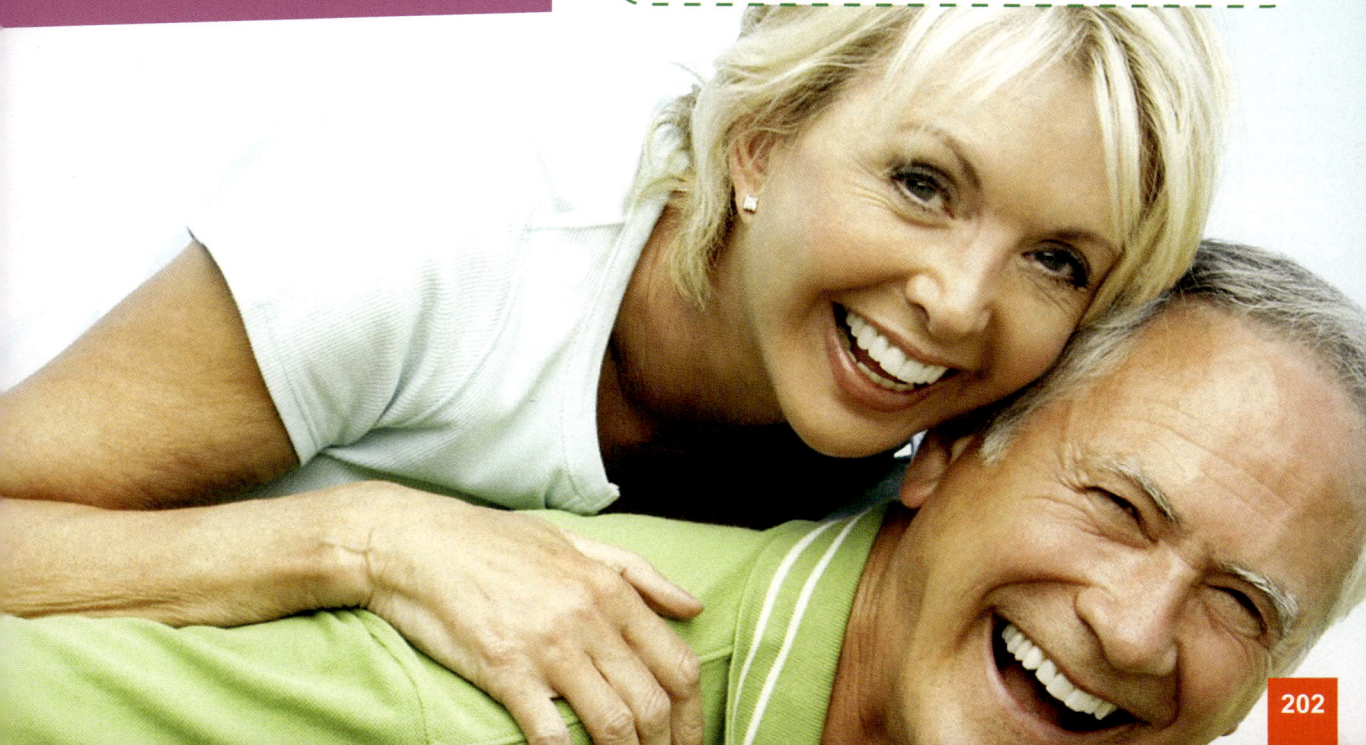

ULTRA MASCULINE

Increase Natural Testosterone

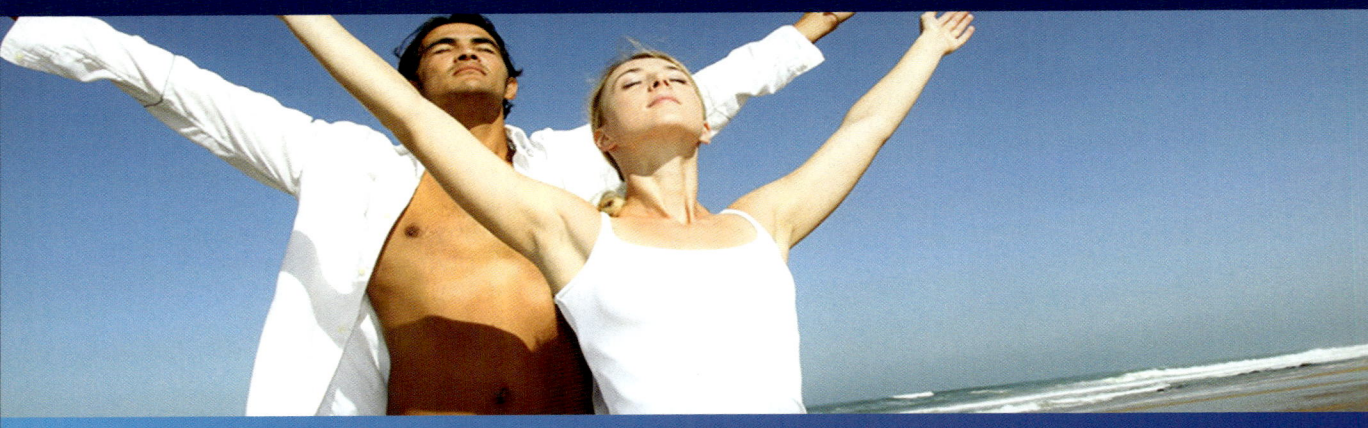

WHAT IS THE IMPORTANCE OF TESTOSTERONE?

Testosterone is a male and female sex hormone essential for sexual stimulation. In addition, testosterone stimulates metabolism, helps build muscle, increases energy and enhances mood. As a man ages, his testosterone levels decline along with all the beneficial effects of the hormone . With its decline, comes emotional instability, loss of muscle mass and decreased or no libido. Erectile Dysfunction, or ED, affects about 30 million men in the United States and is a common health problem.

What can be used to Treat Andropause and Testosterone Deficiency?

In a recent study in the **British Journal of Sports Medicine by Hamzah, S., and Yusof, A., in 2003,** the beneficial effects of eurycoma are impressive. This exceptional ingredient has resulted in increased levels of testosterone in the blood, improved sexual function and increased psychological parameters including mood, energy and a sense of well-being. One of the most significant improvements was the increase in the libido of men and it had given fertility to men that had seemed infertile. Calcium fructoborate, present in fruits, gives an **increase of 12% in testosterone levels**[1] and works alongside eurycoma to quickly pack an even more favorable outcome for your body's health, vitality, increased muscle strength and endurance.[2] After treatment with Eurycoma, an increase in testosterone has ranged from **49% in a 50 year old male to 133% in a 24 year old male.**[3]

Additional Synergistic & Substantial Benefits of Eurycoma and Calcium Fructoborate

Treatment of andropause using eurycoma and calcium fructoborate raises testosterone naturally with no outsource of the hormone, therefore helping your own body produce testosterone. Eurycoma also increases the levels of DHEA and lowers SHBG leaving you with more "free testosterone" to work in your body. Eurycoma has also been proven to raise DHEA, a hormone essential for energy, vitality and youth and considered the grandfather hormone, raising levels by 47% in only a matter of three weeks.[3]   Of 49 men who had been infertile for 5 years, 11 spontaneous pregnancies from spouses had occurred during the first 6 months of a trial.[4]

- Increases blood flow
- Increases testosterone
- Increases DHEA
- Increases libido
- Increases sperm count
- Increases sexual desire
- Increases lean muscle mass
- Increases energy and vitality

Epimedium is a key-holding ingredient that has been used in Asian Medicine for Thousands of years. Only in recent decades has it been catching on in Western Culture as a performance enhancer. Often when I compose customized protocols, I like to include Epimedium for the older men who are beginning to suffer from erectile dysfunction. This is due to the icariin (ICA) in the Epimedium that has been used as a traditional Chinese treatment for ED for years.[1]

When it comes to a natural, safe ingredient for raising testosterone, Tribulus is one of the best contenders. Tribulus increases Luteinizing Hormone (LH) which can indirectly raise both testosterone blood levels and other hormones that may be wasting away with age. LH, produced in the pituitary gland, flips the testosterone switch and triggers natural production.

The use for Tribulus doesn't stop there. This wonderful, anti-aging ingredient helps in a variety of ways for a man's aging body.

- Reduces Triglycerides [2]
- Reduces Cholesterol [2,3]
- Antioxidant Properties [2,3]
- Reduces Serum Glucose Levels [3]
- Helps Hypertension [4]

Panax Ginseng is one of the most well-known herbal ingredients for a reason. It has been used in this Ultra Masculine formulation specifically for it's ability to naturally and incrementally boost nitric oxide levels. It is especially helpful due to it's characteristic of decreasing blood glucose levels in humans. When blood glucose is high, you can bet that Testosterone levels will be next to non-existant.[6]

A double blind study was performed in Korea to test the efficacy of Ginseng. The Placebo group, although enthusiastic, did not experience any changes brought on by the pills. The Ginseng group not only had significant improvement in their erection's quality, both their performance and sexual satisfaction increased compared to the placebo group. In addition, the positive effects were seen in just 8 weeks of usage.[7]

Maca Root may help as a hormone balancer and a booster for the immune system. It is a magnificent ingredient that has successfully increased fertility in both men and women. If that wasn't enough to make me include it in this formulation, I also personally experienced increased energy, memory and focus! What originally called my attention to Shilajit was a double-blind study. In this clinical trial, male volunteers between 45 and 55 were given 250 mg of purified shilajit. After taking the shilajit twice a day for 90 days, those receiving the shilajit had remarkably higher testosterone levels compared to the placebo group! With NO SIDE EFFECTS![8]

Directions:
Take 1 capsule daily for men and women. May increase the dose if needed or recommended by your health practitioner. Male athletes may take 1 capsule twice daily and may discontinue use of supplementation for one week every three weeks.

Ingredients:
Calcium Fructoborate, Tribulus Terrestris, Eurycoma Extract Std., Epimidium Extract, Panax Ginseng

These statements have not been reviewed by the FDA. This product is not intended to diagnose, treat, cure, or prevent any disease.

1. Traish, A.M., et al. "The Dark Side of Testosterone Deficiency: II. Type 2 Diabetes and Insulin Resistance." Journal of Andronology. Vol. 30, No. 1, Jan/Feb 009: 23-32 2.Talbott S, Talbott J, Negrete J, Jones M, Nichols M, and Roza J. Effect of Eurycoma longifolia Extract on Anabolic Balance During Endurance Exercise. Journal of the International Society of Sports Nutrition. 3 (1)S1-S29, 2006.
3. Hamzah, S., and Yusof, A (2003) The ergogenic effects of eurycoma longifolia jack: A pilot study. British Journal of Sports Medicine. 37:464-470.
4. M.I. Tambi, M. Kamarul Imran. Wellmen Clinic, Damai Service Hospital, Kuala Lumpur, Malaysia. Dept of Community Medicine, School of Medical Sciences, Universiti Sains Malaysia, Kbg Kerian, Kelantan. Efficacy of the 'Malaysian Ginseng', US Patented, Standardised Water Soluble Extract of Eurycoma longifolia jack in Managing Idiopathic Male Infertility

Contact our office for extended references

Dr. Tai's Pearl

It wasn't discovered until recently fruits and roots from shrubs could actually increase the testosterone level produced by your own body and have clinical effects. Traditional oral or injectable testosterone therapy causes shrinkage of the testicles in men due to negative feedback. By using this supplement to build your own testosterone, it helps also to normalize testicle size. You can normally see testicular atrophy as a side effect of drugs taken or from old age. Testosterone is very low in these older men.

Clinical Case:
47-year-old plumber noticed severe loss of muscle mass, gaining weight, fat disposition around middle and hips, low libido, and lack of energy. He was diagnosed by family physician on salivary testosterone – very low – in the lower ¼ of the normal range. Physician started in the beginning with subcutaneous pallets, injectable, and plant for 6 months and later changed to prescription Testosterone gel, applied to the testicle area. After an additional 6 months, patient noticed, and doctor confirmed on examination, testicular atrophy, as well as softening of the gland. Doctor changed to Max Andro in conjunction with the continuation with transdermal testosterone – natural, bio-identical – and recovery of the testicular size began in earnest after six weeks, improving in size and firmness well into six months.

Side Effects:
If individual takes a dose that is larger than needed by the body, the body will tell you by offering aggressive behavior, impatience, anger, excessive acne. Lowering the dose to 1 capsule every other day, or even every third day, should be very helpful.

Contraindications:
Over-masculinization, presence of active, known cancer or treatment of cancers. Competitive national/international athletes should check with the governing body of their respective athletic associations to see if the ingredients fall under the guidelines of doping. To our knowledge, there is currently no ruling against any of the ingredients. Do Not Take Product if you are allergic to any ingredients.

Dr. 911 Ultra Skin Gel

Stop Itching/Burning/Pain Immediately

Did you **burn** yourself from too much sun? Stove?
Did you have a **scrape** from a fall or playing sports?
Did you **cut** yourself in the Kitchen?

Well, you get the idea... This extraordinary gel works miracles in helping to reduce or eliminate symptoms fast. Instantaneous results! Hard to believe? I thought so... Until I tried it! It's hard to believe how much relief comes in such a small bottle!

Made with all natural High Energetic Aloe base with homeopathic Arnica, this is not your average run of the mill product, but one that has been tested clinically by doctors, dermatologists, and plastic surgeons. It works everywhere on your body – face, hands, legs, and feet!

The gel is clean and easy to apply, and is specially formulated for the extra dry conditions such as eczema and scaly problems.

Treat inflamed skin this gel to get the relief it deserves.

Try it! You will never forget it!

Dr. 911 Ultra Skin Gel can be used for:

- Skin Pain & Itch
- Sun Burn
- Acid Burn
- Cold Sores
- Diaper Rash
- Eczema
- Dermatitis
- Skin Injury

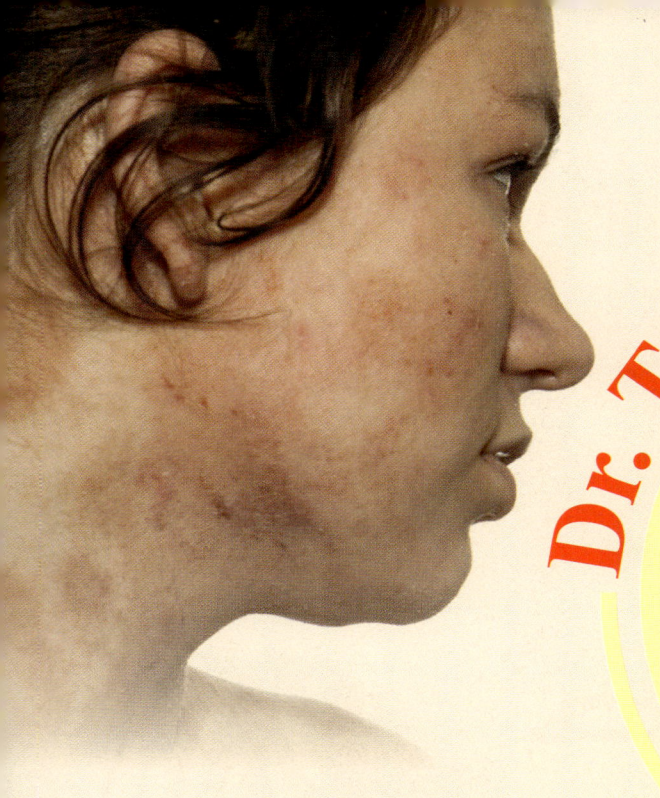

Dr. Tai's Pearl

Do I have a Secret? You bet. Last night my skin on both my arms and backs of my hands were on fire. I do not know why – but it drove me CRAZY! I was scratching to the point of bleeding and breaking skin. In desperation I reached over to the Dr. 911 Ultra Skin Gel and applied it to the affected areas. Without exaggeration – Within 30 seconds I began to feel relief! There were waves of relief where the itching and pain were disappearing and I was left with soothed skin. I quickly fell back to sleep and the night was saved! Thank you Dr. 911 Ultra Skin Gel.

Side Effects: None

Contraindications:
Do not use this product if you are allergic to any of its ingredients

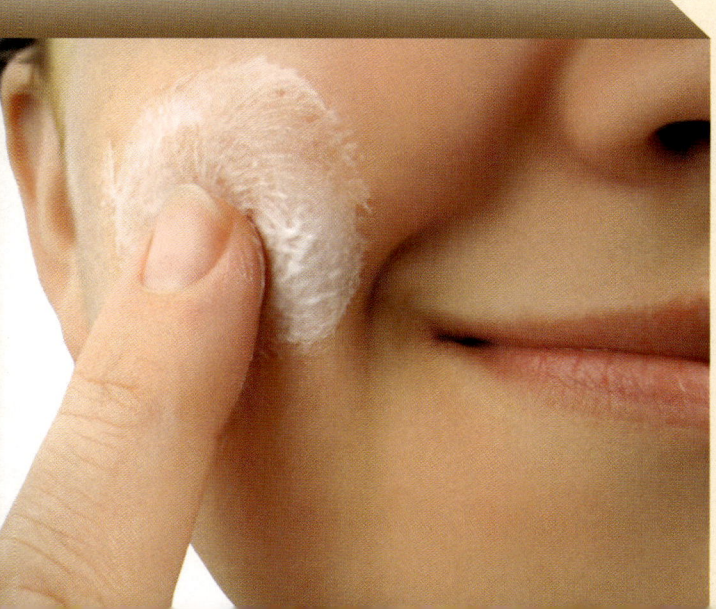

Directions:
Apply to inflamed skin area 3 times daily.

Ingredients:
Energetic Aloe Extract, Homeopathic Arnica 3C

These statements have not been reviewed by the FDA. This product is not intended to diagnose, treat, cure, or prevent any disease.

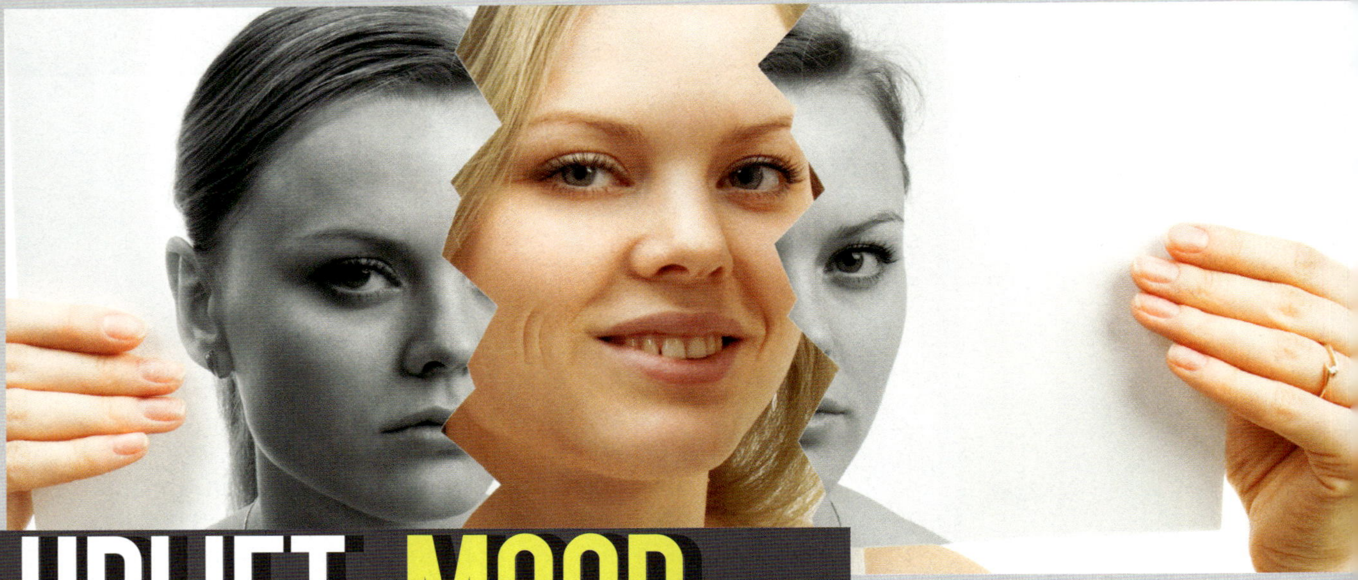

UPLIFT MOOD

Control of Depression – A severe imbalance in the brain!

Depression is a serious illness involving imbalances of the neurotransmitters in the brain. A neurotransmitter can essentially be classified as a chemical messenger, traveling through the brain to send messages from one neuron nerve cell to another. Different neurotransmitters produce different functions ranging from feelings of pleasure to increasing our ability to manage stress. An imbalance in chemical neurotransmitters leads not only to anxiety, stress, anger and depression, but also other health hazardous conditions.

List of some Neurotransmitters and Functions
- Dopamine – pleasure, attachment/love, and altruism.
- Norepinephrine – Arousal, energy, drive, stimulation and fight or flight.
- Serotonin – Emotional stability reduces aggression, sensory input, sleep cycle, appetite control.
- GABA – Controls anxiety, arousal, convulsions and keeps brain activity balanced.

Depleted serotonin has been viewed as a major cause of depression.[1] Worse yet, diminished activity of serotonin was seen in suicide victims with major depression.[2] When levels are low, symptoms may include irritability, over sensitivity to sights and sounds, increased anxiety and impulsive or abusive behavior. The ratio of dopamine and serotonin activity is very important. Keeping them balanced is the key to anxiety, worries and depression.[3]

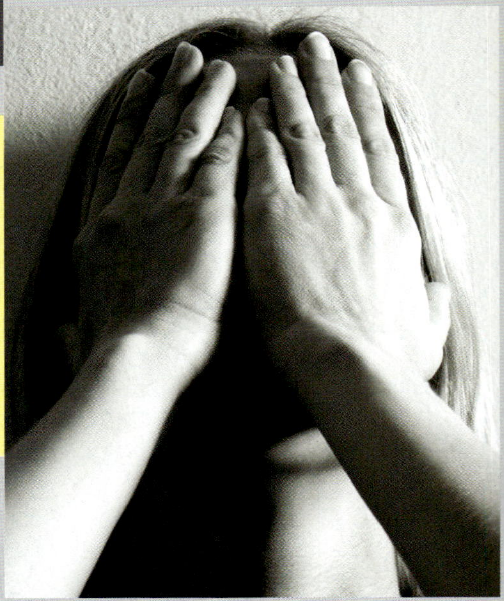

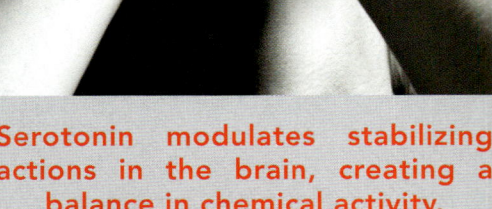

Serotonin modulates stabilizing actions in the brain, creating a balance in chemical activity, allowing those suffering from depression to be emotionally stable and serene. With sufficient amounts of serotonin, our brain is better able to approach stressful situations and determine if there is a threat present in a more logical manner.

Uplift Mood consists of selected plant extracts of wheat grass, corn, bamboo and other young grass leaves by a proprietary patent-pending process. Many studies at renowned research centers such as the University of Utah and Rhodes University indicate the extracts to be safe with no known side effects. It has been shown to improve mood, feelings of well-being, and help coping with stress, as they are a precursors to serotonin.

Dosage is the Key! Dosage may need to be adjusted to individual needs. After beginning intake, dosage may be increased given individual circumstances and beneficial effects for each individual.

People who have used Serotonin Adaptogens are reporting the following benefits:

- **Enhanced mood & energy**
- **Better mental focus**
- **Improved sleeping patterns**
- **Lessened anxiety**
- **Heightened self confidence**

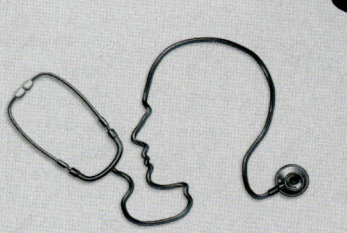

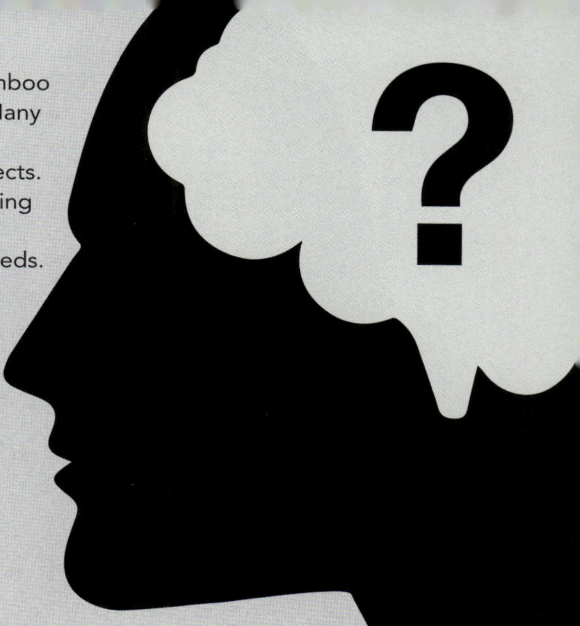

"I finally found a natural supplement worthy of my praise. I've tried everything from St. Johns wort, 5HTP, Rhodiola, sceletium, valerian, passion flower, tryptophan, l-theanine, picamilon, and in my opinion none of these compare to the benefits I've been getting. My anxiety is about 90% gone and my moderate depression is almost nonexistent. I was wary at first but decided what the heck, I've tried everything else. It started working the first day I took it. I highly recommend this product if you have serotonin problems."

Directions:
Take 1-2 full droppers twice daily. Dosage must be adjusted for individual needs. Consult with your health care professional.

Ingredients:
Cordyceps Extract, Grass Leaf Extract, Virgin Coconut Oil, Mint Flavors, Stevia

These statements have not been reviewed by the FDA. This product is not intended to diagnose, treat, cure, or prevent any disease.

1. Arthur J. Prange, Jr., of the University of North Carolina at Chapel Hill, Alec Coppen of the Medical Research Council in England. 1960

2. Stockmeier CA, Shapiro LA, Dilley GE, Kolli TN, Friedman L, Rajkowska G. Increase in serotonin-1A autoreceptors in the midbrain of suicide victims with major depression-postmortem evidence for decreased serotonin activity. J Neurosci. 1998 Sep 15;18(18):7394-401.

3. H. Soderstrom, K. Blennow, A-K Sjodin, and A. Forsman. New evidence for an association between the CSF HVA:5-HIAA ratio and psychopathic traits. Journal of Neurology, Neurosurgery and Psychiatry, Vol. 74, 2003, 918-21.

Dr. Tai's Pearl
Anti-Depressants are by nature, also depressants. This is not double-talk - it is well researched that when you are taking anti-depressants you may actually have lower serotonin levels at the end of your treatment than you did in the beginning! Therefore, anti-depressants must be constantly changed after time to continue to have significant value and provide the desired therapeutic effects. However, Depression Specialist is very different because of its natural ability to cross the brain-barrier to provide a sense of peace and hope that is often stolen away by depression. I love this product for the natural and soothing way of which it approaches Depression – Gentle and Steady without interfering with other medications.

Side Effects: None

Contraindications:
Do not take if you are allergic to any ingredients. Can be used together with anti-depressant medication.

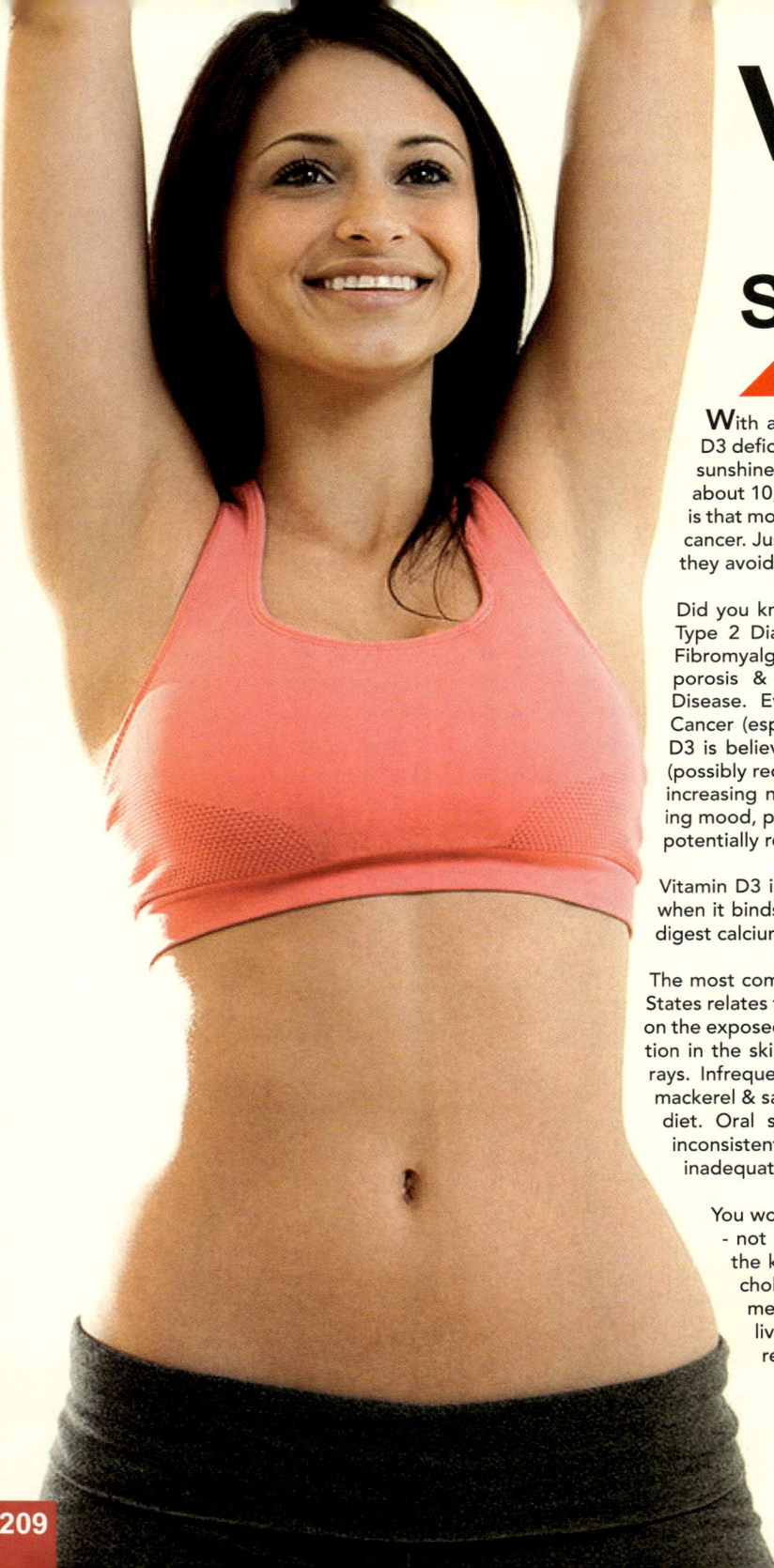

Vitamin D3-K2 Specialist

Most POWERFUL Vitamin Combinatio

With all the medical advances in the 20th century, Vitami D3 deficiency is still an epidemic. Fifteen to twenty minutes sunshine each day, in the nude, helps your body manufactu about 10,000 to 15,000 iu's of vitamin D3 per day. The proble is that most people avoid the sun these days due to fears of ski cancer. Just think about plants and what happens to them whe they avoid the sun. They wither & die.

Did you know that vitamin D3 deficiency can result in Obesit Type 2 Diabetes, High Blood Pressure, Depression, Psoriasi Fibromyalgia, Chronic Fatigue Syndrome, Kidney Stones, Oste porosis & Neuro-degenerative disease including Alzheimer Disease. Eventually, Vitamin D deficiency may even lead t Cancer (especially breast, prostate, and colon cancers). Vitami D3 is believed to play a role in controlling the immune syste (possibly reducing one's risk of cancer and autoimmune disease increasing neuro-muscular function and decreasing falls, impro ing mood, protecting the brain against toxic chemicals, and potentially reducing pain.

Vitamin D3 is both a vitamin and a hormone. It acts as a vitam when it binds with calcium for proper absorption. Humans cann digest calcium without adequate amounts of Vitamin D3.

The most common reasons for Vitamin D3 deficiency in the Unite States relates to lack of exposure to sunlight. High utilization of SF on the exposed areas for skin protection prevents Vitamin D produ tion in the skin. Vitamin D is only produced in the skin from UV rays. Infrequent consumption of cold water fish such as wild salmo mackerel & sardines are the only good sources of Vitamin D for o diet. Oral supplementation of Vitamin D3 proves to be ve inconsistent in absorption from the GI tract resulting inadequate serum levels.

You won't get sufficient D3, technically a hormone precurs - not a vitamin, from foods. Sunlight and supplements a the keys. The sun's UBV rays on exposed skin mixes wi cholesterol, yes cholesterol, in your skin to start a series metabolic biochemical changes that culminate in yo liver and kidneys to produce D3 for those VDR receptors.

When you take natural animal or plant based suppl ments, you bypass the sunlight exposure phase th creates the vitamin D3 precursor. Instead, you g naturally derived precursors that go directly in the liver and kidneys for processing.

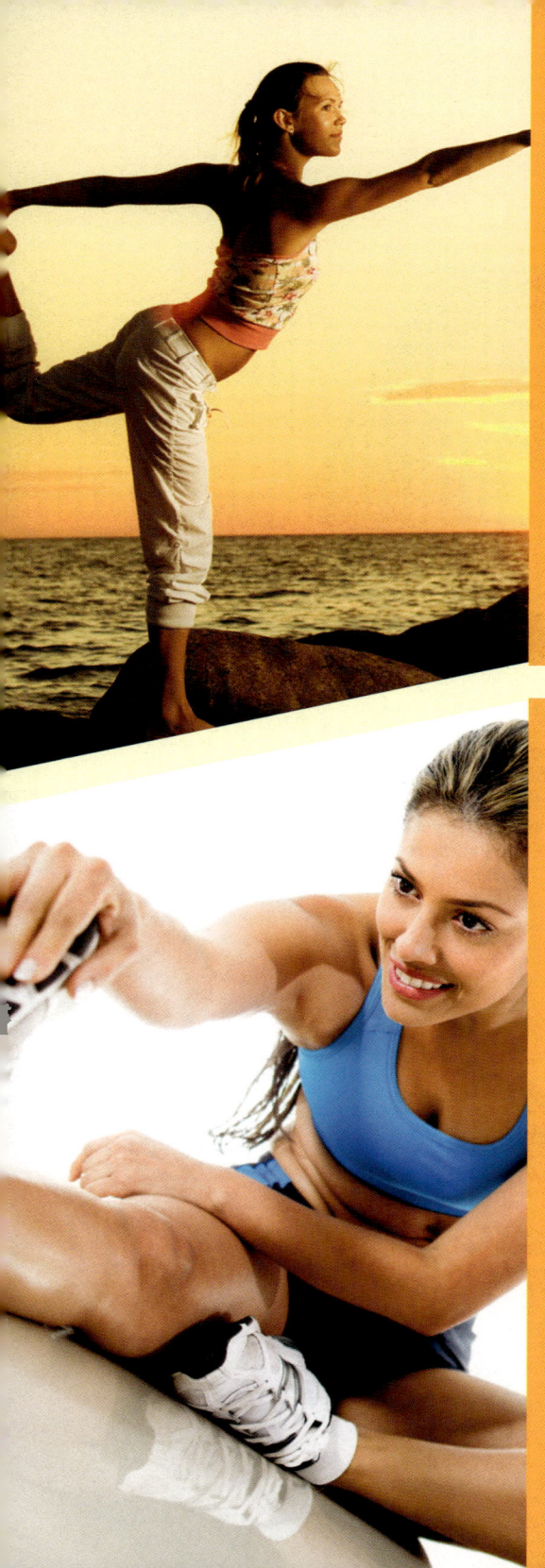

The health benefits of D3 are numerous, from preventing or reversing Alzheimer's (with curcumin), cancer, and minor flus and colds. It is an anti-inflammatory compound and immune system regulator that increases or decreases the immune system as needed.

Vitamin K is a fat-soluble vitamin required for blood coagulation and metabolic pathways in bone and other tissue. The group of vitamins known as Vitamin K actually consists of two natural vitamers: vitamin K1 and vitamin K2[3]. Vitamin K is essential for normal cell formation and maintenance of a healthy cardiovascular system.

Vitamin K, known as phylloquinone, are found in the highest amounts in green leafy vegetables because it is directly involved in photosynthesis. Animals may also convert it to vitamin K2, also called menaquinones. Menaquinone-4 (MK-4) has four isoprene residues & is the most common type of vitamin K2 in animals as well as the most studied.

Bacteria in the colon (large intestine) converts K1 into vitamin K2, lengthening the isopreneoid side chain of vitamin K2 and produce forms MK-7 & MK-11.

Vitamins K3, K4 & K5 are all synthetic types of vitamin K. K3 (menadione) has shown toxicity[4], while K4 & K5 have been discovered to be non-toxic.

Conversion of Vitamin K1 in the testes, pancreas, and arterial walls results in vitamin K2[5]. Conversion is not dependent on gut bacteria[6,7].

Mk-7 consumption reduces the risk of bone fractures and cardiovascular disorders. MK-7 may be converted from phylloquinone (k1) in the colon by E. coli bacteria[8]. Mk-4 has been shown to decrease the incidence of fractures up to 87%[9]. For the prevention and treatment of Osteoporosis, the Ministry of Health in Japan has approved 45mg of MK-4 daily[10]. Vitamin K2 exerts a more powerful influence on bone than does vitamin K1.

Vitamin K2 as MK-4 prevents bone loss and/or fractures:

- Caused by corticosteroids (e.g., prednisone, dexamethasone, prednisolone)[11,12,13,14]
- Anorexia nervosa,[15]
- Cirrhosis of the liver,[16]
- Post Menopause Osteoporosis,[10,17,18,19,20,21]
- Disuse from Stroke,[22]
- Alzheimer's disease,[23]
- Parkinson disease,[24]
- Primary biliary cirrhosis,[25]
- Leuprolide treatment,[26]

In animals, the carboxylation of certain glutamate residues in proteins to form gamma-carboxy glutamate (Gla) residues involves Vitamin K. Gla residues, involved in binding calcium, are essential for the biological activity of all known Gla proteins27.

210

Recommended Amounts:
Vitamin K for a 25-year old male is 120 micrograms (μg) daily.
Adult women is 90 μg/day.

Food sources of vitamin K2 include fermented or aged cheeses, eggs, meat such as chicken and beef and their fat, livers, and organs, and in fermented vegetables, especially natto, as well as sauerkraut and kefir[46].

We have discovered an increased prevalence of vitamin K deficiency in those who suffer from liver damage or disease and cystic fibrosis. Secondary vitamin K deficiency occurs with bulimics, stringent diets, and taking anticoagulants, salicylates, barbiturates, and cefamandole. Deficiency can result in coagulopathy (a severe bleeding disorder)[47].

Vitamin K2's function in the animal cells is the addition of a carboxylic acid functional group to a glutamate amino acid residue in a protein - forming a gamma-carboxyglutamate (Gla) residue, or "Gla protein". This protein allows it to chelate calcium ion. This binding of calcium ion triggers the function of Gla-protein enzymes like vitamin K dependent clotting factors.

Within the cell vitamin K undergoes electron reduction to reduced form called vitamin K hydroquinone by the enzyme vitamin K epoxide reductase (VKOR)[48]. Vitamin K hydroquinone then oxidizes and allows carboxylation of Glu to Gla resulting in the enzyme gamma-glutaml carboxylase – or – vitamin K-dependent carboxylase[49, 50]. Carboxylation reaction only proceeds if the carboxylase enzyme is able to oxidize vitamin K hydroquinone to vitamin K epoxide. Carboxylation and epoxidation reactions are coupled. Vitamin K epoxide is then reconverted to vitamin K by VKOR. Reduction and reoxidation of vitamin K, coupled with carboxylation of Glu is called the vitamin K cycle[51]. Vitamin K1 is continuously recycled in cell making a deficiency extremely rare[52].

Gla domains have been discovered in 16 different human proteins and play key roles in the regulatin of three physiological processes:
- Blood coagulation: prothrombin (factor II), factors VII, IX, and X, and proteins C, S, and Z.[28]
- Bone metabolism: osteocalcin, also called bone Gla protein (BGP), matrix Gla protine (MGP)[29], periostin[30], and the recently discovered Gla-rich protein (GRP)[31,32]
- Vascular biology: growth arrest-specific protein 6 (Gas6)[33]
- Unknown function: proline-rich g-carboxy glutamyl proteins (PRGPs) 1 and 2, and transmembrane g-carboxy glutamyl proteins (TMGs) 3 and 4.[34] Vitamin K, a lipid-soluble vitamin, is stored in the fat tissue of the human body. When the intestine (small bowel) is heavily damaged resulting in malabsorption of the molecule, it can result in a rare dietary deficiency. Risk group for this deficiency were subject to decreased production of K2 by normal intestinal microbiota, seen in broad spectrum antibiotic use[35]. Broad-spectrum antibiotics reduces vitamin K production by 74%[36]. Diets low in vitamin K decrease the body's vitamin K concentration[37]. Chronic kidney disease increases the risks of Vitamin K deficiency, as well as vitamin D deficiency, especially those with the apoE4 genotype[38]. The Elderly will also experience a reduction in vitamin K2 production[39].

Research demonstrates that the small intestine and the large intestine (colon) seem inefficient at absorbing vitamin K supplements[40,41]. This is reinforced by human cohort studies where subjects showed inadequate vitamin K. The presence of large amounts of incomplete gamma-carboxylated proteins in the blood, which is primarily an indirect test for vitamin K deficiency[42, 43, 44]. Animal Model MK-4 prevented arterial calcifications, showing potential to prevent other such calcifications[45]. Vitamin K1 was tested & connected to vitamin K1 intake and calcification reduction. Only vitamin K2 influenced warfarin-induced calcification.

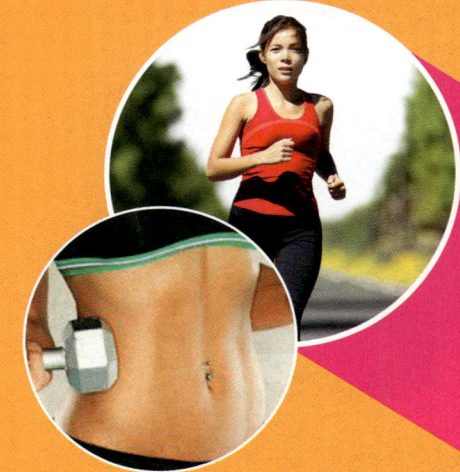

Vitamin D3-K2 Specialist

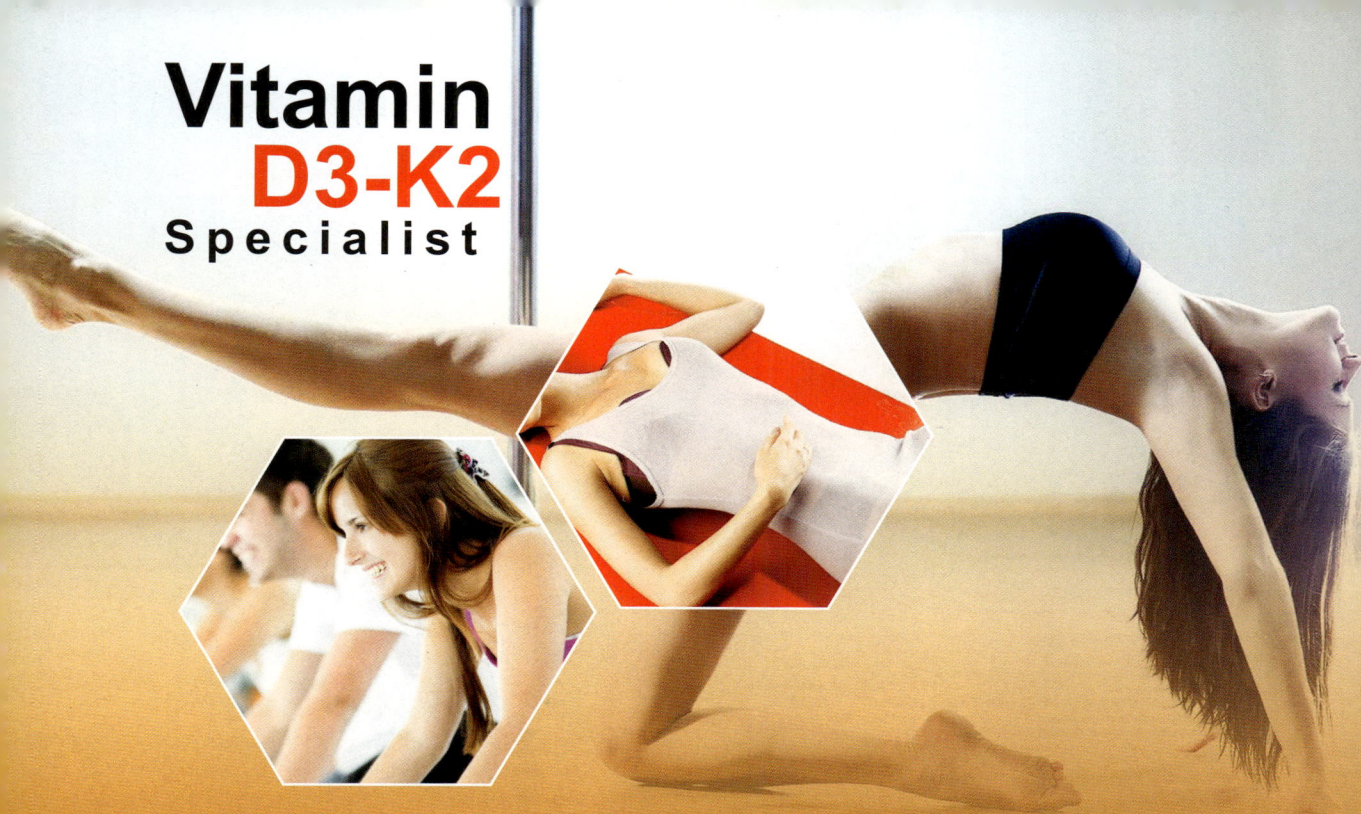

Warfarin blocks the action of the VKOR[53]. As a result, the carboxylation reaction catalyzed by the glutamyl carboxylase is inefficient. In turn the production of clotting factors will have inadequate GLA. Without GLA on the amino termini they no longer have binding stability to the blood vessel endothelium, and cannot activate clotting to allow formation of a clot during tissue injury.

Vitamin K status assessed:

The prothrombin time (PT) test measures the time required for blood to clot[54]. Biophysical studies suggest that supplemental vitamin K promotes osteoblastic processes and slow osteoclastic processes. Atkins et al[55] revealed menatetrenone (MK-4) promote mineralization by human primary osteoblasts. Vitamin D is reported to regulate the OC transcription by osteoblast, showing that vitamin K and vitamin D work in tandem for the bone metabolism and development. Lian discovered two nucleotide substitution regions they named "osteocalcin box" in the rat and human osteocalcin genes[56].

The 1998 Nurses Health Study indicates an inverse relationship between dietary vitamin K1 and the risk of hip fracture. 110 micrograms/day of Vitamin K significantly lowered the risk of hip fractures in women. The Framingham Heart Study showed subjects in the highest quartile of vitamin K1 intake (254 µg/day) had 35% lower risk of hip fracture[57]. 254 µg/day is above the US Daily Reference Intake (DRI) of 90 µg/day for women and 120ug/day for men.

Menoaquinone-7 (MK-7) stimulates osteoblastic bone formation and inhibits osteoclastic bone resorption[58]. MK-7 also inhibited the bone-resorbing factors parathyroid hormone and prostaglandin E2[59]. February 19, 2011, HSA (Singapore) approved a health supplement that contains vitamin K2 (MK-7) and vitamin D3 for increasing bone mineral density[60].

Vitamin K2 (MK-7) and Coronary Heart Disease

Gast et al. (2009), [61] reported "an inverse association between vitamin K(2) and risk of CHD with a Hazard Ratio (HR) of 0.91." Authors concluded that " a high intake of menoquinones, especially MK-7, MK-8 and MK-9, could protect against CHD.

Vitamin K2 (MK-7) and Alzheimer's Disease

Antioxidant properties of vitamin K show the concentration of vitamin K is lower in the circulation of carriers of the APOE4 gene. These properties also show the ability to inhibit nerve cell death due to oxidative stress. Vitamin K may reduce neuronal damage, benefitting the treatment of Alzheimer's disease[62].

Vitamin K may be applied topically and has been shown when applied to help treat broken capillaries (spider veins), rosacea, and to aid in the fading of hyperpigmentation and dark under-eye circles[63, 64].

After studying 21 women with viral liver cirrhosis, it was found that women in the group with supplementation of vitamin K2 as (MK-4) were 90% less likely to develop liver cancer[65, 66]. A German Study found a significant inverse relationship between vitamin K2 consumption and advanced prostate cancer[67].

In 2006, a clinical trial discovered K2 as the menaquinone-4 (MK-4) was able to reduce the recurrence of liver cancer[68].

Diabetes risk was 51% lower in the highest circulating levels of vitamin K & showed a reduced risk of type 2 diabetes[69].

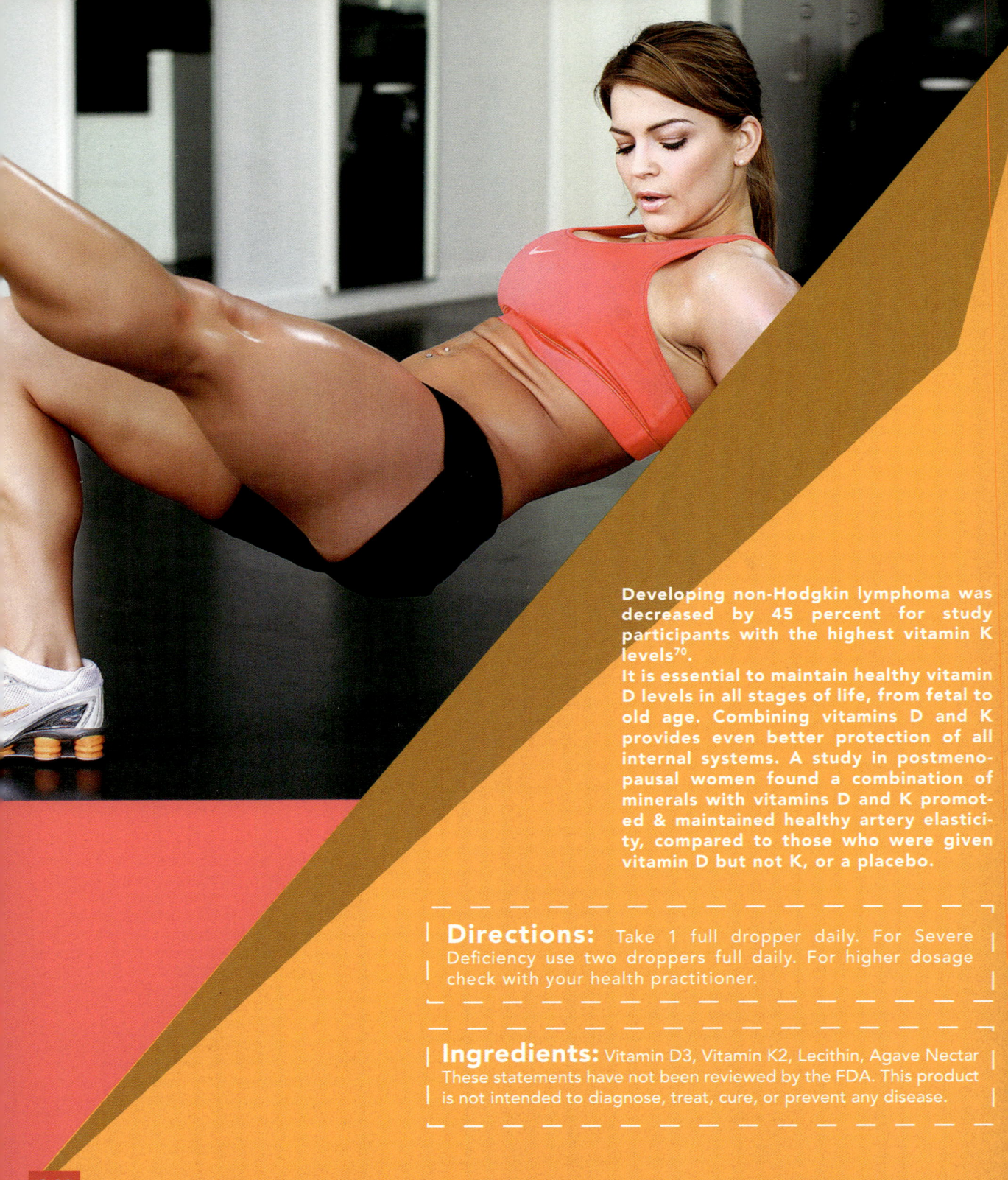

Developing non-Hodgkin lymphoma was decreased by 45 percent for study participants with the highest vitamin K levels[70].

It is essential to maintain healthy vitamin D levels in all stages of life, from fetal to old age. Combining vitamins D and K provides even better protection of all internal systems. A study in postmenopausal women found a combination of minerals with vitamins D and K promoted & maintained healthy artery elasticity, compared to those who were given vitamin D but not K, or a placebo.

Directions: Take 1 full dropper daily. For Severe Deficiency use two droppers full daily. For higher dosage check with your health practitioner.

Ingredients: Vitamin D3, Vitamin K2, Lecithin, Agave Nectar
These statements have not been reviewed by the FDA. This product is not intended to diagnose, treat, cure, or prevent any disease.

Vitamin D3 - Clinical Applications:

1. Are you getting enough Vitamin D3?, P. Egan et.al
2. Are stress and high cortisol depleting your vitamin D?, PF Louis, Natural News.com, September 3, 2012
3. Dam H. (1935). "The Antihaemorrhagic Vitamin of the Chick.: Occurrence And Chemical Nature". Nature 135 (3417): 652-653. doi: 10.1038/135652b0
4. Higdon (February 2008). "Vitamin K". Linus Pauling Institute, Oregon State University. Retrieved 12 April 2008.
5. Newman P., Shearer MJ; Newman, Paul (2008). "Metabolism and cell biology of vitamin K". Thrombosis and Haemostasis: 530-547. Doi: 10.1160/TH08-03-0147.
6. Davidson, RT; Foley AL, Engelke JA, Sutie JW (1998) " Conversion of Dietary Phylloquinone to Tissue Menaquinone-4 in Rates is Not Dependent on Gut Bacteria1". Journal of Nutrition 128 (2): 220-223. PMID 9446847
7. Ronden, JE; Drittij-Reijnders M-J, Vermeer C, Thijssen HHW. (1998). "Intestinal flora is not an intermediate in the phylloquinone-menaquinone-4 conversion in the rat". Biochimica et Biophysica Acta (BBA) – General Subjects 1379 (1): 69-75. Doi: 10.1016/S0304-4165(97)00089-5. PMID 9468334
8. Vermeer, C; Braam L (2001). "Role of K vitamins in the regulation of tissue calcification". Journal of bone and mineral metabolism 19 (4): 201-206. Doi:10.1007/s007740170021. PMID 11448011
9. Sato, Y; Kanoko T, Satoh K, Iwamoto J (2005). "Menatrenone and vitamin D2 with calcium supplements prevent nonvertebral fracture in elderly women with Alzheimer's disease". Bone 36 (1): 61-8. Doi: 10.1016/j.bone.2004.09.018. PMID 15664003
10. Iwamoto, I; Kosha S, Noguchi S-1 (1999). " A longitudinal study of the effect of vitamin K2 on bone mineral density in postmenopausal women a comparative study with vitamin D2 and estrogen-progestin therapy". Maturitas 31 (2): 161-164. Doi: 10.1016/S0378-5122(98)00114-5. PMID 10227010

Dr. Tai's Pearl

After many years of research and studying deficiencies of the body, I have come to learn one very startling fact: The body will very rarely have a single deficiency. It is much more likely that the deficiencies are complex and multiple. If we have a deficiency of Vitamin D3, which is known as an epidemic all over the world, we certainly also have a deficiency of Vitamin K2. I say this because research shows we know very little about Vitamin K2. We used to think of it as being involved in only coagulation but we now know it is extremely powerful and essential for thousands of biochemical reactions and our nutritional metabolism that bodies depend on. I was so excited to be able to create a German Lyposome Vitamin D3 and K2 together so that we may wipe out these severe epidemic deficiencies — one such benefit is improvement & reversal of Osteoporosis - with one stroke, one product, where they work synergistically with each other to enhance absorption and benefits that you may derive from Vitamins D3 and K2.

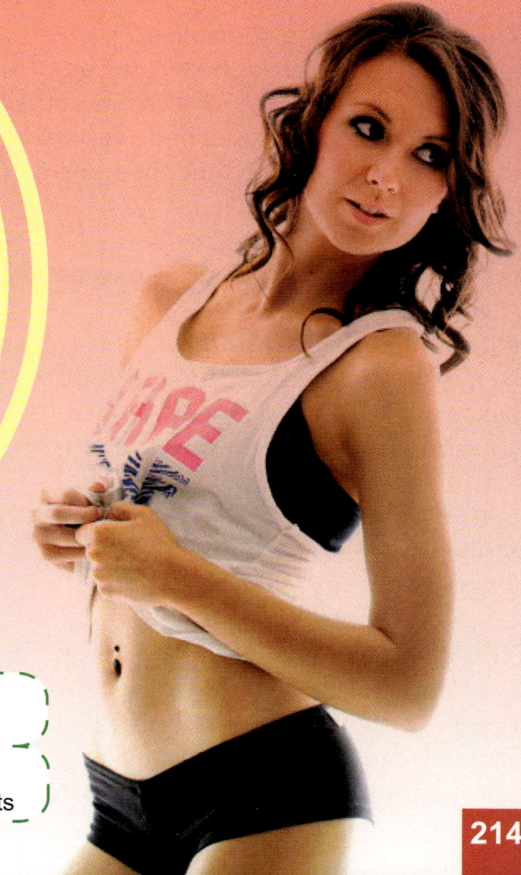

Side Effects: None

Contraindications:
Do not use this product if you are allergic to any of its ingredients

Water Specialist

Come to your KIDNEY'S Rescue!

Do you wake up with swollen eyelids?
Are your ankles so swollen you cannot see your toes?
Having problems just removing your wedding ring from your finger?

These changes to your body are all special signs and symptoms of not only water retention, but failing Kidneys. These changes can be hormonal, such as a lack progesterone, but could also be caused by sluggish kidneys and toxified from poor diet and environmental chemicals.

When the food that you eat breaks down, it leaves waste that accumulates in your blood. Removing this excess waste from the blood and balancing electrolytes is essential to sustaining life. Electrolytes like Potassium and Magnesium are frantically running around your body in order to help keep YOU in balance.

The Kidneys are a specialized pair of organs in your body that sit slightly above mid-waist. They are connected through two tubes of ureters going down to the bladder and out of your body through the urethra. Kidneys are actually large organs made up of tiny little kidneys inside. These "smaller kidneys" are called Nephrons. There are at least 1 million tiny little nephrons inside of every single kidney, connected to small capillary blood vessels that run directly from your arteries and veins.

Kidneys produce three essential hormones that are made nowhere else in the body.[1]

#1 is called **Erythropoietin**. This is a special hormone that stimulates all of the flat bones in your body to manufacture the red blood cells that carry the oxygen from your lungs to enrich your tissues. **#2** is called **Renin**, whose importance lies in its job of regulating the blood pressure in your body. **#3**, the last and the most important, is a vitamin that is made active only in the kidney – and this is **Vitamin D3**. Although Vitamin D2 is commonly supplemented, the forms that you take by mouth are NOT ACTIVE. Vitamin D is only activated after ingestion & absorption. The Kidneys are where Vitamin D3 finally "clocks in for work" and continues on to maintain the minerals in your body, such as Calcium that aids in bone health!

You may not have drawn the connection between extreme Stress, periods of P.M.S., or Allergic reactions from pollen, pets, or food. During these difficult periods, your kidneys react by slowing down. When this happens, the extra fluid that is usually excreted is backed up into your blood stream, causing you to swell. In every instance your body becomes uncomfortable, puffy and unrecognizable. What you mark off as 'just a little fluff' or 'puffiness' can actually be a very serious emergency flare, signaling that *something is not right*.

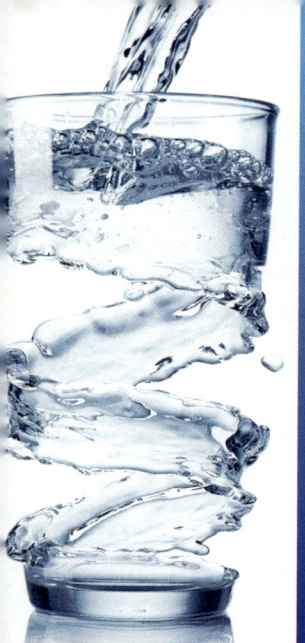

Your blood vessels can only hold a set volume of fluid. The excess fluid overflows into the lymphatic vessels. These vessels actually work together with all the tissues in your entire body. When the kidneys aren't working properly, the lymphatics are backed up and all the excess swelling goes to the foot, ankle and legs during the day when you are most active. Although it appears harmless, swelling causes major complications around your foot and ankle. In some cases, swelling has been so severe that the ankle can get to be the size of a thigh. As the swelling increases, the skin, blood vessels and nerves are all breaking down – creating major ulcers and complications that can threaten your life.

Early in the morning when you stumble out of bed and into your bathroom, you can clearly see the state of your lymphatics when you look into your mirror. Those bags under your eyes aren't designer, they're a result of the excess fluid accumulated in your face. You touch them and go to inspect, only to realize that your hands are so swollen that you may not be able to remove your wedding ring. You now have two warning signs that your kidneys are not up to par. If you wait for a third, you could be dealing with Kidney Disease.

I've created an extraordinarily important supplement to keep your kidneys functioning at their peak.

Water Specialist is gentle, yet extremely powerful, comprised of several important natural herbs:

Asparagus – When organically grown, Asparagus acts as a special, natural extract that detoxes the kidneys. It is wonderful not only to cleanse the kidneys, but the liver as well as the spleen. Because of its ability to rejuvenate major organs, it is also very important to the foundation of your immunity. By cleaning your blood system and removing all of the excess toxins, your immunity is given a special grace to be able to spend all of it its time neutralizing and attacking the Cancer cells, viruses, bacteria and funguses that are growing in your body. Asparagus extract is essential to lowering the stress put on your cardiovascular system. Therefore, it is especially important to those individuals who have a family history of Cardiovascular Disease and Stroke. Asparagus has natural micro minerals that are excellent for the tissues of your body. These micro minerals include Selenium, Zinc, Organic Folic Acid, Asparaginase, Asparamide, Histone, and other microscopic elements that are essential to the health and strengthening of your kidneys, liver, and body. Asparaginase is a special SUPER enzyme that the body uses to cleanse the kidneys as well as kill Cancer Cells that are present in the blood system, such as Lymphocytic Leukemia, Hodgkin's Lymphoma, Non-Hodgkin's Cancer, etc. Cancer Cells depend on Aspargine, an amino acid that is produced from Aspartic acid, to grow into a mass. Asparaginase comes in on horseback, saving your body by breaking down Asparagines and putting a stop to unwanted cell growth.

Of course, Asparagus Extract is also a wonderful source of Glutathione. As you all know, Glutathione is one of the most important and essential antioxidants in the human body, without which we cannot live and a myriad of diseases would be free to deteriorate our bodies. As we grow older our bodies produce less and less Glutathione! We are SAVED by Asparagus Extract, restoring us to Optimum Glutathione levels that fend off disease and protect our organs.

I created this very specific formula for the extraordinary rejuvenation of your kidneys. **Water Specialist** begins working immediately at cleaning your Blood System and strengthening your body with a healthy and more powerful immune system. For added protection, I've added a wonderful tree from the Amazon Rainforest. This Herb, called **Chuchuhuasi** is a key indigenous herb from the Natives which used Chuchuhuasi for rejuvenation of the body and combating Arthritis, Rheumatism and Back Pain. Chuchuhuasi can be found as a popular drink in the Amazon that they call **"The GO Juice"** because it keeps you going with boundless energy. Chuchuhuasi is a tonic that helps to speed up healing as it cleanses your kidneys and rejuvenates your liver. We now know that the Chuchuhuasi plant is extremely potent in triterpenes, flavonoids and very special herbal Catechin that can help to rejuvenate your body and create a powerful anti-inflammatory and an anti-algesic affect. Much of the research published in the United States as well as Japan shows that Chuchuhuasi is a wonderful anti-inflammatory, anti-arthritic as well as anti-tumor for the rejuvenation of the body. It is wonderful to help relax your muscles, stops menstrual abnormalities and has a powerful effect on hormonal disorders and imbalances in women as well as men while also being a powerful helper to the adrenal glands.

In this formula's extraordinary combination, I've also included the famed **Poria Mushroom**. Poria is an exotic mushroom from Asia that has been scientifically proven to help people who suffer from fatigue, urinary fluid retention, kidney disorders, insomnia, or spleen problems. The publications both in the Chemical Pharmaceuticals in Tokyo, as well as the Herbal Journals in China, have shown that Poria is extremely powerful in helping with rejuvenation of the kidney, anti-inflammatory, and improving immunity.

Water Specialist was designed especially for those of you who suffer from that painful and uncomfortable Swelling of the Ankle & Leg, Swelling in the face, Hangovers, Diabetes, Hypertensive Complications, Kidney Problems, Sluggishness, Water Retention, Liver Complications & Low Immunity.
Water Specialist was also designed with those individuals suffering from Heart Disease and High Cholesterol in mind.

Directions:
Take 1 capsule 3 times daily. You may take higher or more frequent dosages as needed or recommended by your health practitioner.

Ingredients:
Proprietary Formula - Asparagus Ext., Chuchuhuasei, Poria Ext., Lobelia Ext.

These statements have not been reviewed by the FDA. This product is not intended to diagnose, treat, cure, or prevent any disease.

Dr. Tai's Pearls:

Maria Teresa said to me in tears:
"When I looked in the mirror that morning and saw my face swollen almost beyond recognition, I knew it wasn't just water retention, it was a cry out from my kidneys for an effective detox."

I meet many patients that exhibit all the signs of a toxic circulatory system. It is often overlooked that we have waste accumulating in our blood. From our poor diet to environmental chemicals, the majority of us cannot naturally filter these super-toxins in our over-worked kidneys without a little nutritional help.

Water Specialist is a winning combination of Asparagus, Chuchuhuasi and Poria Mushroom that not only rejuvenates the kidney, but battles against inflammation that comes from toxic-buildup in the body.

An additional little known secret not even your doctor will tell you...
If you want a little extra fast water removal, use Progesterone Lyposome cream on your body, rubbing vigorously on the skin along with taking Water Specialist capsules for the Best Natural Dynamic Duo against toxic water retention EVER!

Mission accomplished!!
Without all those synthetic drugs prescriptions that cause horrible side effects.

Clinical Case:
67-year-old Dr. Charles P. is a pediatric physician who battled Chronic Kidney Failure for a number of years. He attempted multiple prescription drugs at the hand of his physician, but his condition continued to deteriorate with rising BUN and excess proteinuria in his urine analysis. In true "kidney-failure-fashion", Dr. Charles quickly noticed that his ankles had started to swell, his regular morning puffiness had gotten out of hand, and his blood pressure was more and more difficult to control with the drugs he was presently taking. Dr. Charles began a protocol composed of Water Specialist, Lung Specialist, Ionic Micro Minerals & Max Performance in Higher doses. Within three months he saw a marked improvement and within six months he was seeing a return to a normal BUN and diminishing proteinuria. Extremely happy with the results, he swore to me that Water Specialist was a miracle supplement.

Side Effects: None

Contraindications:
Do not take if you are allergic to any of the ingredients. Those with Gout should **NOT** take **Water Specialist**, as the Asparagus Extract may increase uric acid.

REFERENCES

1. "The National Institute of Diabetes and Digestive and Kidney Diseases of The National Institutes of Health. Your Kidneys and How They Work. NIH Publication: 98-4241. March 1998. Last updated April 8, 1998. (Online) http://www.niddk.nih.gov/health/ kidney/pubs/yourkids/index.htm
2. Human Physiology: From Cells to Systems, by Lauralee Sherwood
3. Gullett NP, Ruhul Amin AR, Bayraktar S et al. Cancer prevention with natural compounds. Semin Oncol. 2010 Jun;37(3):258-81. Review. 2010.
4. Phillips KM, Rasor AS, Ruggio DM et al. Folate content of different edible portions of vegetables and fruits. Nutrition and Food Science. Bradford: 2008. Vol. 38, Iss. 2; pg. 175. 2008.
5. Jones DP, Coates RJ, Flagg EW et al. Glutathione in foods listed in the National Cancer Institute's Health Habits and History Food Frequency Questionnaire. Nutr Cancer. 1992;17(1):57-75. 1992.
6. Pompella, A; Visvikis, A; Paolicchi, A; Tata, V; Casini, AF (2003). "The changing faces of glutathione, a cellular protagonist". Biochemical Pharmacology 66 (8): 1499–503. doi:10.1016/S0006-2952(03)00504-5. PMID 14555227
7. Gonzalez, J. G., et al. "Chuchuhuasha—a drug used in folk medicine in the Amazonian and Andean areas. A chemical study of Maytenus laevis." J. Ethnopharm. 1982; 5: 73–7
8. Morita, H., et al. "Triterpenes from Brazilian medicinal plant "chuchuhuasi" (Maytenus krukovii)." J. Nat. Prod. 1996; 59(11): 1072-75.
9. Bruni, R., et al. "Antimutagenic, antioxidant and antimicrobial properties of Maytenus krukovii bark." Fitoterapia. 2006 Dec; 77(7-8): 538-45.
10. Shao Y, Chin CK, Ho CT et al. Anti-tumor activity of the crude saponins obtained from asparagus. Cancer Lett. 1996 Jun 24;104(1):31-6. 1996.
11. Cuellar MJ, Giner RM, Recio MC, et al. Effect of the basidiomycete Poria cocos on experimental dermatitis and other inflammatory conditions. Chem Pharm Bull (Tokyo) 1997;45:492-4. View abstract.
12. Prieto JM, Recio MC, Giner RM, et al. Influence of traditional Chinese anti-inflammatory medicinal plants on leukocyte and platelet functions. J Pharm Pharmacol 2003;55:1275-82.

WEIGHT & INCHES SPECIALIST

Stop Accumulation of Fat!

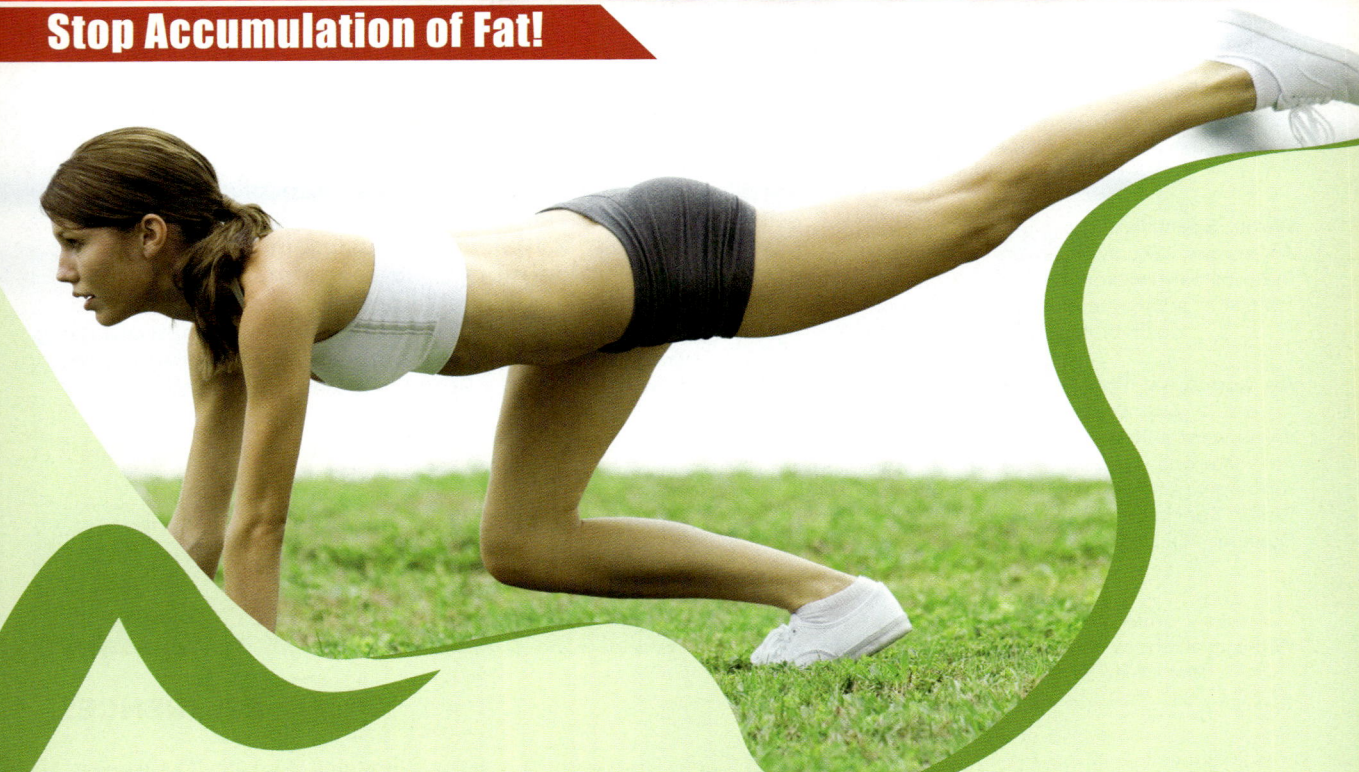

HAVE YOU EVER FOUND YOURSELF IN A SITUATION WHERE YOU CONTINUE TO EAT EVEN THOUGH YOU'RE ALREADY FULL?

Have you ever searched for comfort at the bottom of a bag of potato chips or at the bottom of an ice cream container? Has your chronic overeating left you feeling overweight, sluggish and depressed? If you long to look in the mirror and see the person you once remember being, look no further than Dr. Tai's Weight and Inches Specialist. This special formula, which contains only the highest-quality, natural ingredients, is your secret weapon in the battle of the bulge.

Health Risks Associated With Obesity

Appearance means a lot to everybody. However, where obesity is concerned, there is more at stake than just your vanity. Excess weight might make you feel and look unattractive, but it can also be a precursor to more serious health complications such as Type II Diabetes. Using fermented, soybean-derived Touchi Extract, Dr. Tai's Weight and Inches Specialist formula may regulate cortisone and sugar levels. Touchi Extract has been proven to be a naturally safe and effective way to regulate and control borderline and mild- Type II Diabetes. Reference: Fujita, Yamagami and Ohshima (American Society for Nutritional Sciences—2001).

A diet high in sugars and carbohydrates is highly unhealthy and potentially dangerous to the system. High sugar levels create a two-part problem within the body. First, when sugar levels rise, the body responds by over-stimulating the pancreas and producing too much insulin. Second, when sugar peaks, it is converted to fat. In response, the pancreas drops insulin down below the normal level and the body begins to enter hypoglycemic, or starvation, mode. The Touchi Extract contained in Dr. Tai's Weight and Inches Specialist formula may work to calm down the overreaction of high and low insulin levels.

The Keys to Effective Weight Loss

Appetite and craving suppression are the keys to weight loss. The phenomenon of overeating has long been believed to be due to a lack of "control" on the part of a person. However, this is far from the truth. Most often, overeating is due to a Dysfunctional Satiety Center (DSC).

When a person consumes food, the hypothalamus (a small gland located at the base of the brain) registers when the stomach is full. Once food enters the stomach, the stomach secretes a hormone that sends a message to the brain that it has received food. Unfortunately, however, an abnormal hypothalamus does not register when food has entered the stomach. There is a non-functioning circuit between the stomach and the brain. As a result of this lapse in communication between body and brain, those with an abnormal hypothalamus are prone to overeating.

Dr. Tai's Weight and Inches Specialist formula may regulate an abnormal hypothalamus. Using Ginsenosides, a specific extraction that may normalize the internal "switch" and allow the stomach to quickly respond when you eat- this formula may regulate a dysfunctional system and virtually eliminate the possibility of overeating.

Jumpstart Your Metabolism the Natural Way

Sometimes diet and exercise are just not enough. When this is the case, Dr. Tai's Weight and Inches Specialist formula goes to work using Green Tea Extract that may give your metabolism the "jumpstart" it needs. Green Tea Extract may improve metabolic rate with Polyphenols and EGCG, which contain powerful antioxidant properties and may help stimulate and improve your metabolism while neutralizing the damage done by free radicals that come through dieting.

Next, Eleutherococus (Siberian Ginseng) and Spirulina (a natural sea vegetable) go to work, imparting natural, anti-fatigue properties. Finally, Rhodiola Rosea may modulate mood swings that are a commonplace occurrence among dieters. All ingredients contained in Dr. Tai's Weight and Inches Specialist formula are non-stimulatory and gentle to the system.

Directions:
Take one capsule three times a day a half hour before eating.

Ingredients:
Ginsenosides, Touchi Extract, Green Tea Extract, Eleutherococus, Rhodiola Rosea, Spirulina

These statements have not been reviewed by the FDA. This product is not intended to diagnose, treat, cure, or prevent any disease.

Dr. Tai's Pearl

I love this product myself, as I have used it in my own journey in the quest for better health and lower abdominal fat. Abdominal fat had been a hallmark of my unhealthy days - I was extremely inflamed and toxic from it. Weight & Inches helped me obtain the belly fat-loss I was desperately looking for.

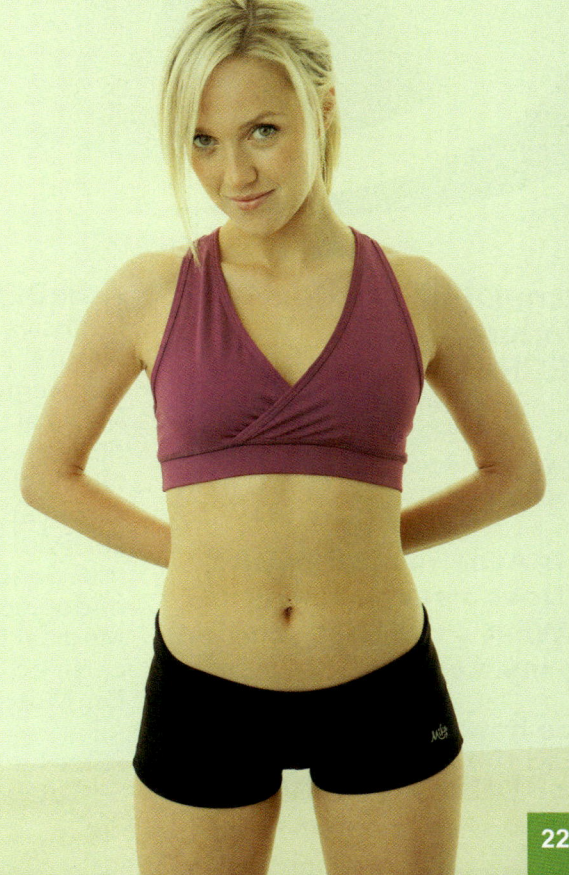

Side Effects: None

Contraindications:
Do not use this product if you are allergic to any of its ingredients

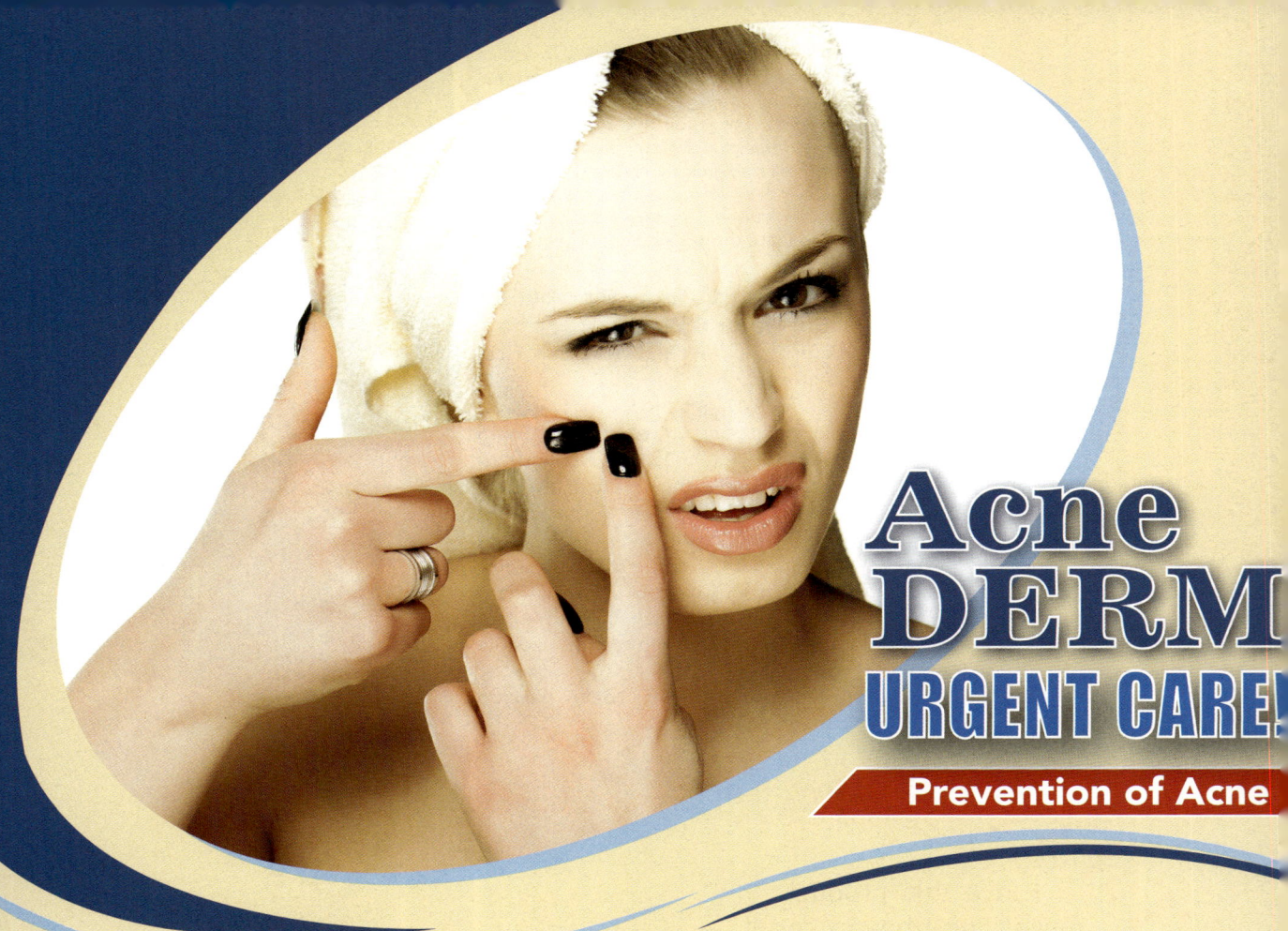

Acne DERM URGENT CARE!
Prevention of Acne

AcneDERM - Understand the SECRETS of Acne!

All new & unique ingredients not available in any other products even by prescription!

- Is Acne related to diet?
- Does stress cause acne?
- What's the best solution to my Acne?

See how AcneDERM works; read the 2-Step Program with DUAL POWER Action.

AcneDERM
Intensive Acne Treatment Natural Herbal Ingredients & Recommended by Prestigious Medical Journal "Health Science Institute" Newly developed and formulated by the renowned **Dr. Paul Ling Tai** & Independently tested and endorsed by a Yale Trained Medical Doctor & Board certified Dermatologist **Dr. Morris Westfried**

After he evaluated Health Secrets' AcneDERM products,

Dr. Morris Westfried, MD (Dermatologist) said in his letter:

- "In patients with postural acne, I have noted significant improvement..."

- "This regimen is superior to over the counter products and similar in efficacy to topical prescription acne medications..."

The Steps:
Step One
Apply **Smart Skin** to dry face and rub briskly until dead skin deposits have formed on the surface.
Step Two
Apply a small amount of **AcneDERM Urgent Care**, to pimples only, twice daily.

DUAL POWER Action
- May attack pustules – and kill P. Acne bacteria that cause acne pustules
- May attack inflammation Anti-inflammatory
- May reduce hormone levels on the skin
- May attack oiliness – and diminish oiliness of the skin

Key Features
The exact science of what causes acne remains unknown. The issue of when a person develops acne or grows out of acne is highly personalized. You may not be able to totally avoid the acne outbreak, but today you are able to find effective treatment due to scientific advancement.

AcneDERM is the "Definitive Approach" to the acne problem. It uses powerful yet natural, herbal ingredients. Fast acting, it may work within four weeks. AcneDERM is simple to use, non-drying/non-peeling and contains natural, herbal ingredients.

Ingredients:
Acne Derm Urgent Care - Allantoin, Aloe Vera, Butylparaben, Carbopol, A. Dahurica, A. Lappa, R. Coptidis, G. Glabra, U. Barbata, Curcumin Longa, Citrus Extract, Fragrance, D. Panthenol, Propylene Glycol, SD Alcohol 40, Sodium Hyaluronate, Triethanolamine, Water

These statements have not been reviewed by the FDA. This product is not intended to diagnose, treat, cure, or prevent any disease.

Side Effects: None

Contraindications:
Do not use this product if you are allergic to any of its ingredients

The Simple Secret
AcneDERM Urgent Care should be used ONLY at the beginning of a pimple. Place the product on pimples before they have come to a head to fight against bacteria.

Skin Patrole:
Check you skin first thing in the morning and last thing at night. Utilize Smart Skin and AcneDERM Urgent Care for 4 days until budding pimples are gone. Prevention is EVERYTHING! AcneDERM Urgent care is intented on NEW Pimples. Once these pimples have broken to the surface they are infected!

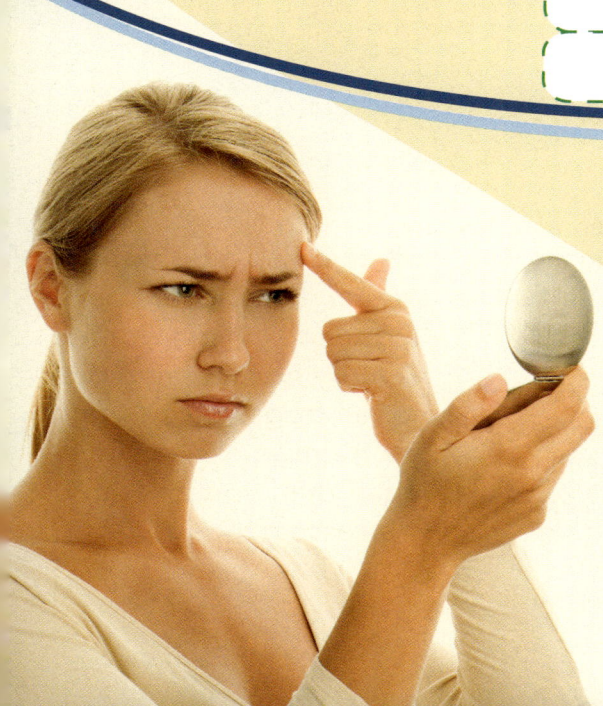

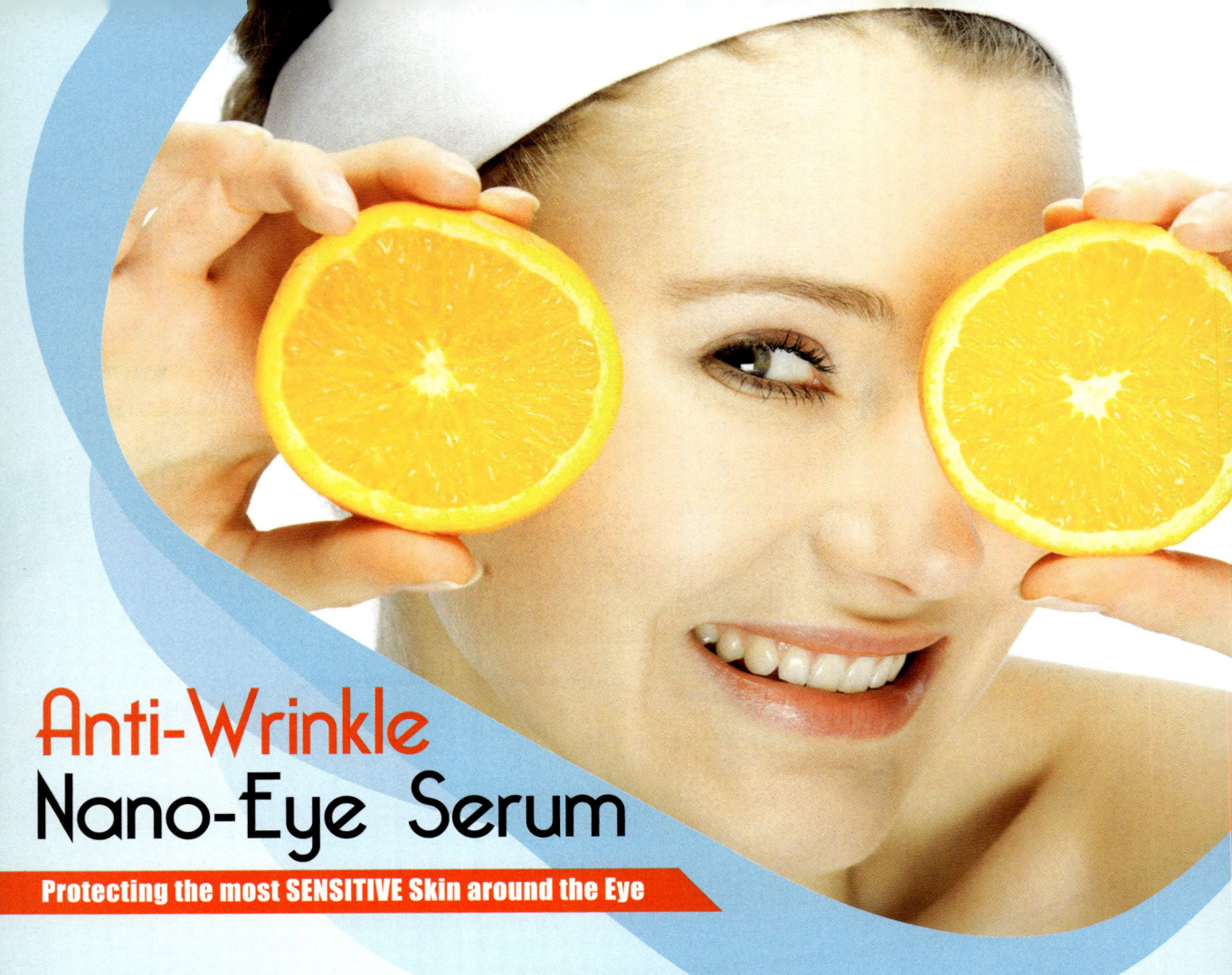

Anti-Wrinkle Nano-Eye Serum

Protecting the most SENSITIVE Skin around the Eye

Pampering yourself is not something that should be left to every other weekend, not even every other day; it must be done daily! Take a couple of daily minutes to give something back to yourself with our Advanced Nano-Eye Serum, containing Algae and Mugwort.

You might be familiar with the tale of the Princess and the Frog. Legend has it that, after kissing the frog down by the waters edge, the Princess later washed the algae from her face and noticed that her fine lines and wrinkles improved. She immediately ran back to the lake and collected bunches of algae for her beauty routine. And she was the fairest in all the land…

OK so that's a bit of a stretch, but it could have happened! Most women have by now learned that not all frogs you kiss turn into Princes. That doesn't mean that women aren't Princesses, though.

How can Anti-Wrinkle Nano-Eye Serum make me the fairest of them all?

The serum works in three ways. First, it replenishes the empty reservoir of phyto-hormones with extract of Pueraria. This may improve the appearance of wrinkles from around your eyes and reveal the sparkling brightness just waiting to shine. Second, it provides essential multi-peptide nutrients from marine collagen that may reduce the appearance of premature lines, loss of elasticity and sagging.

The third and most important aspects is the harnessed benefits of algae and mugwort, so that wrinkles may vanish and free radicals are prevented from causing further damage to your delicate eye area by the vitamin A (retinol A).

Q: I am using Anti-Wrinkle Nano-Eye Serum and I love it! But sometimes I wonder what else can I do for my skin to protect it from free radicals in the environment from the sun's ray.

A: Free radicals are a primary culprit in aging. The molecules (missing electron) bind to and destroy body cells; free radicals can derive from external sources such as smoke, sunlight and food, but they are mostly produced in the body as byproduct of energy production and waste. To get the most out of your Anti-Wrinkle Nano-Eye Serum, complement it with our high quality special antioxidants for anti-aging!

Hard working cream, so that you don't have to!

Our Advanced Nano-Eye Serum works as a system in three ways. Sounds impressive, yes? All you have to do is apply a small amount around the eyes in the morning and evening. Some redness and tingling may occur to increase skin circulation and remove stagnant toxins locked by the skin and increase the supply to nutrient needed to rejuvenate the tired cells.

It is important to remember that we live in a polluted world and our bodies have not had time to evolve "thicker skin", so to speak. Because of this it is necessary to give added protection.

You're not only keeping the bad stuff out, but keeping the good stuff in, while giving added nourishment to boot!

Looking after the fine lines around you eyes is just one step in a holistic skincare routine:
1. Cleanse
2. Tone
3. Protect & Moisturize

Pamper Procedure:
Apply a small amount around the eyes morning and evening.

Dr. Tai's Pearl
Help your body to keep free radicals at bay from the inside by eating fresh fruit and vegetables daily. These are rich in antioxidants, which form a strong front-line against these culprits in aging produced in your body. Use our Ancient Chinese Secrets called Royal Ling Zhi made especially for this problem.

Ingredients:
Water, Ionic Water, NaEDTA, Glycerin, K-Sorbate, Aloe Vera, Bamboo Ext, Peapod Ext, Glucosamine, Deep Sea Peptide, Pueraria, Marine Collagen, Algae Ext, Mugwort Ext, Vitamin A, Sodium Hyaluronate, Ascorbyl Palmitate, D-Panthanol, Vitamin E, DPHP, Bisabolol, Matrixyl Peptide, Kukui Nut, Prodew, Phenoxyethanol, Allantoin, Xanthan Gum, Deer Antler Extract, Epidermal Growth Factor (EGF), Triethanolamine

These statements have not been reviewed by the FDA. This product is not intended to diagnose, treat, cure, or prevent any disease.

Active Element: Pueraria
This Asian plant is also known as Kwao Krua Kaao in its native northern Thailand. Kaao means "white", as there are several species of Kwao Krua and this one has delicate white flowers. Anti-Wrinkle Nano-Eye Serum is enriched with a root extract from the Pueraria "white". Among its many benefits, it possesses anti-aging properties, reduces the appearance wrinkles and stimulates blood circulation.

Active Element: Algae Extract
Algae is often cruelly labeled as "pond scum". It is created from naturally present cyanobacteria in bodies of still water. Algae is rich in fatty acids and protein, which benefit the skin in two ways:
1. Repair damaged skin cells
2. Replace old cells and assisting in the production of new ones

There is nothing more beautiful than feeling good on the inside. What our eye serum system can give you is just that: increased self-esteem and confidence.

Side Effects: None

Contraindications:
Do not use this product if you are allergic to any of its ingredients

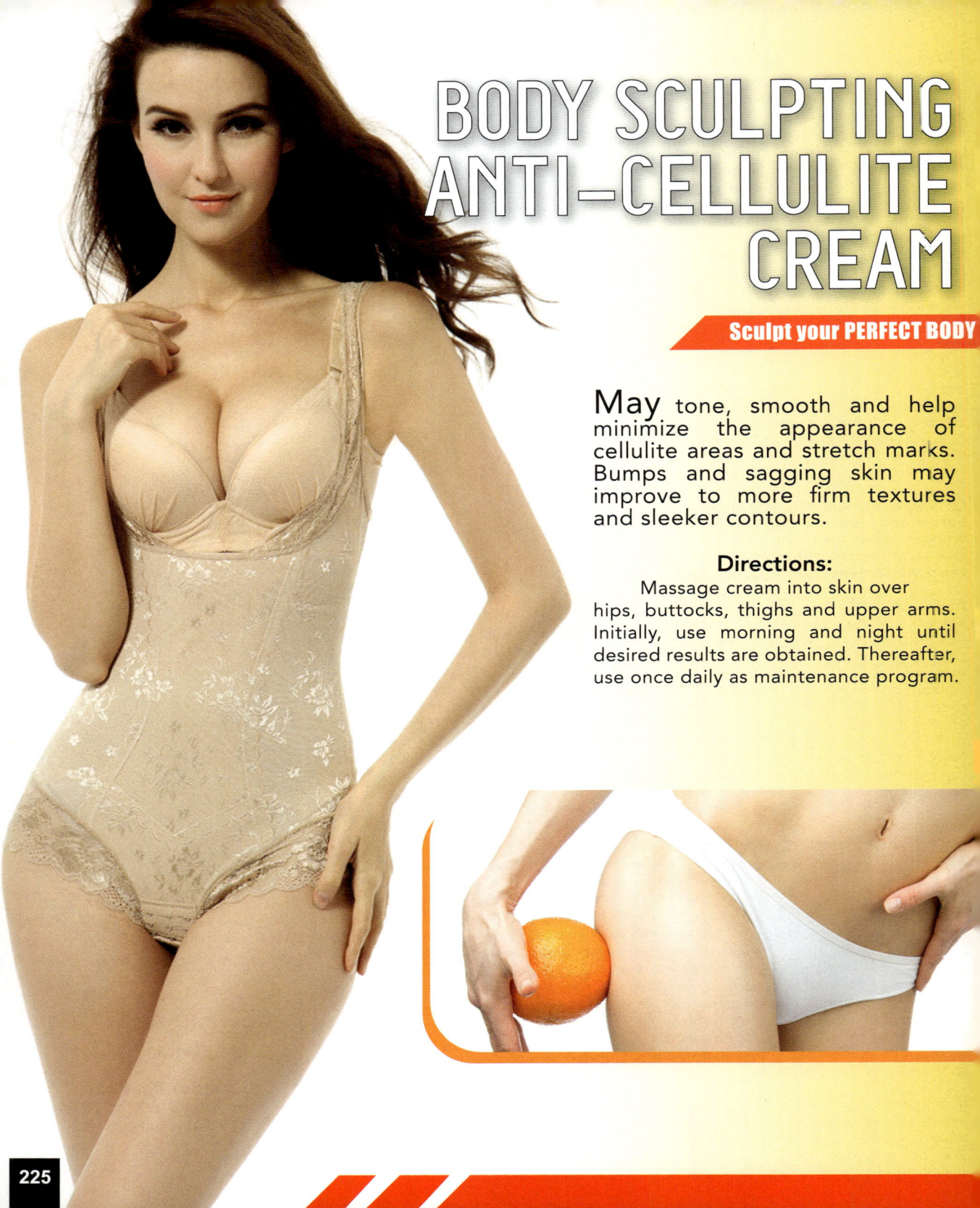

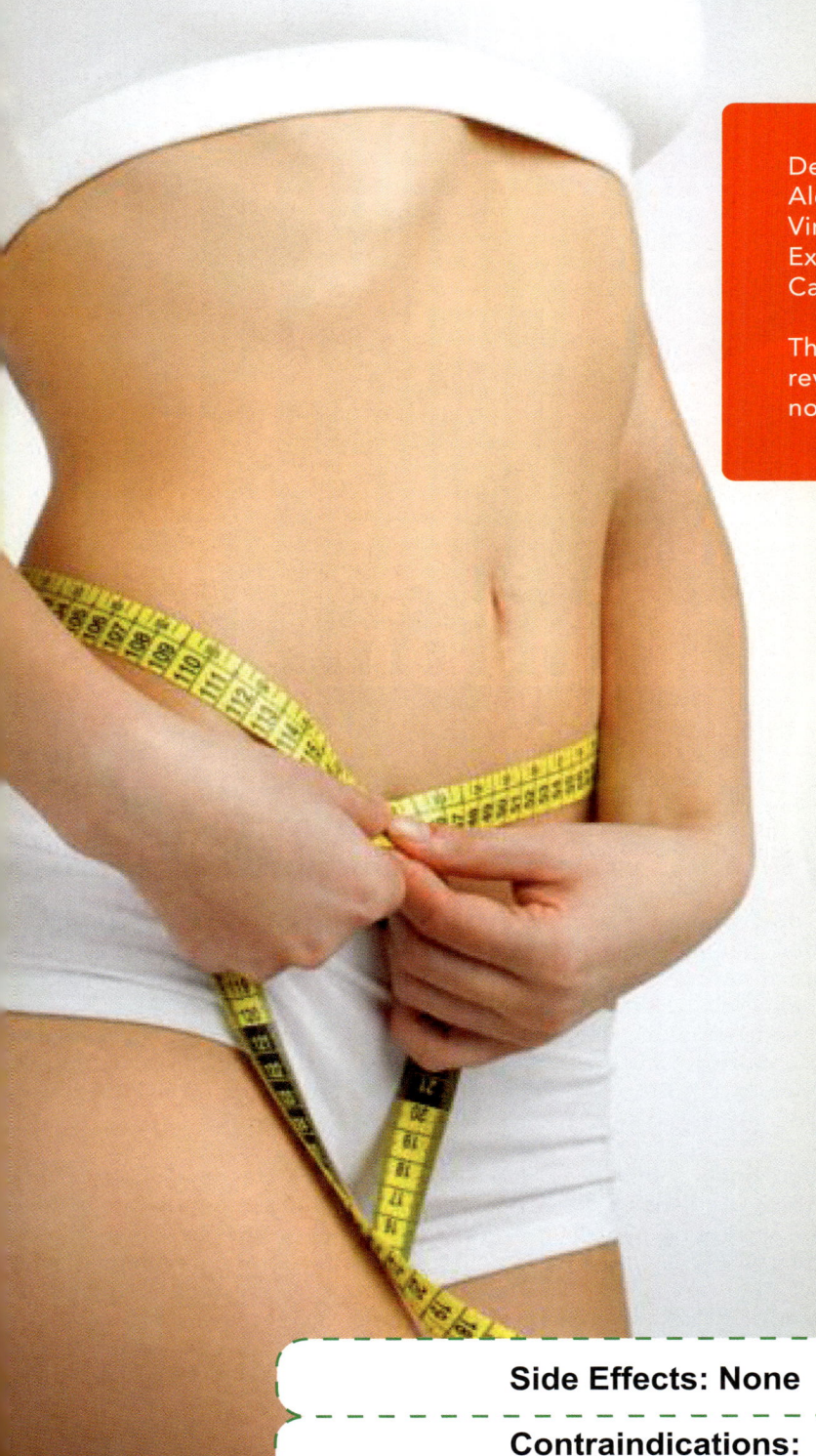

Ingredients:
Deionized Water, Glycerin, Cetearyl Alcohol, Maltodextrim, Cupana Extract, Virgin Caffeine, Carnitine, Sea Lettuce Extract, Ginseng Extract, Squalene, Carbomer, Xanthan Gum, Phenoxyethanol, Triethanolamine

These statements have not been reviewed by the FDA. This product is not intended to diagnose, treat, cure, or prevent any disease.

Side Effects: None

Contraindications:
Do not use this product if you are allergic to any of its ingredients

226

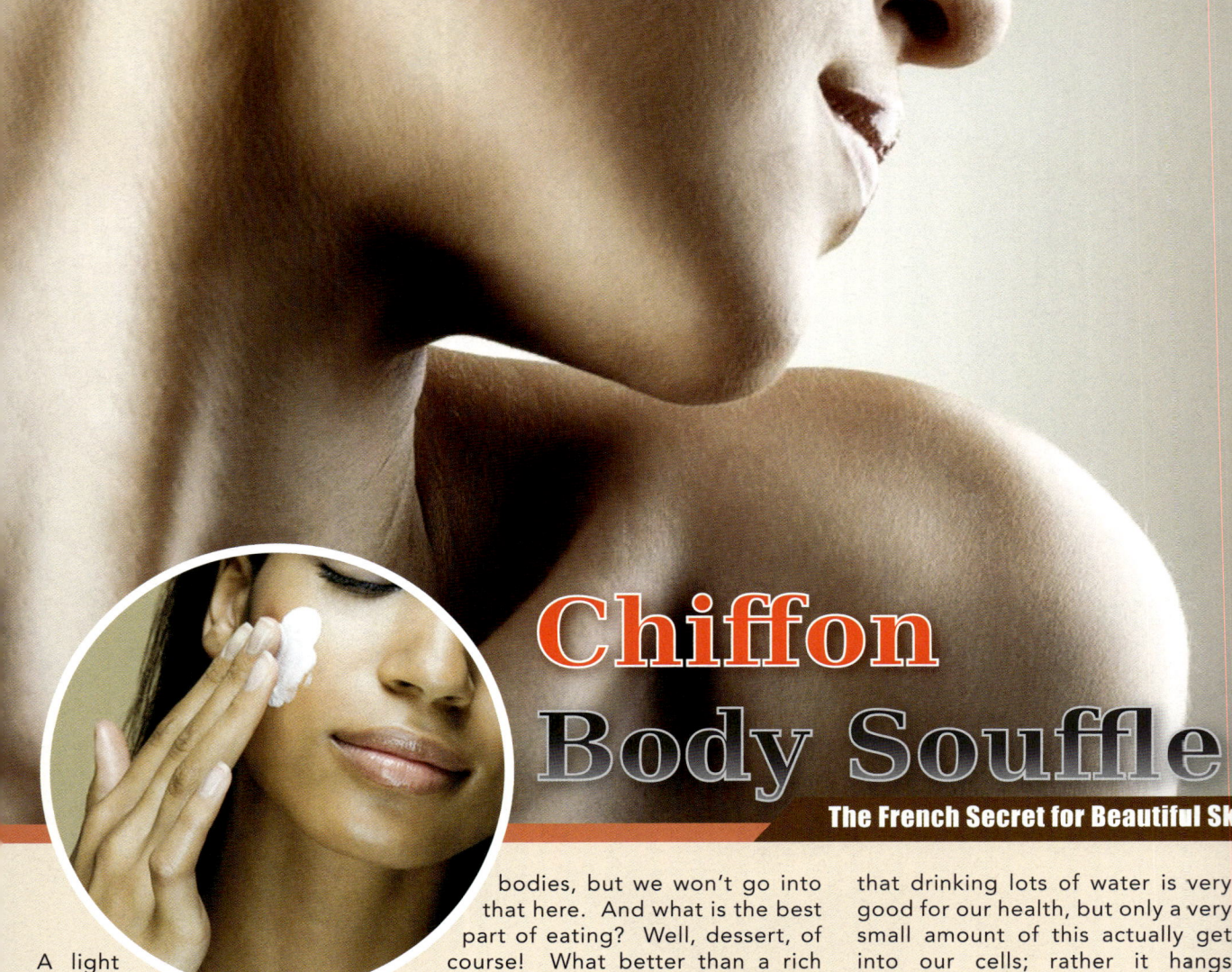

Chiffon Body Soufflé

The French Secret for Beautiful Skin

A light mousse containing exotic butters and rare tropical essence oils whipped to make a perfect dessert for your skin, a dessert that may hydrate and quench trillions of thirsty cells on our body. Miraculously airy, light CHIFFON BODY SOUFFLE is made for especially easy application on your body, and may penetrate like magic into your skin with micro-minerals for immediate nourishment.

Food isn't just something to put in your body, but also on your body - and sometimes on other peoples bodies, but we won't go into that here. And what is the best part of eating? Well, dessert, of course! What better than a rich but light mousse whipped with exotic butters and rare tropical essence oils? Stop drooling; it's for your skin!

Chiffon Body Soufflé may quench the thirst of trillions of cells in your body, hydrating you from the inside out.

I drink a lot of water, and yet I still struggle with skin problems. Why?

Is this you? You're not the first person to ponder this puzzle. The science behind hydration tells us that drinking lots of water is very good for our health, but only a very small amount of this actually get into our cells; rather it hangs around extracellular. At a cellular level, you are still dehydrated. Surprised to learn this? We were too!

That's why we developed Chiffon Body Soufflé to get that nourishing hydration flowing where it's needed. Micro-minerals may improve your cells up take of water, increasing hydration at the cellular level. Don't be surprised if you hear something sloshing around as you move, it's just your cells soaked in water; you'll get used to it! OK...maybe I was kidding.

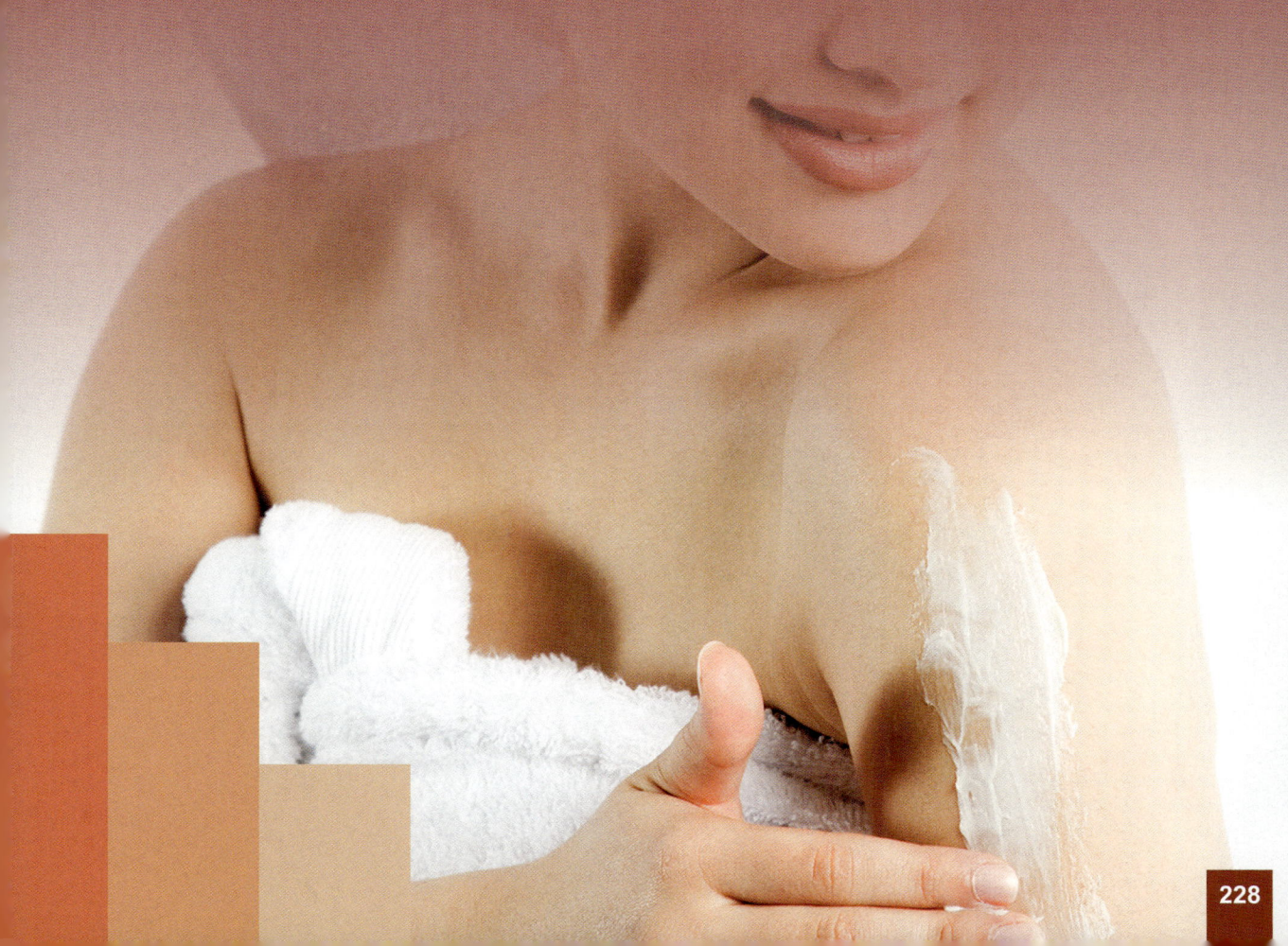

Active Element: Micro-Mineral Ions

Micro-minerals, also known as "trace minerals", are required in every living organism. In humans, micro-minerals are essential for healthy daily cell function. Human are essentially electrical beings (proof by the EKG and EEG electric signals).

Micro-minerals aid your body in many ways, including teeth and bone health, immune function, essential enzyme function, connective tissue, arterial strength and antioxidant production. Antioxidants are your front line defense against aging! But it cannot do their jobs fully without the help of micro-minerals nudging the cascades of chemistry needed by our body to carry vital electrical signals throughout our body to be healthy and alive. Micro-minerals absorb better into skin layers to rejuvenate the skin.

Active Element: Kukui Nut Oil

Kukui Nut Tree, though not native to Hawaii, has become its official tree! "Kukui" means "enlightenment" in Hawaiian; we consider this a good omen! The oil has long been used for massaging, its benefits to the skin lauded even among royalty. It has a creamy quality that absorbs quickly into the skin without blocking pores, leaving it feeling soft to the touch, but without being greasy.

All of this is making me hungry! Are there foods that can help to hydrate my skin?

Why, indeed there are! Treat yourself to Fatty Acids rich foods, berries and leafy greens, particularly spinach and extracts of Royal Ling Zhi for the ultimate "Baby soft" skin. Try to reduce your alcohol and caffeine consumption as these can dehydrate. Sounds like a lot of work, eh? Reward yourself with a yummy veggie soufflé.

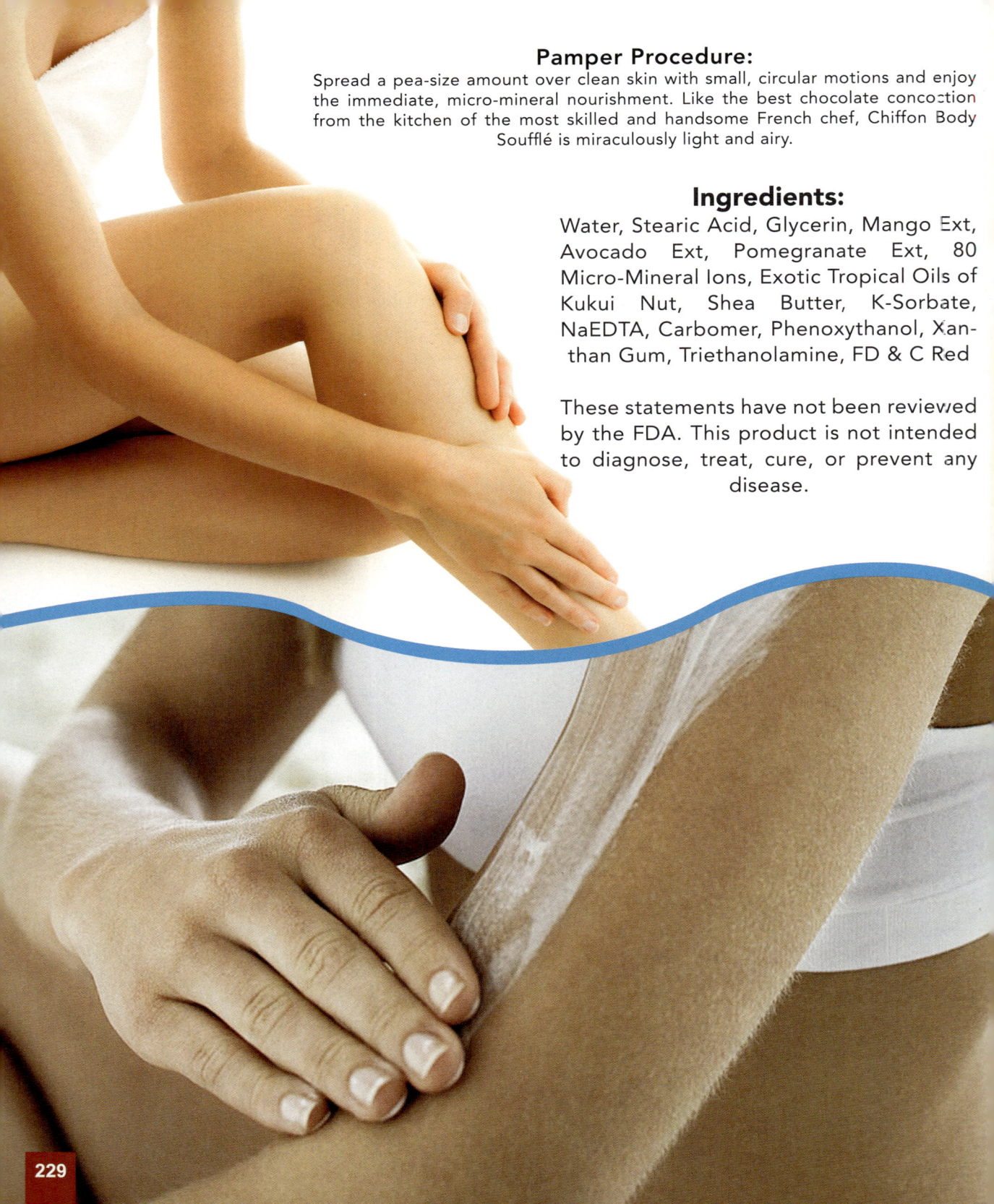

Pamper Procedure:
Spread a pea-size amount over clean skin with small, circular motions and enjoy the immediate, micro-mineral nourishment. Like the best chocolate concoction from the kitchen of the most skilled and handsome French chef, Chiffon Body Soufflé is miraculously light and airy.

Ingredients:
Water, Stearic Acid, Glycerin, Mango Ext, Avocado Ext, Pomegranate Ext, 80 Micro-Mineral Ions, Exotic Tropical Oils of Kukui Nut, Shea Butter, K-Sorbate, NaEDTA, Carbomer, Phenoxythanol, Xanthan Gum, Triethanolamine, FD & C Red

These statements have not been reviewed by the FDA. This product is not intended to diagnose, treat, cure, or prevent any disease.

Dr. Tai's Pearl

By now you're familiar with micro-minerals, but there are also major-minerals that are important for overall health. Some major-minerals contribute to overall fluid balance in your body. A balanced, healthy diet can ensure you have sufficient micro and major mineral levels. And yes, chocolate is a source! Choose dark or bitter 70% chocolate for a low-sugar option. But beware of the fat content!

Side Effects: None

Contraindications:
Do not use this product if you are allergic to any of its ingredients

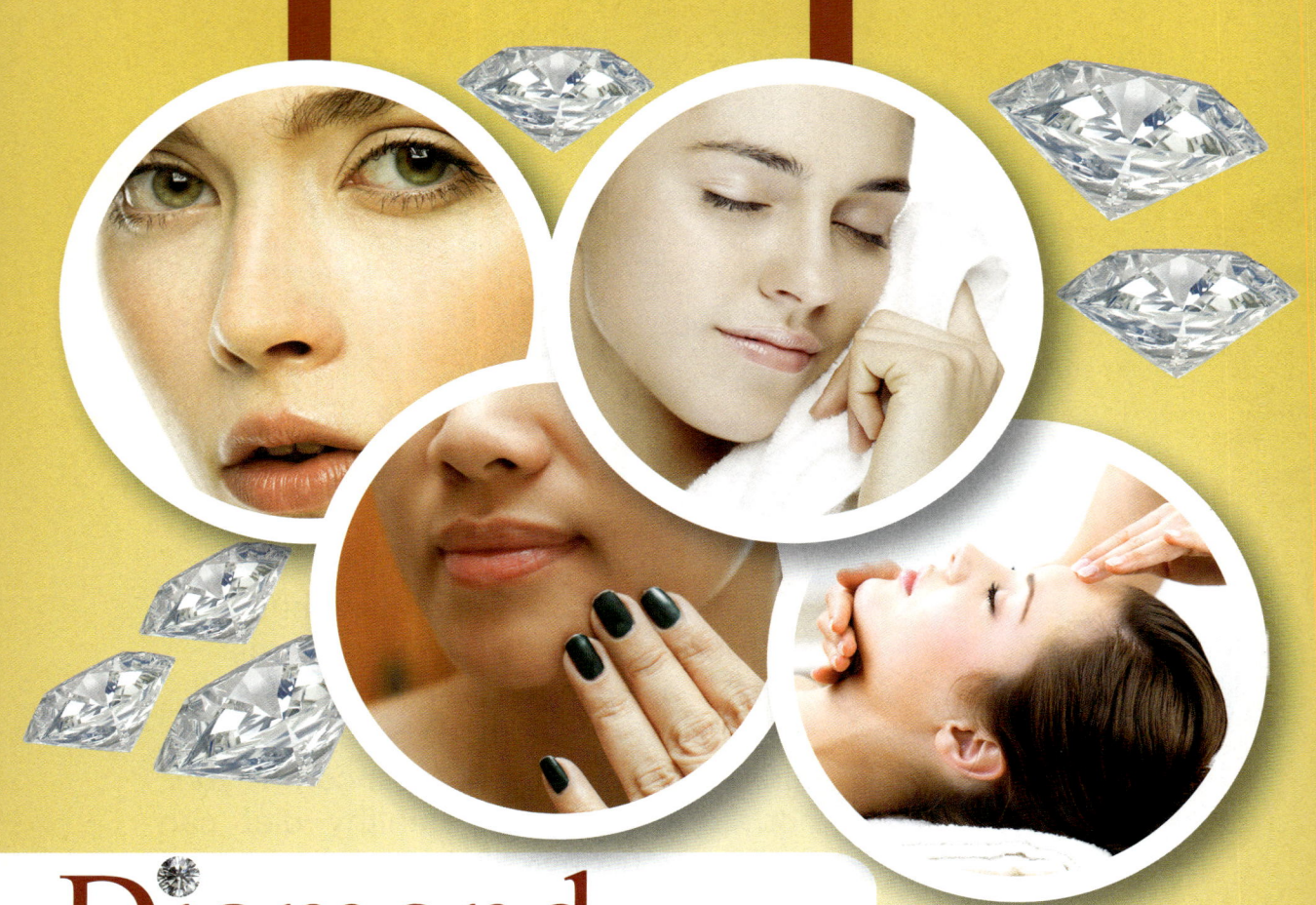

Diamond Microdermabrasion
Natural Skin Exfoliation Without Abrasion

They say that "Diamonds are a girl's best friend."

Diamond Microdermabrasion was created to leave your skin feeling as dazzling as the gem itself. The product is natural, non-allergenic and the Diamonds pulverized to half of a micron to exfoliate skin. It has the extraordinary capability of lifting dead skin cells that have accumulated over time and have caused your skin to dull. For that extra special experience we've added Papaya and Pineapple Enzymes to achieve a soft buffed glow.

Every day there is an accumulation of dead skin on your body. Sure, it sounds a bit "icky", but it is a perfectly normal part of your bodys natural rejuvenation self-spa process. As with any spa experience, a little expertise goes a long way; that's why polishing your skin with Diamond Microdermabrasion as part of your holistic skincare routine is a small investment with big return.

Q: "Abrasion sounds a bit rough. Is it safe to use every day?"

- Jake, 25

A: The diamonds used in this product is 5 Nano, it is only 1/10 the size of your skin pores so they cannot cause irritation. The purpose is to finely polish your skin and perfectly tightens the pores for that perfect, warm glow you see in the movie star's face as they are walking down the red carpet.

The Benefits of Microdermabrasion

Polishing has two major benefits. Firstly, it helps you to slough off these dead skin cells to reveal the fresh and smooth surface beneath. Washing with a regular cleanser gets some of these flakes, but you need a diamond polishing schedule to get in under those stubborn ones and expose the fresh cells and increase the appearance of firmer skin. Diamond Microcrystals cleans and tighten enlarged pores and help to reduce the formation of comedones, or blackheads, and may reduce the severity of acne.

Squeaky Clean

Secondly, your skin is now polished clean and poised to best absorb the lotions and potions of your skincare routine. Dirt, including dead skin cells, stand in the way of the benefits your skin can be afforded by your repairing and rejuvenating creams. The diamonds in Diamond Microdermabrasion refers to the polished sparkle that your skin will radiate thanks to its extraordinary capability that may lift dead skin cells that have accumulated over time and cause your skin to dull. As if diamonds weren't enough, we've added papaya and pineapple enzymes for a soft buffed glow.

Active Element: Bromelain

Pineapple enzyme goes by the street name, bromelain. It also has anti-inflammatory properties, a feature it shares with papaya enzyme. Anti-inflammatory action may help to reduce redness and has been shown to be beneficial for skin conditions including acne, psoriasis and eczema.

Adding pineapple to your diet can aid in digestive function, which is a sure fire way to get maximum toxin expulsion from your system. It also works as a blood thinner by breaking down certain amounts of the protein fibrin, allowing blood to course more freely through your veins. This benefits the circulatory system and may be associated with lower chances of circulatory disease, heart attack

Active Element: Papain

Papaya enzyme – or papain – gets to work on debriding dead skin cells. Debriding means to break down. In essence, the papaya enzyme works on breaking up the layer of radiance-blocking dead skin cells and dirt, allowing the microdermabrasion beads to do their job most effectively.

Pamper Procedure:

After exfoliating your face with Smart Skin, apply a small amount of the natural, non-allergenic Diamond Mirodermabrasion to your face in a circular motion. Let it sit or 10 minutes then rinse with warm water. Apply Essence Flash Toner to tighten the pores.

Directions:
Apply a small amount onto damp face in circular motion. Rinse with warm water.

Ingredients:

Water, Cetearyl Alcohol, Glycerin, Diamond Microcrystals, Papaya Enzymes, Pineapple Enzymes, Vitamin E, D-Panthanol, Allantoin, Cyclomethicone, Carbomer, Phenoxyethanol, Xanthan Gum, Triethanolamine

These statements have not been reviewed by the FDA. This product is not intended to diagnose, treat, cure, or prevent any disease.

Dr. Tai's Pearl

Clean skin helps the body to expel toxins. Your body works to expel toxins through the skin barrier. Sweating not only pushes dirt out of the pores, but toxins from the body. Clean surface area, i.e. skin, allows for maximum expulsion efficiency.

Side Effects: None

Contraindications:
Do not use this product if you are allergic to any of its ingredients

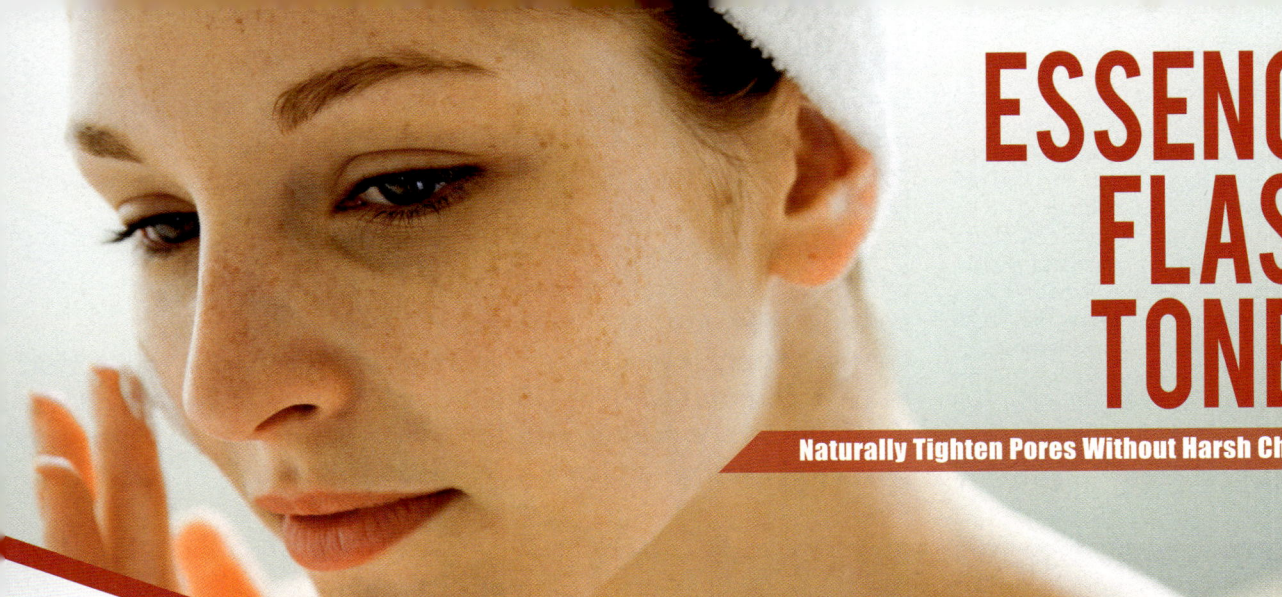

ESSENCE FLASH TONER

Naturally Tighten Pores Without Harsh Chemicals

With Broassonetia Papyrifera extract, a native plant from the highlands of Asia, this special toner may tighten and brighten your face. It's a slightly mild astringent that may leave your skin feeling as smooth as silk. This is a very rare combination of toner that may brighten the skin. Many women report clean, silky and glowing skin along with looking and feeling younger and more energized!

If you can, washing your face with warm water will help in your efforts of cleansing. Why? Well, warm water encourages your pores to open and therein shall you find the dirt! Your holistic skincare routine may be of the highest quality, but if toxins and accumulated pollutants are trapped within the pores behind closed, well, doors, you may be setting yourself up to fail. Now that you have successfully opened and cleaned your pores, to leave them in this way is only to allow more dirt and pollutants in as you go about your day! This won't do at all. Cold is now required to close the pores and increase the feeling of firmness in the skin.

Why can't I close my pores with a splash of cold water?

Unless you are living at the source of pure water high up on a mountaintop, chances are your water is treated with chemicals and impregnated with impurities. A splash of this water only serves to introduce toxins to your skin once again. Besides, you would need to endure a splash of extremely cold water to achieve the desired results. If you don't live near a frozen lake in Finland, what you need is an astringent.

After exfoliating your face with Smart Skin and polishing it with Diamond Microdermabrasion, apply the Essence Flash Toner to tighten and brighten your face. It's so simple and yet so effective! Our toner contains nourishing elements, making it second only to a pure mountain spring.

The special ingredient in Essence Flash Toner is Broassonetia Papyrifera extract, a native plant from the highlands of Asia, which, in laymans terms, is a mild astringent that may leave your skin feeling as smooth as silk.

The Toner Secret: Astringents

Astringent means, "to bind fast". It is a substance that serves to shrink or constrict body tissues, such as pores. Thus, it can protect the skin.

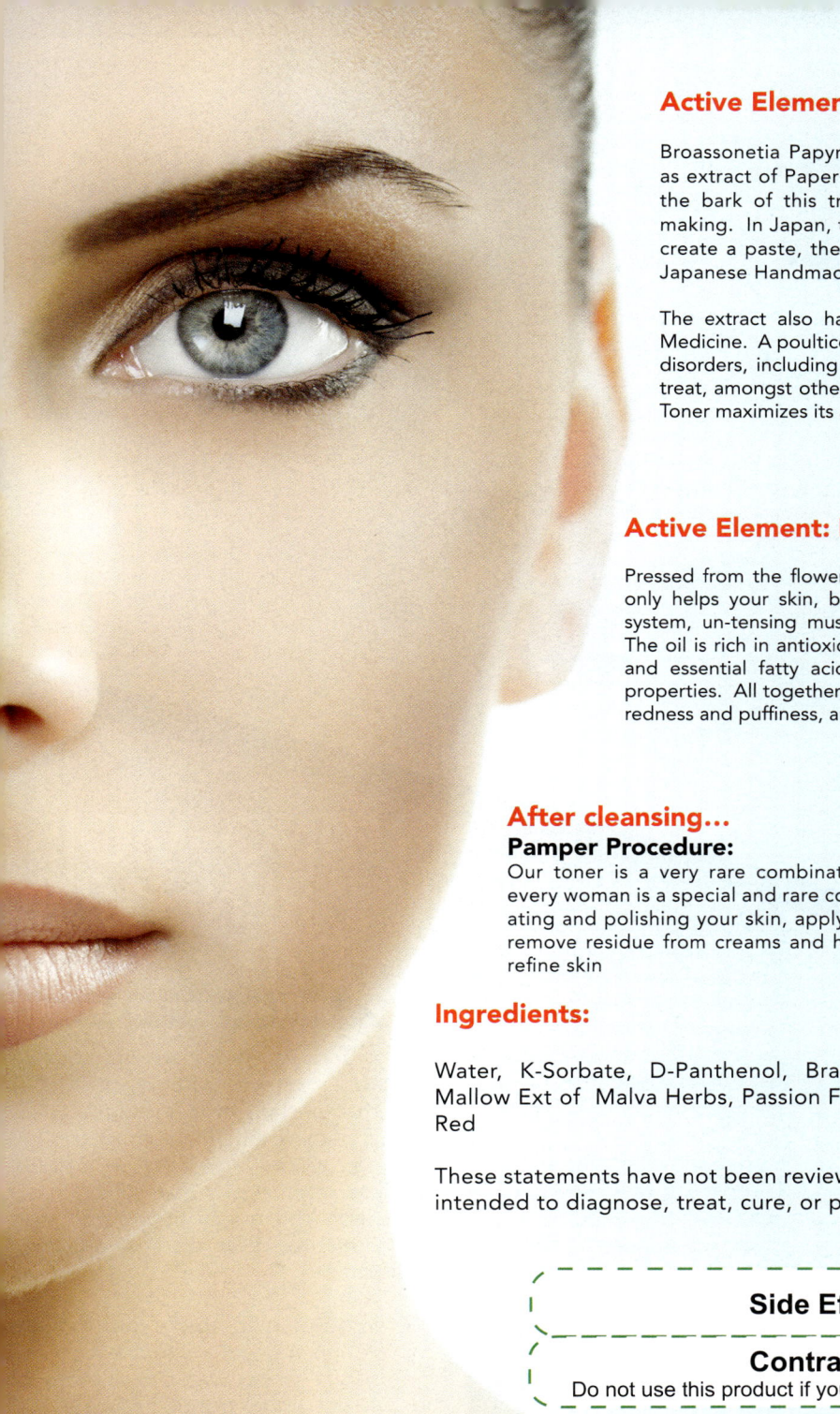

Active Element: Broassonetia Papyrifera

Broassonetia Papyrifera extract is more commonly known as extract of Paper Mulberry Tree. As the name suggests, the bark of this tree is used in paper, as well as cloth making. In Japan, the inner bark is pounded with water to create a paste, then spread on wire mesh to make washi, Japanese Handmade Paper.

The extract also has a long history in Chinese Traditional Medicine. A poultice of leaves is used to treat a variety of skin disorders, including bites, and a juice of the leaves used to treat, amongst other ailments, dysentery. Our Essence Flash Toner maximizes its astringent qualities.

Active Element: Passion Flower Oil

Pressed from the flower of the plant, Passion Flower Oil not only helps your skin, but is known for relaxing the nervous system, un-tensing muscles, and promoting peace of mind. The oil is rich in antioxidants (our free radical fighting friends) and essential fatty acids; it also contains anti-inflammatory properties. All together, the oil may reduce the appearance of redness and puffiness, and help skin to stay soft and supple.

After cleansing...
Pamper Procedure:
Our toner is a very rare combination of special ingredients, because every woman is a special and rare combination unto herself. After exfoliating and polishing your skin, apply our toner with a soft cotton pad to remove residue from creams and hard water to tighten the pores to a refine skin

Ingredients:

Water, K-Sorbate, D-Panthenol, Brassonetia Papyrifera, D-Panthanol, Mallow Ext of Malva Herbs, Passion Flower Oil, Phenoxyethanol, FD & C Red

These statements have not been reviewed by the FDA. This product is not intended to diagnose, treat, cure, or prevent any disease.

Side Effects: None

Contraindications:
Do not use this product if you are allergic to any of its ingredients

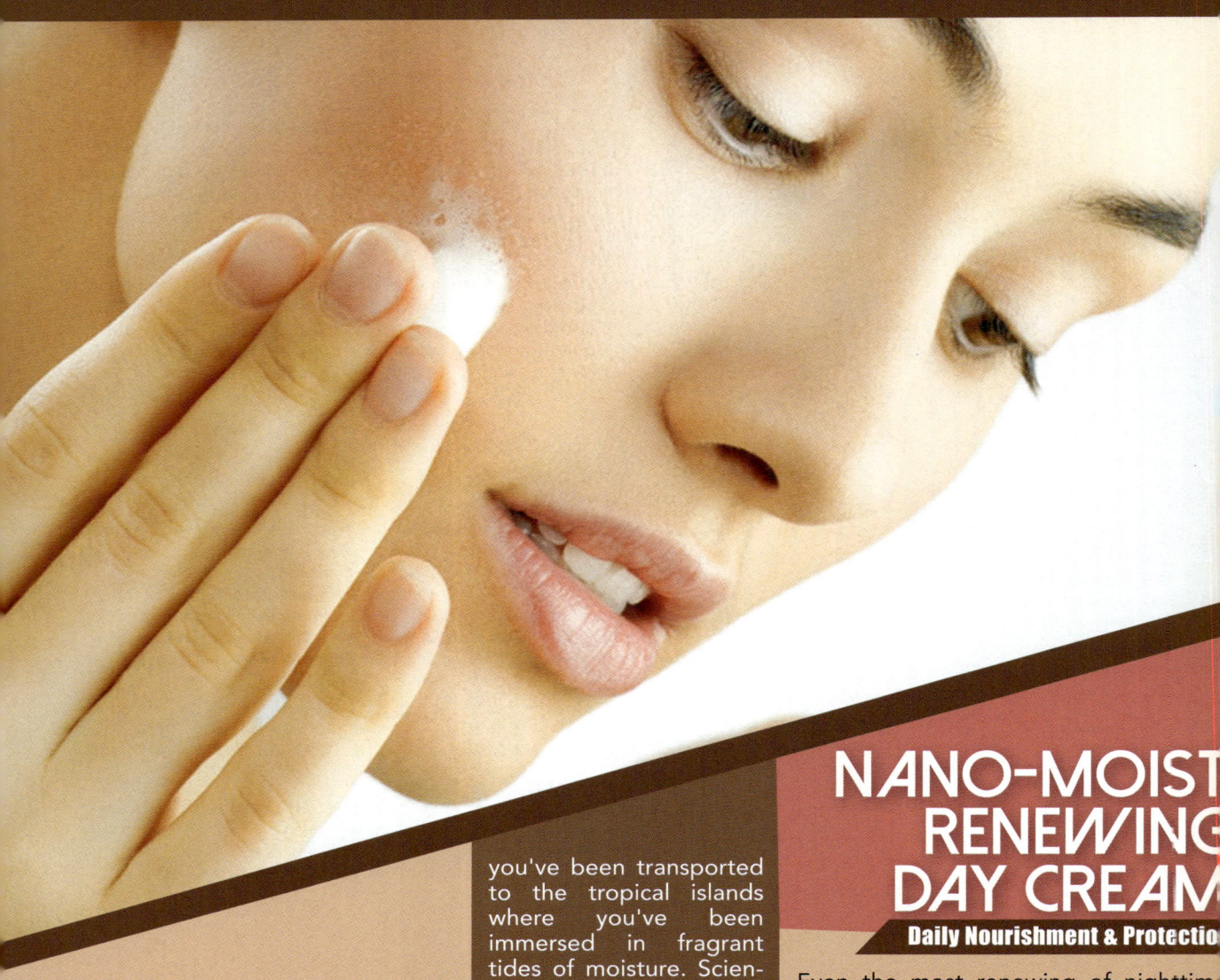

NANO-MOIST RENEWING DAY CREAM
Daily Nourishment & Protection

This non-greasy, light and naturally rich formula may protect against aging skin and stress pollutants. Nano-Moist Renewing Day Cream has what others do not- Nano Liposomes, a formulation made to increase skin oxygenation that may allow your skin to absorb our powerful plant extracts. With nano-encapsulated technology we've been able to pack microscopic bundles of Prodew, a nourishing skin humectant that may promote moisture retention in your skin and may increase moisture and nutrient uptake and storage. The infused with Kukui Nut Oil will make you feel as if you've been transported to the tropical islands where you've been immersed in fragrant tides of moisture. Scientific research has proven that our combination of oils and herbs may give your skin 500% more moisture than any other lotion or cream you've used. The driving force behind our moisturizer is the Phyto-hormone of Pueraria Extract. It may repair damaged collagen and reconstruct elastin allowing a newer and more vitally active looking skin. This may result in a warm, healthy, and youthful glow.

Even the most renewing of nighttime skin-care routines cannot protect u from the onslaught of pollutants jus waiting outside our front door the nex morning. A key ingredient in a holisti skin-care regime is a quality day crean to protect from nasty toxins and main tain nourishment as we move throug our lives.

Unless you plan to apply your make-u atop a layer of saran-wrap, ou Nano-Moist Renewing Day Cream ha the perfect light, non-greasy, naturall rich formulation that may form a barrie of protection against stress pollutants i the environment.

Modern Girl: Nano-Technology

Don't worry; you do not need to be a rocket scientist in order to enjoy the benefits of science-fiction-sounding gizmos. Nano technology simply means working on the super-duper incredibly teeny-weeny scale. You can't see them without a very, very powerful and expensive microscope and a very knowledgeable scientist. Luckily, we've done the hard work for you; so just smooth it onto your skin and reap the benefits.

Active Element: Pueraria

This Asian plant is also known as Kwao Krua Kaao in its native northern Thailand. Kaao means "white", as there are several species of Kwao Krua and this one has delicate white flowers. Anti-Wrinkle Nano Renewing Day cream is enriched with a root extract from the Pueraria "white". Among its many benefits, it possesses anti-aging properties, reduces the appearance wrinkles and stimulates blood circulation.

What this day cream has that others do not is Nano-liposomes. This unique addition is made to increase skin oxygenation that may allow it to absorb our powerful plant extracts. Thanks to nano-encapsulated technology we've been able to pack microscopic bundles of Prodew – a nourishing skin humectant that may promote moisture retention so that your skin can soak up and save nutrients.

The driving force behind our moisturizer is the Phyto-hormone of Pueraria Extract, which may lift damaged collagen and reconstruct elastin back into new and vitally active skin. Kukui Nut Oil is the final touch in our recipe. Supported by scientific research, our combinations of oils and herbs may give your skin 500% more moisture than other lotions and potions you may have tried over the years in the hunt for truly supportive skin-care products.

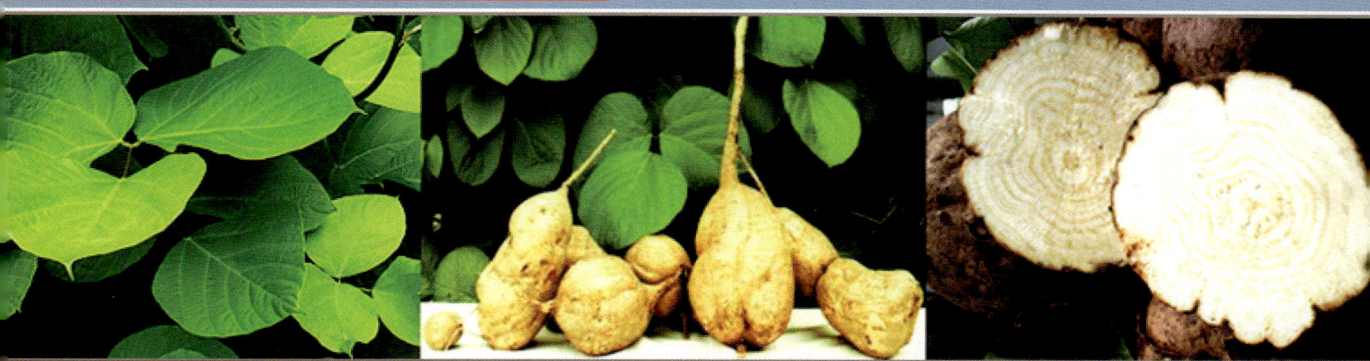

Phyto-what-now?

Phytohormones are nothing more exotic than a hormone-like substance produced by plants. They are completely naturally occurring phenomenona. In plants, these hormones regulate or control various physiological functions, such as growing tall and strong; particular phytohormones determine the loveliness of the plants flowers.

Active Element: Silica

The bamboo extract in our Nano-Moist Renewing Day Cream naturally contains silica. Most beneficial is its tendency to absorb toxins, helping to keep those environmental baddies from doing damage. While doing this, silica is double tasking at helping the body to absorb essential minerals. Bamboo extract has a soothing effect on the skin, reducing the appearance of blemishes and acne, increasing firmness and elasticity. To top it all off, a natural antioxidant presence may give a warm, healthy and youthful flow.

Beauty transported directly into your cells

To put it in its most basic incarnation, liposomes serve to transport water-soluble and fat-soluble substances. In this case, they transport beneficial ingredients in skincare products into the skin. Their remarkable dual action is due to their double-layer membrane; the inner layer is lipophilic (fat-soluble substances can pass through), and the outer layer is hydrophilic (water-soluble substances can pass through). Since liposomes are a component in your cells, the liposome technology carrying fat and water-soluble goodness has no problem slotting right in, with minimal risk of adverse reaction. And the best part is that liposomes can be designed to contain just about anything, so you can rest assured that you are getting active ingredients delivered to where they are needed most.

Active Element: Extract of Camellia sinensis

Pressed from the tealeaves known for their phenomenal antioxidant properties, Green Tea Extract has long been used in traditional medicine for its many healing effects. Applied to the skin, green tea extract has anti-inflammatory properties, reducing redness and puffiness, and works against the action of collagenase. Collagenase is an enzyme that breaks down collagen, which is a sort of scaffolding within your cells. With green tea extract working to maintain the health of collagen, your skin may benefit from increased firmness and elasticity.

Pamper Procedure:

Your day is filled with activities and exposure to the damaging elements from the sun, wind and rain. To keep your skin in tip-top condition throughout the day, start it with an application of Nano-Moist Renewing Day Cream. After Smart Skin, Diamond Microdermabrasion and Essence Flash Toner, apply a small amount of Nano-Moist Renewing Day Cream over entire face every morning to seal in the moisture in the skin all day long.

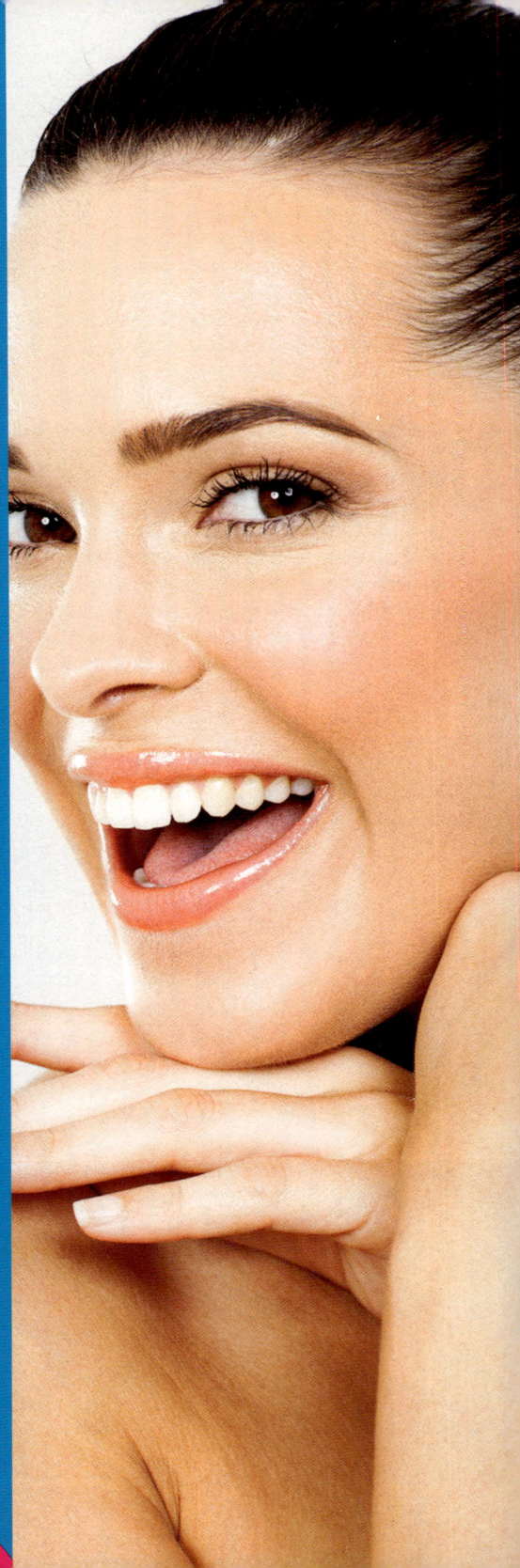

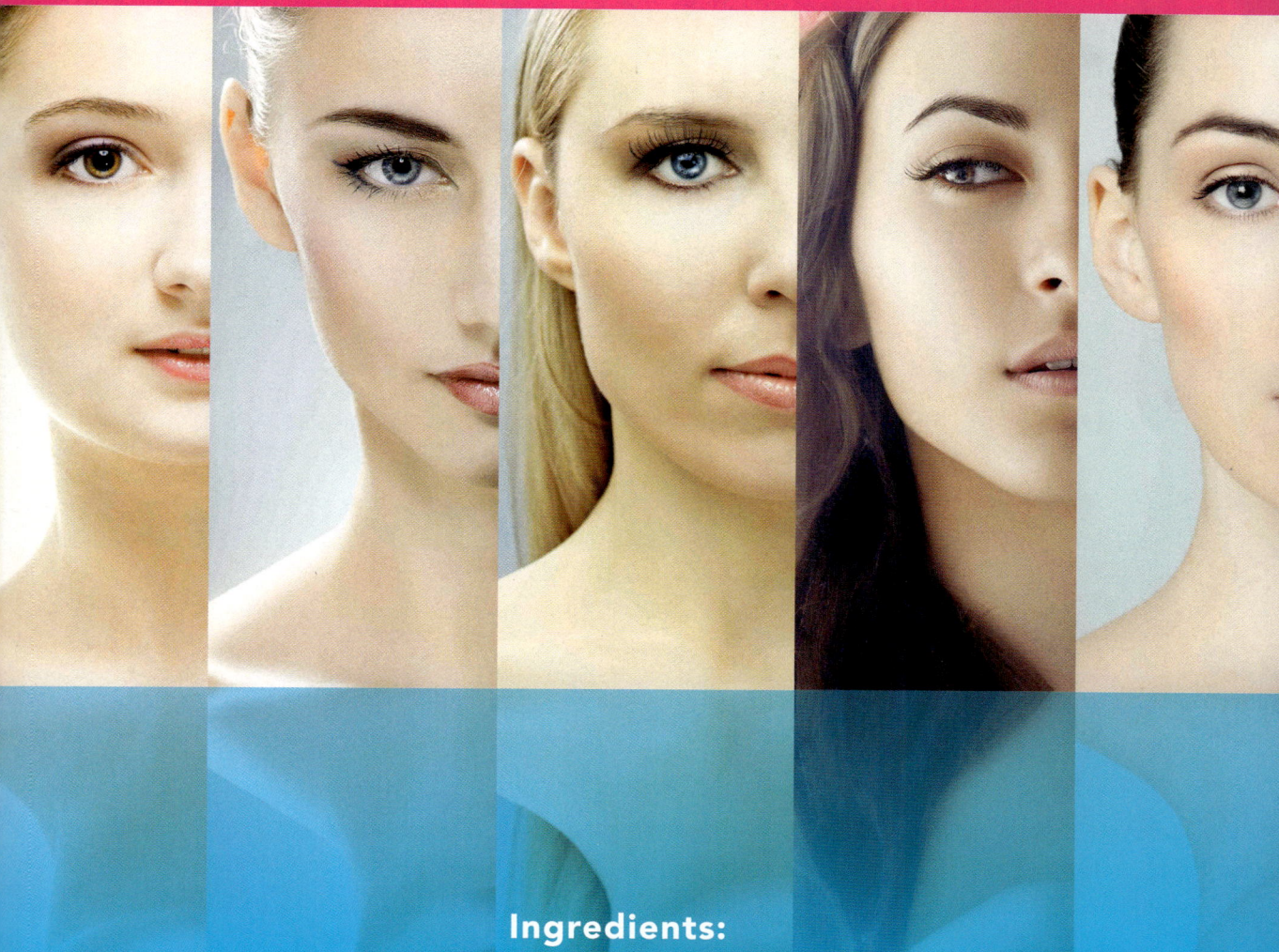

Directions:
On clean skin, apply over entire face in the morning.

Ingredients:
Water, Cetyl Ethylhexanoate, Bamboo Ext, Peapod Ext, Glucosamine, Deep Sea Peptide, Kukui Nut Oil, Pueraria Ext, Prodew, Niacinamide Compound, Hyaluronic Acid, Green Tea Ext, Alpha Lipoic Acid, Vitamin A, 80 Micro-Mineral, Lecithin, NaEDTA, Carbomer, Phenoxythanol, Xanthan Gum, Triethanolamine

These statements have not been reviewed by the FDA. This product is not intended to diagnose, treat, cure, or prevent any disease.

Side Effects: None

Contraindications:
Do not use this product if you are allergic to any of its ingredients

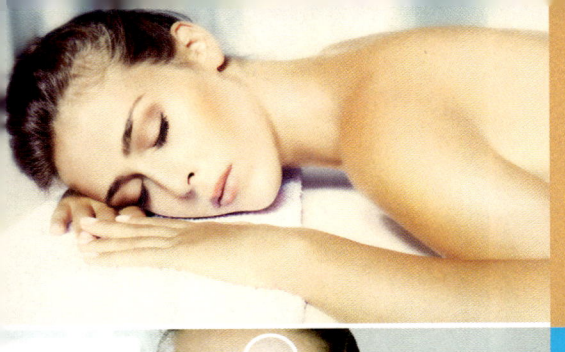

Nano-Restoring Night Caviar

Most Powerful Night-Time Treatment

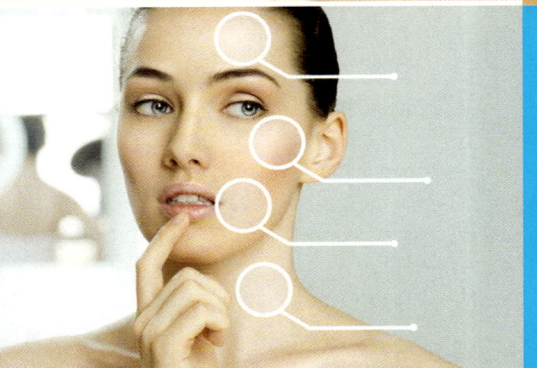

Most creams lose their freshness while sitting on store shelves for months at a time, but not our Nano-Restoring Night Caviar. The special bio-available Isoflavones of Pueraria extract contain natural ingredients that may stimulate the development of your tissues to tighten and firm your skin. Nano-Restoring Night Caviar also has Prodew to replenish lost moisture and may help smooth away wrinkles, restore elasticity, and firm your skin. Some redness and tingling may occur.

As you power down and prepare to sleep, your body is preparing to do essential housekeeping. That is why it is essential have a strong morning skincare routine and doubly essential to give your skin all the help you can in its own natural nighttime routine. This is where Nano-Restoring Night Caviar cream comes in.

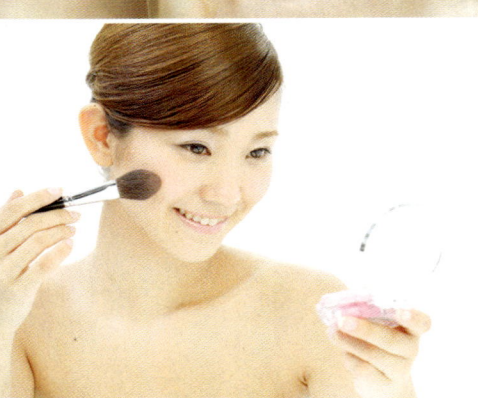

A key component of this cream, Pueraria extract – a flower native to Asia and long used in traditional medicines - contains natural ingredients that may stimulate firmness in your skin, reduce the appearance of wrinkles and freckles, and stimulate blood circulation.

Unlike other creams that lose their freshness over time while sitting on store shelves just waiting to be taken to their forever homes, the bio-available isoflavones of Pueraria extract in our Nano-Restoring Night Caviar do not.

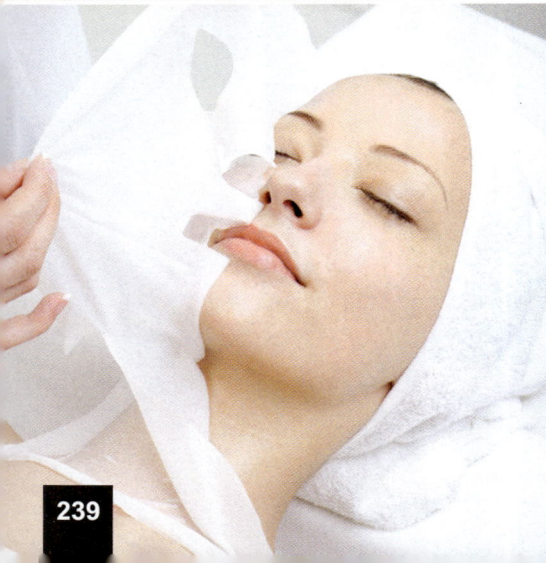

Bio-Available Isoflavones for the "Tinman" in all of us

Isoflavones have been shown to have antioxidant properties, comparable to that mainstay in skin health, vitamin E. The body does not produce its own vitamin E, so it is sourced externally through foodstuffs, supplements and extracted from natural compounds. Antioxidants work to neutralize free radicals, which slows the appearance of aging by preventing those free radicals from "rusting" cells and defeating the Wicked Witch of the West!

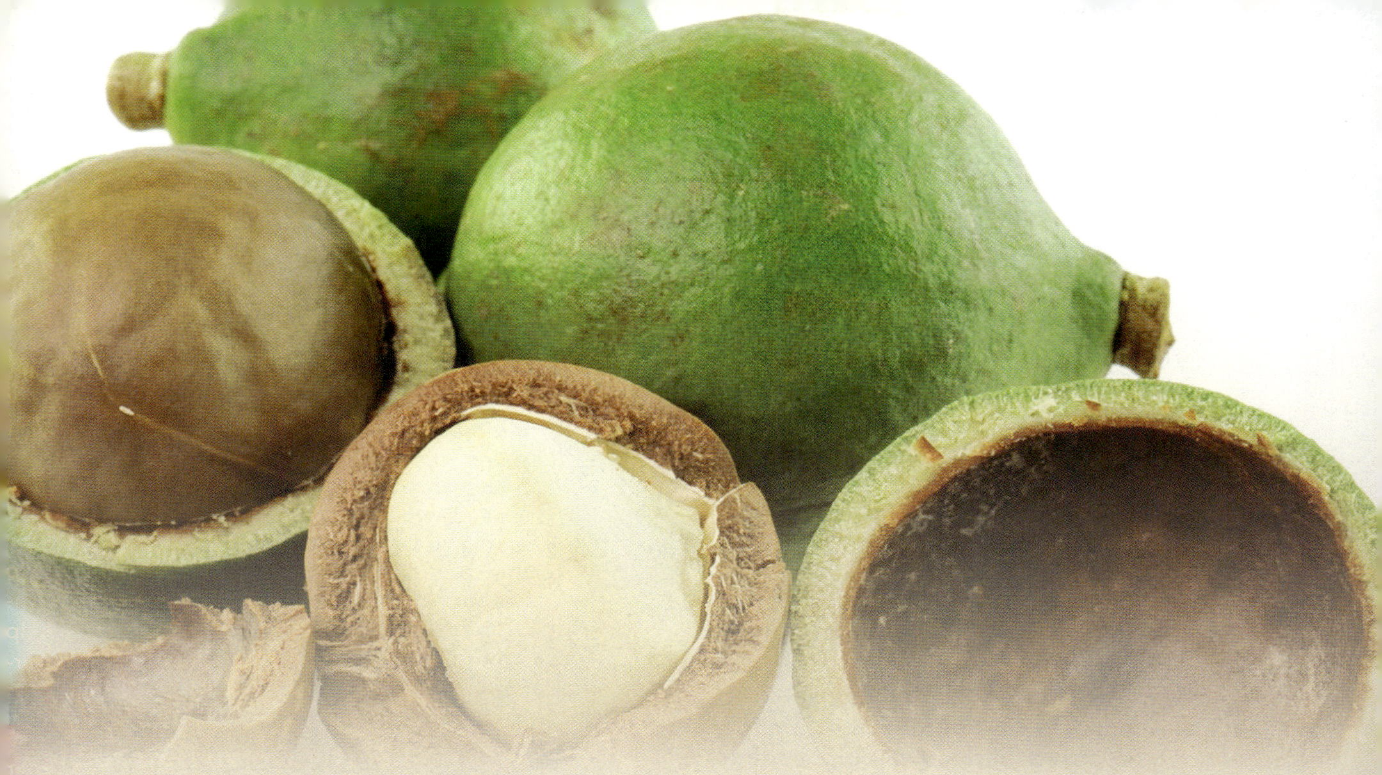

Active Element: Sodium PCA
Sodium PCA – that's a fancy way of saying salt - is a humectant – that's a fancy way of saying a substance that keeps things moist. Humectants form loose bonds with water, and, when used in a cream, can increase the solubility of the active ingredient by elevating skin penetration. Sodium PCA contains essential vitamins D and E, for skin health and firmness.

Active Element: Deep Sea Peptide
This important element is also found in our complementary daytime cream, Nano-Moist Day Renewing Cream. Peptides are the building blocks of proteins, which are the building blocks of humans! More specifically, they play a role in the cellular function of the skin and may prove effective in repairing damaged and aging skin. These little wonders may also reduce the appearance of dark circles under the eyes. Enjoy the benefits of Deep Sea Peptides round the clock, delivered to you in both day and night nano-beneficial creams, which we have optimized to give your skin the nourishment and protection it needs, exactly when it needs it.

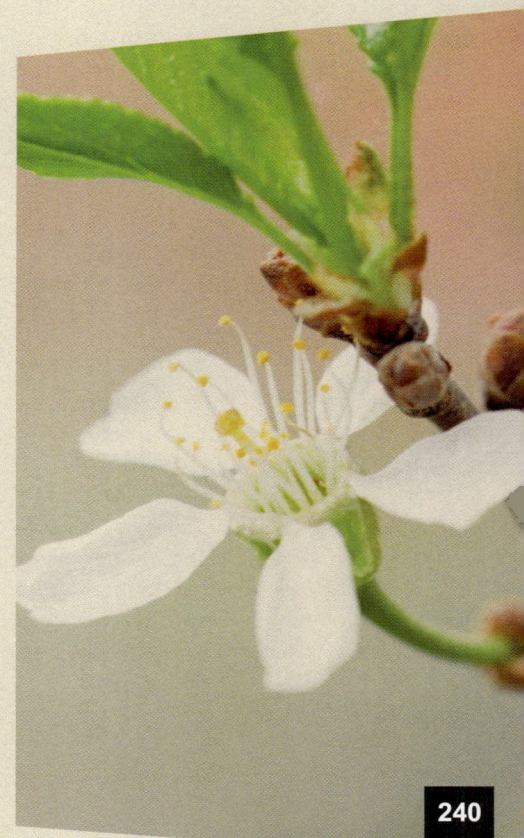

This cream is also rich in Prodew to replenish lost moisture with the added bonus that it may help to restore elasticity and firm your skin, smoothing away wrinkles. Some redness and tingling may occur, but this is just the sparkle doing its thing to increase circulation for nourishment of the repairing cells.

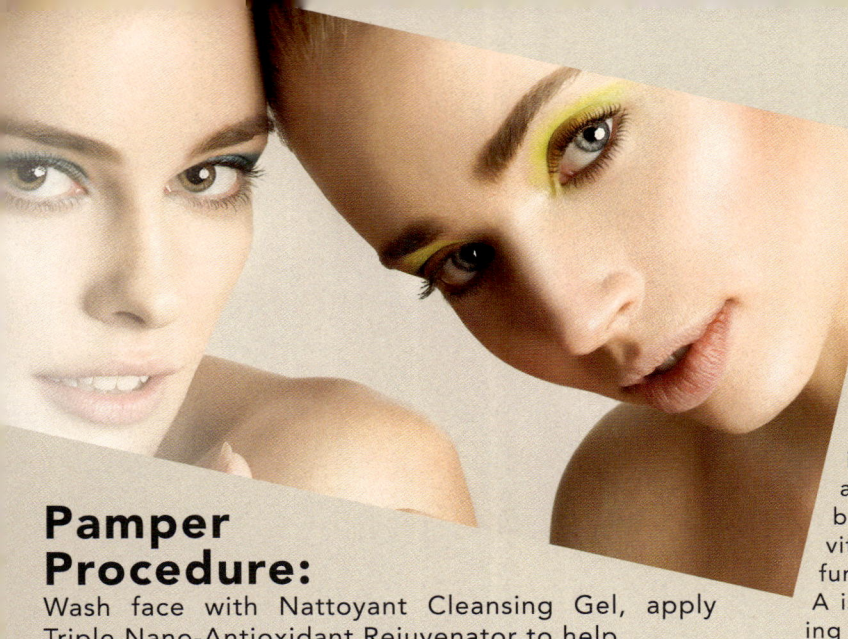

Active Element: Vitamins E & A

Vitamins E & A are absolutely essential for health of any part of your body, not least the biggest organ, skin. Vitamin A has calming, healing effects, and has been shown to reduce the symptoms of psoriasis; it plays a role in wound healing. Like vitamin A, vitamin E is a powerful antioxidant, meaning it can have anti-aging effect on skin cells. Antioxidants are our front-line defense against free radicals, which attack and break down cells. Eating foods with vitamins E & A can help you get further benefits. In particular, vitamin A is required for the proper functioning of many bodily systems, including eyes and immune system.

Pamper Procedure:

Wash face with Nattoyant Cleansing Gel, apply Triple Nano-Antioxidant Rejuvenator to help delaying the aging of your skin. Then apply a small amount of Nano-Restoring Night Caviar over the entire face and neck at night before bedtime for that final touch of repairing and rebuilding collage on your face. Then cozy up with your favorite squeeze and get a good nights rest. If you fail to get adequate sleep, or keep your brain buzzing with TV in bed or playing games on your tablet after you've turned out the light, your brain and body will be too jazzed to fall into restorative REM sleep.

Settle Down Before Sleep

Now that you know the importance and very real nature of "beauty sleep", switch off your appliances an hour before bed time and instead choose a good book or some quiet meditation time

Directions:
Apply over the entire face and neck at night before bedtime

Ingredients:
Water, Cetyl Octanoate, Sorbitol, Sodium PCA, Glycerin, Bamboo Ext, Peapod Ext, Pueraria Ext, Glucosamine, Deep Sea Peptide, Sodium Hyaluronate, 80 Micro-Mineral, Bisabolol, Kukui Nut Oil, Niacinamide, Vitamin A, Nano-Vitamin C, Vitamin E, Flora Blanca, Phenoxyethanol, NaEDTA, Carbomer, Xanthan Gum, Triethanolamine

These statements have not been reviewed by the FDA. This product is not intended to diagnose, treat, cure, or prevent any disease.

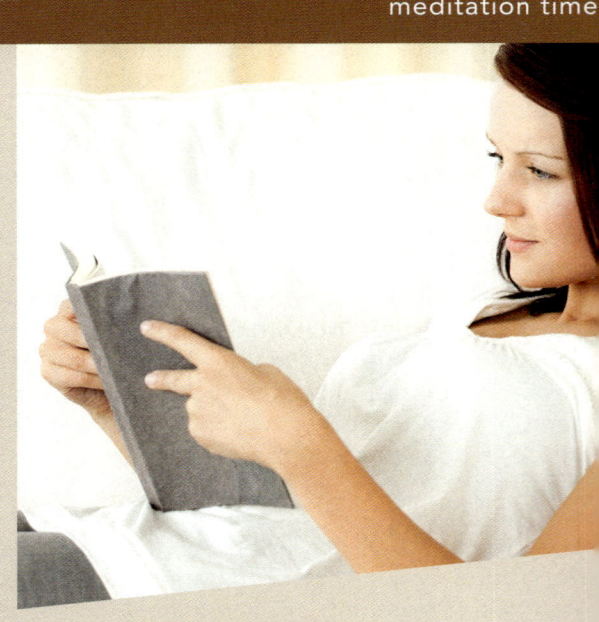

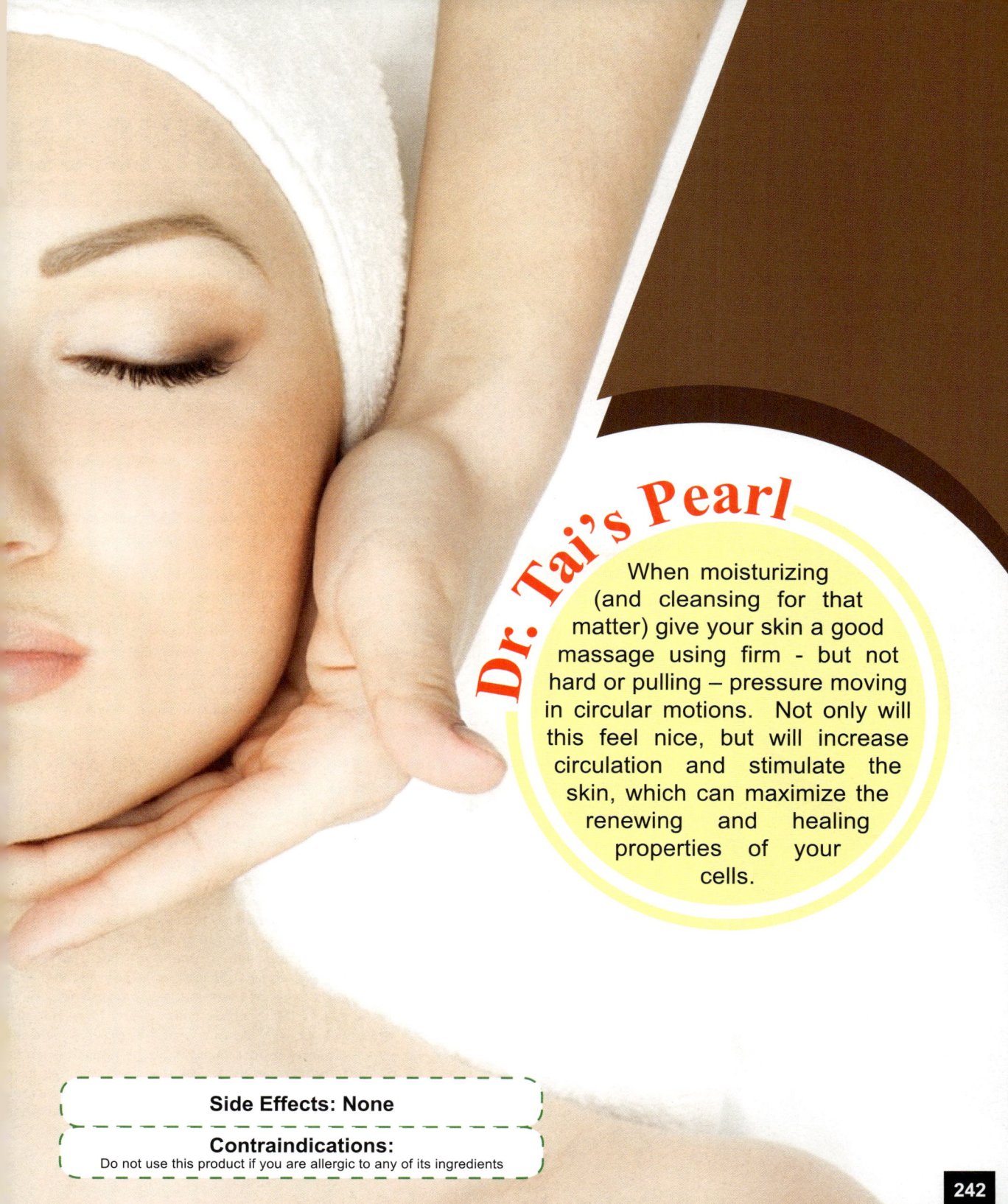

Dr. Tai's Pearl

When moisturizing (and cleansing for that matter) give your skin a good massage using firm - but not hard or pulling – pressure moving in circular motions. Not only will this feel nice, but will increase circulation and stimulate the skin, which can maximize the renewing and healing properties of your cells.

Side Effects: None

Contraindications:
Do not use this product if you are allergic to any of its ingredients

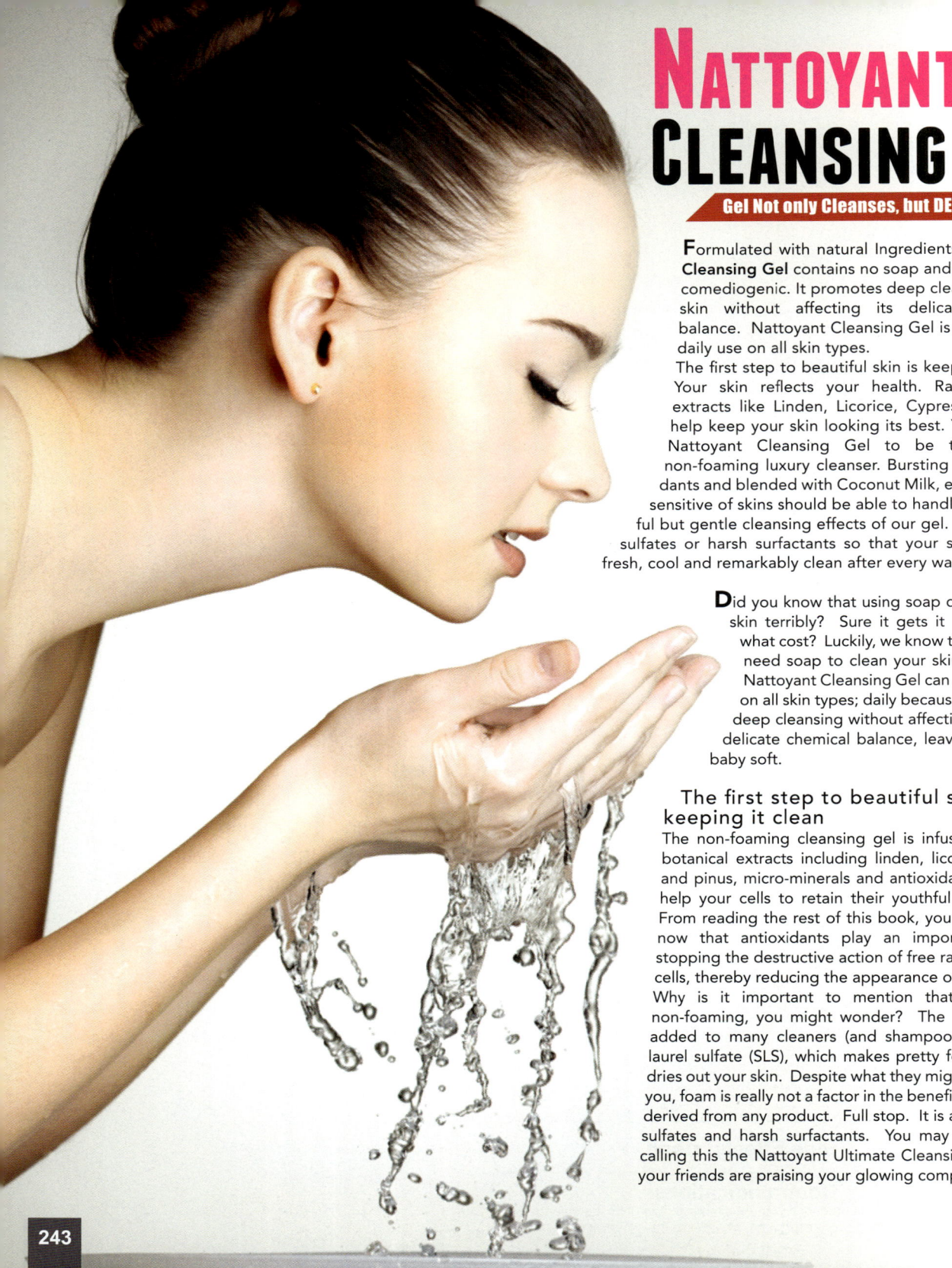

Nattoyant Cleansing Gel

Gel Not only Cleanses, but DETOXIFIES Ski

Formulated with natural Ingredients, **Nattoyant Cleansing Gel** contains no soap and is non-comediogenic. It promotes deep cleansing of the skin without affecting its delicate chemical balance. Nattoyant Cleansing Gel is intended for daily use on all skin types.

The first step to beautiful skin is keeping it clean. Your skin reflects your health. Rare botanical extracts like Linden, Licorice, Cypress and Pinus help keep your skin looking its best. You may find Nattoyant Cleansing Gel to be the ultimate non-foaming luxury cleanser. Bursting with antioxidants and blended with Coconut Milk, even the most sensitive of skins should be able to handle the powerful but gentle cleansing effects of our gel. There are no sulfates or harsh surfactants so that your skin may feel fresh, cool and remarkably clean after every wash

Did you know that using soap dries out your skin terribly? Sure it gets it clean but at what cost? Luckily, we know that you don't need soap to clean your skin! Soap free Nattoyant Cleansing Gel can be used daily on all skin types; daily because it promotes deep cleansing without affecting your skins delicate chemical balance, leaving your skin baby soft.

The first step to beautiful skin is keeping it clean

The non-foaming cleansing gel is infused with rare botanical extracts including linden, licorice, cypress and pinus, micro-minerals and antioxidants that may help your cells to retain their youthful appearance. From reading the rest of this book, you will know by now that antioxidants play an important role in stopping the destructive action of free radicals in your cells, thereby reducing the appearance of aging.

Why is it important to mention that this gel is non-foaming, you might wonder? The agent that is added to many cleaners (and shampoos!) is sodium laurel sulfate (SLS), which makes pretty foam but also dries out your skin. Despite what they might try and sell you, foam is really not a factor in the benefits that can be derived from any product. Full stop. It is also free from sulfates and harsh surfactants. You may find yourself calling this the Nattoyant Ultimate Cleansing Gel when your friends are praising your glowing complexion.

Ancient (Botanical) Man

Since ancient man started smearing lotions and potions on the skin, the benefits of botanicals – fruits and flowers - have been the active ingredient. These naturally growing organisms contain necessary vitamins and minerals. As science progressed, hash chemicals began to replace natural substances due to their seeming ability to do a better job. However, it soon became clear that though they act fast with good results, these chemicals over time cause more harm than good. Modern science began to think again; they rediscovered the benefits of botanicals but this time they were able to isolate and extract the beneficial compounds and combine them to produce a cream or gel that has concentrated botanical extract benefits.

Soapy Secrets

What makes soap "soap" is sodium laurel sulfate (SLS). SLS is a known comediogenic, which is a fancy term for something that exacerbates acne and blackheads. If your skin is too dry, it compensates by producing more natural oils. However, these oils, combined with a heavy "dry skin" moisturizer, contribute only to the exact opposite of what you are aiming for! This means that Natoyant Cleansing Gel – free from SLS - can work well for even the most sensitive skin should be able to endure the powerful cleansing effects of the gel.

Get Sweating

Supplement your cleansing routine with a good sweat. Not only will exercise that makes you sweat help to clear your pores from their very depth, but will also help add a natural brightness to your skin and overall feeling of vitality and self-confidence.

Active Element: Licorice

Licorice contains the compound Glycyrrhizinate, which has proven effective in reducing puffiness and redness, as well as increasing moisturization. It is often used in products aimed at reducing the effects of Rosacea, a skin condition causing redness and blotchiness. Licorice extract may reduce hyper-pigmentation, which is the darkening of skin, resulting in a brighter, lighter complexion.

Active Element: Cypress

Cypress oil has long been lauded for its ability to clear oily, congested pores. It is also known for its relaxing properties, soothing anger and promoting feelings of calm. As you wash your face, breathe in the aroma and create a momentary bubble of peace, before pop goes your day!

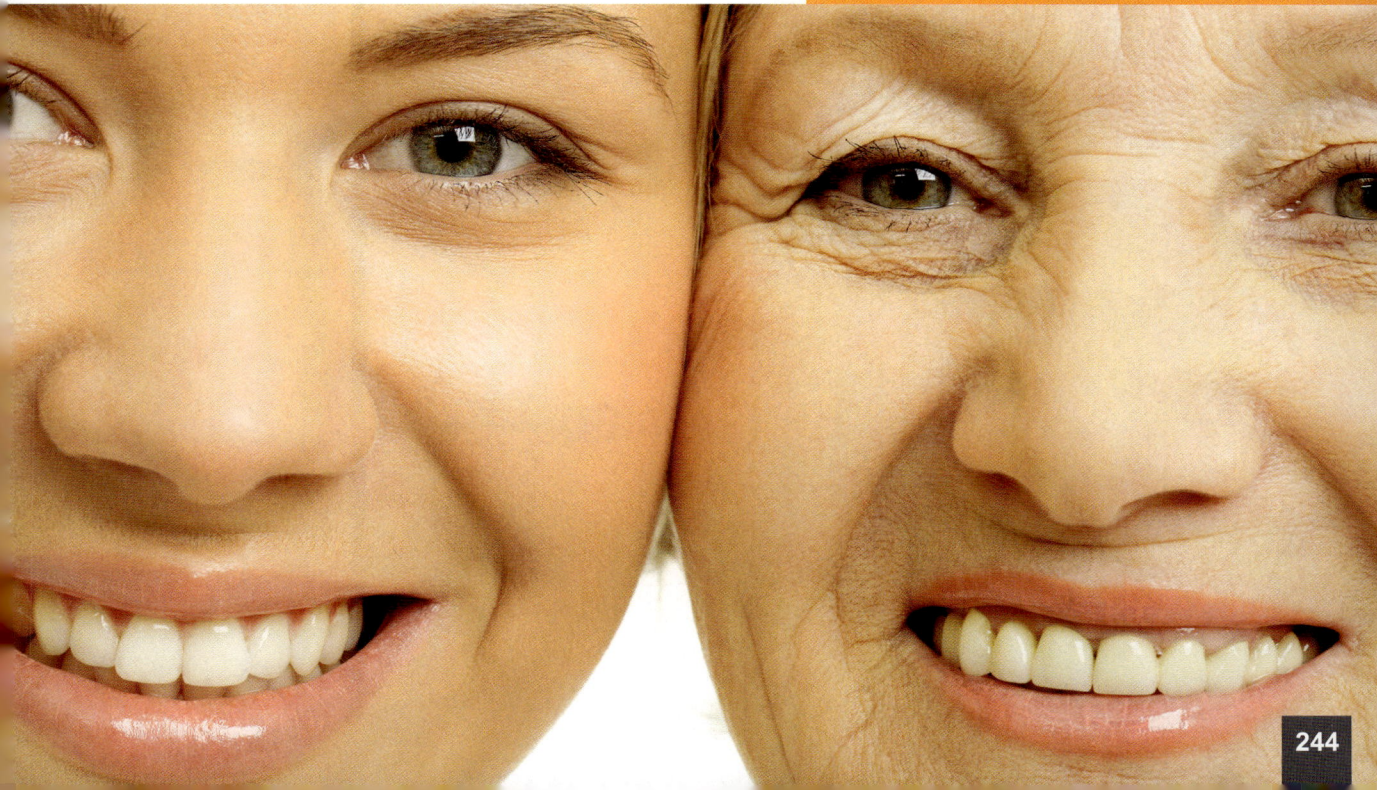

Q: So, what you're saying is that using normal soap to dry to clean my skin and reduce my acne problem actually makes the problem worse, thanks to the SLS?
Joanne, 18

A: In short, yes! It is a common misunderstanding that drying out skin will make it less oily.

Pamper Procedure:

Morning and evening, apply a few drops of the Nattoyant Cleansing Gel and massage in a clockwise circular motion, tissue off and Rinse face with cold water. Your skin may feel "Baby soft" and remarkably clean after every wash. Continue with your holistic skin-care routine.

Ingredients:

Water, Glyceryl, Stearate, Glycerin, Linden, Licorice, Cyress, Pinus Ext, 80 Micro-Mineral Ion Water, Xanthan Gum, Phenoxyethanol, Vitamin E, D-Panthanol, Marine Algae Ext

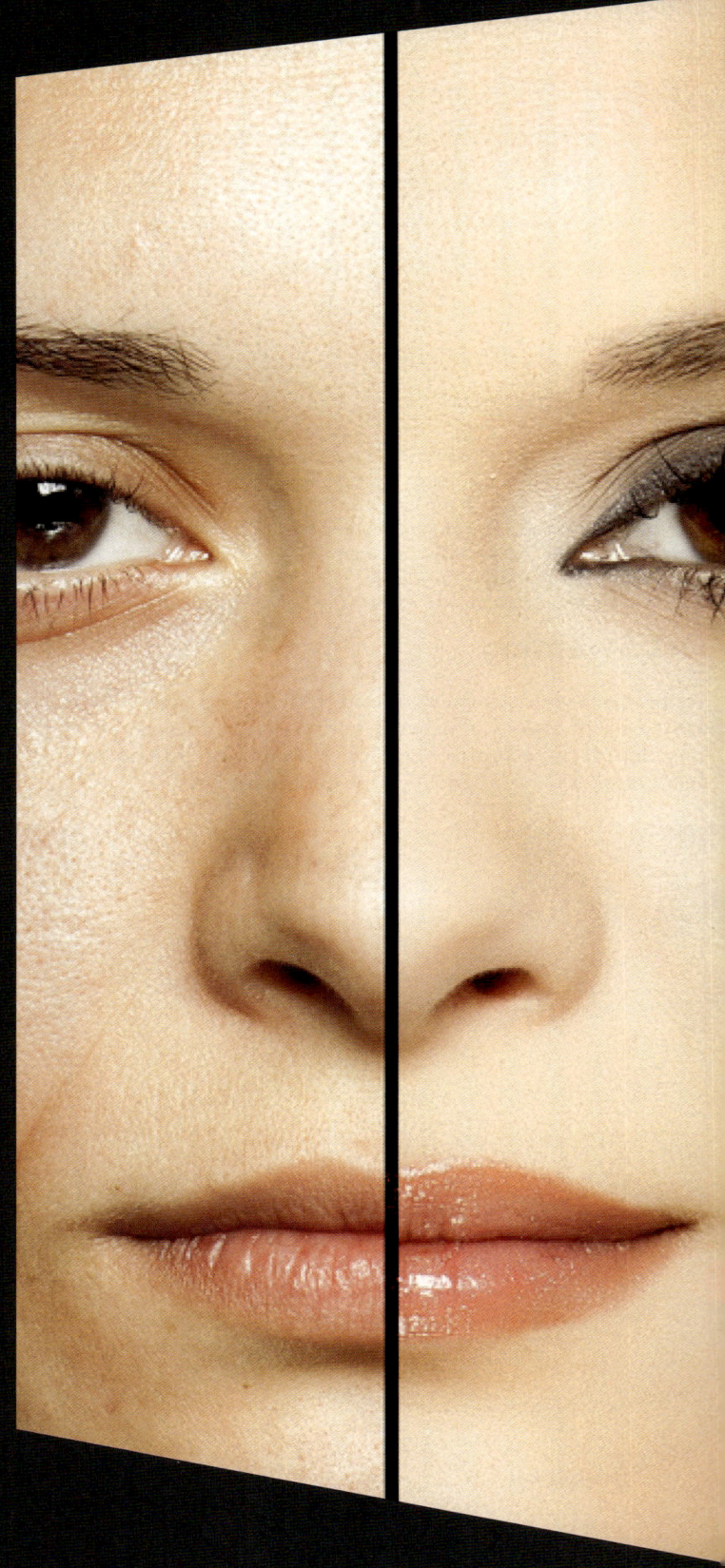

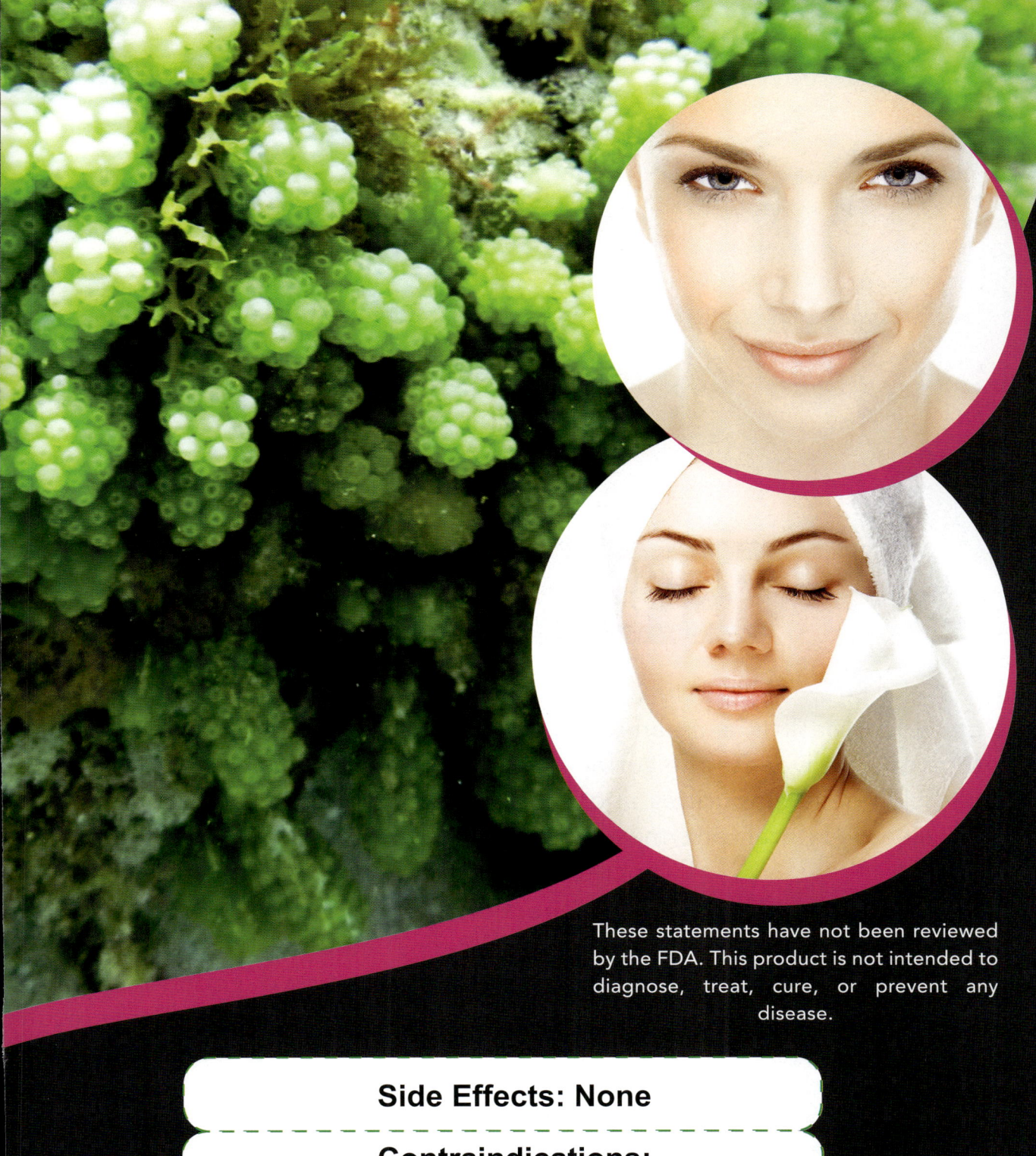

These statements have not been reviewed by the FDA. This product is not intended to diagnose, treat, cure, or prevent any disease.

Side Effects: None

Contraindications:
Do not use this product if you are allergic to any of its ingredients

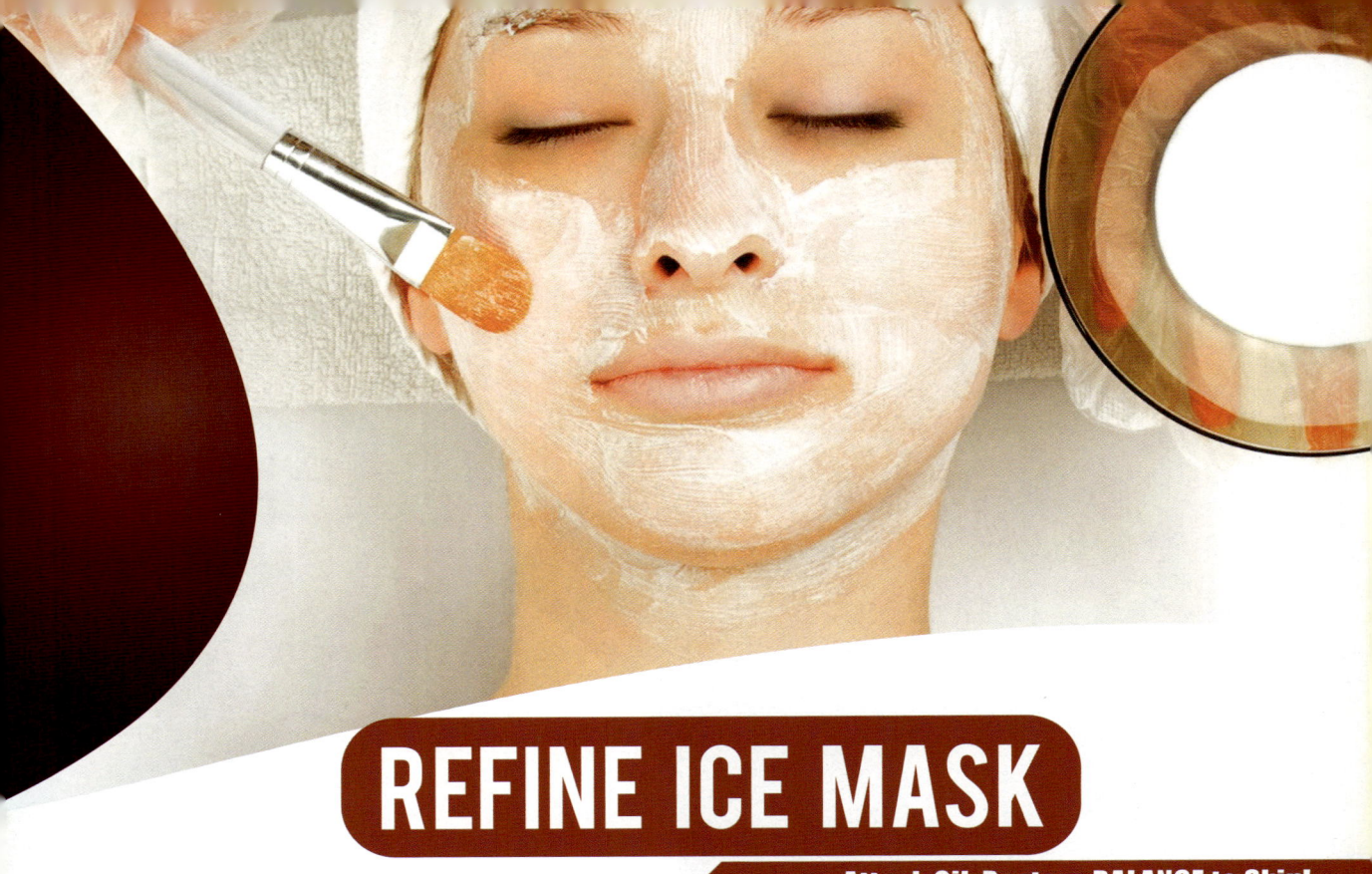

REFINE ICE MASK

Attack Oil, Restore BALANCE to Skin!

Refine Ice Mask is a creamy, soothing and cooling clay mask that may purge and rejuvenate the surface of the skin. Refine Ice Mask may remove dead skin cells, impurities and excess oil leaving your skin glowing, soft and clear. Natural enzymes from exotic tropical fruits may stimulate increased circulation.

Directions:

Gently massage mask into skin. Use of Refine Ice Mask weekly may result in the tightening of pores, the increase and promotion of younger skin and may leave your skin looking radiant. The use of Refine Ice Mask may result in the experience of temporary redness and tingling because of the increased microcirculation and cleaning of toxins from the skin.

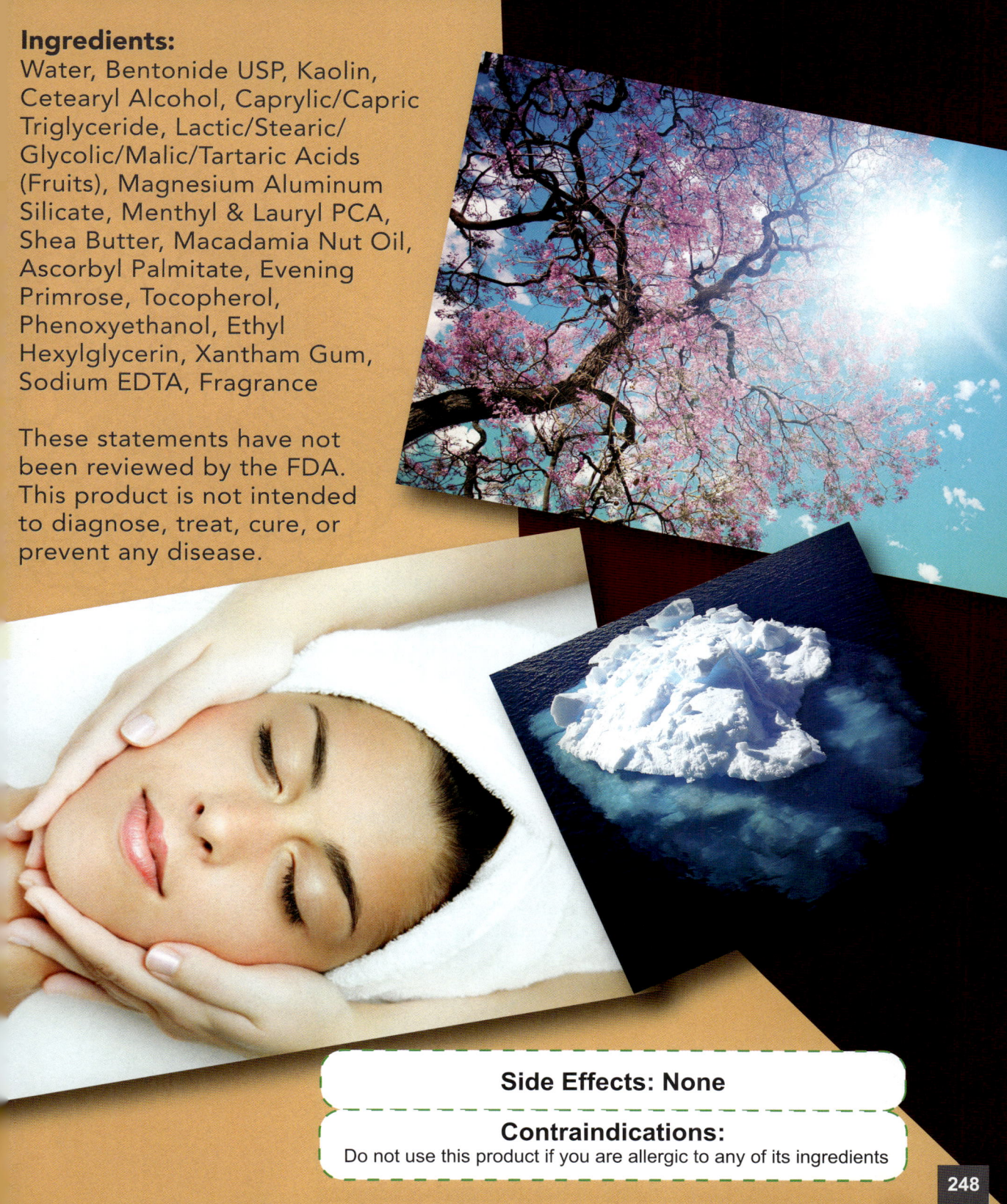

Ingredients:

Water, Bentonide USP, Kaolin, Cetearyl Alcohol, Caprylic/Capric Triglyceride, Lactic/Stearic/Glycolic/Malic/Tartaric Acids (Fruits), Magnesium Aluminum Silicate, Menthyl & Lauryl PCA, Shea Butter, Macadamia Nut Oil, Ascorbyl Palmitate, Evening Primrose, Tocopherol, Phenoxyethanol, Ethyl Hexylglycerin, Xantham Gum, Sodium EDTA, Fragrance

These statements have not been reviewed by the FDA. This product is not intended to diagnose, treat, cure, or prevent any disease.

Side Effects: None

Contraindications:
Do not use this product if you are allergic to any of its ingredients

SKIN RENEW

DNA Repair of Skin Cells

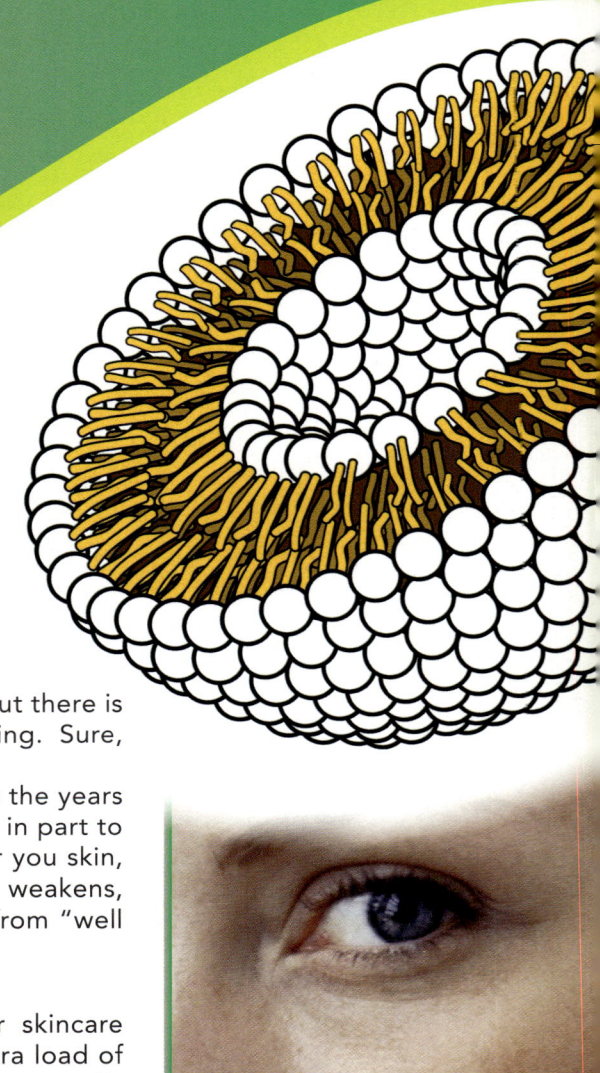

This all-in-one liposome formula may deliver cellular repair power to new cells with an extra load of collagen and elastin.

As you age you can take the best care of your skin but there is one thing you will never halt, and that is the effects of aging. Sure, you can slow it down by nourishing and protecting your skin, but its ability to renew will lessen as the years fly by. The main culprit is loss of elasticity in the skin due in part to breakdown of collagen. Collagen is a sort of scaffold for you skin, keeping the structure firm and pert. When the scaffold weakens, skin can sag and wrinkles creep in places that take you from "well seasoned" to "overdone".

Vitamins and minerals are essential to your skincare routine. As you get older, Skin Renew serum with an extra load of collagen and elastin may deliver cellular repair power to new cells and firm you up in all the right places. Elastin allows body structures (on the teeny tiny level) to bounce back after they have been stretched. This can even be a non-invasive, natural alternative to botox!

Pamper Procedure:

After exfoliating your face with Smart Skin, apply a small amount of Skin Renew to face and neck. Leave on the skin for 10-15 minutes to allow for activation to occur, then rinse well with water and continue with your holistic skin-care routine.

Active Element: Micro-Minerals

Micro-minerals, also known as "trace minerals", are required by every living organism. In humans, micro-minerals are essential for healthy daily cell function. Micro-minerals aid your body in many ways, including teeth and bone health, immune function, essential enzyme function, connective tissue, arterial strength and antioxidant production. Antioxidants are your front line defense against aging!

Active Element: Retinotretin

Vitamin A acids, salicylic acids and fruit acids are all essential elements in the renovation of the dermis (skin) cells. Skin cells naturally depend on these acids to cleanse, revitalize and stimulate new cell production with higher collagen and elastin content. Skin Renew is enriched with retinotretin. In fact, retinotretin, with its properties promoting skin peeling and cell renewal, is effective – and often prescribed - in treating sunburned skin. Skin cells simply thrive on the positive effect of Skin Renew.

Directions:
After a skin sensitivity test on your forearm, apply in equal amounts Skin Renew and Ultra Lightener to the face and neck. Leave on for 5 minutes to allow activation to occur and rinse well with water.
Use every night.

Ingredients:
Deion Water, Carbopol, Retinotretin, Phenoxyethanol, Ethylglycerin, Xanthan Gum, Microminerals

These statements have not been reviewed by the FDA. This product is not intended to diagnose, treat, cure, or prevent any disease.

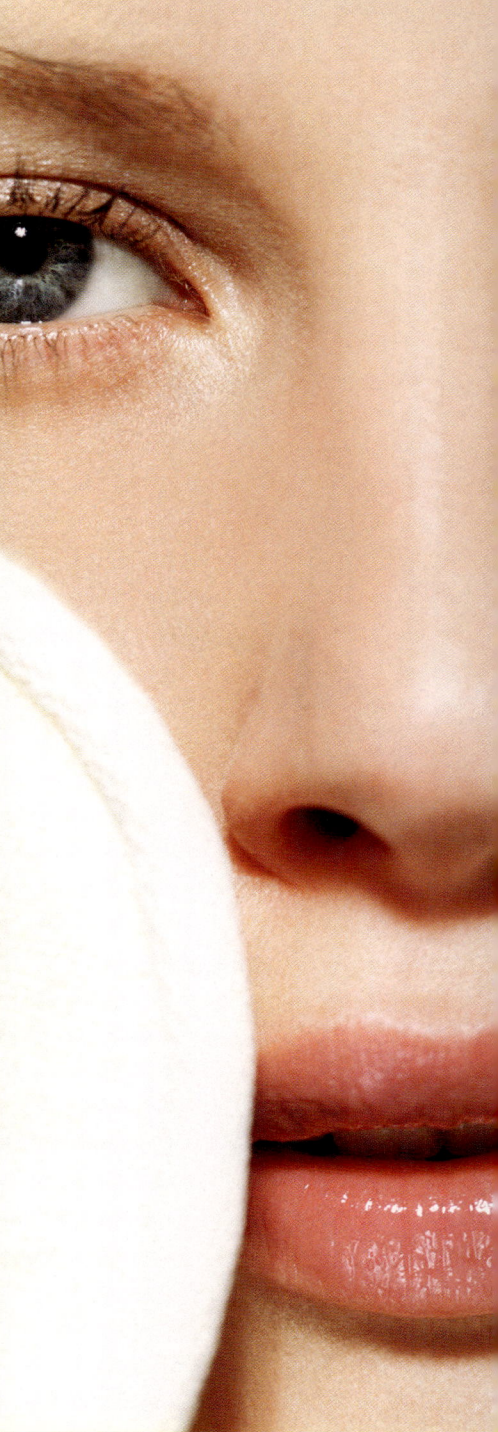

Side Effects: None

Contraindications:
Do not use this product if you are allergic to any of its ingredients

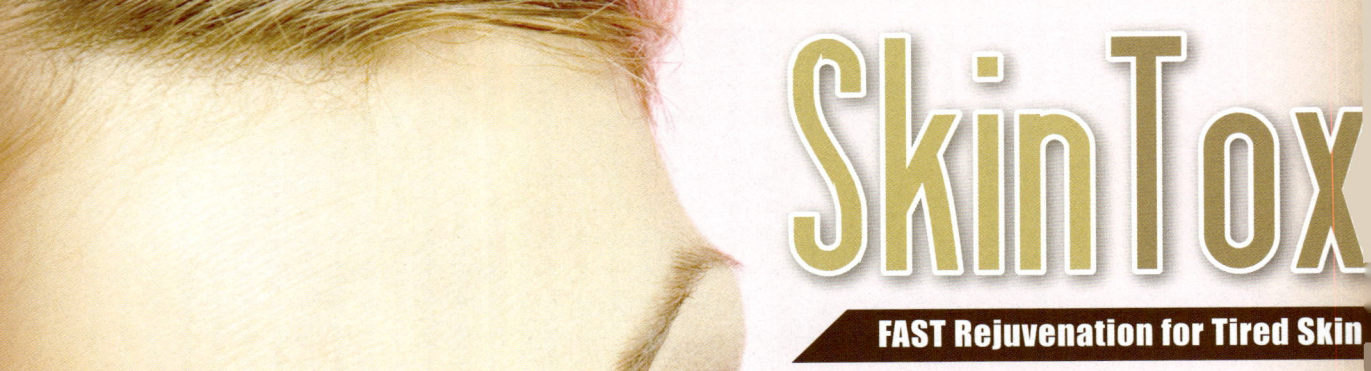

SkinTox

FAST Rejuvenation for Tired Skin

Have you ever thought of the idea of receiving 20 injections all over your face just to help diminish those pesky little wrinkles? **Yes,** along with some improvement, you will have that "special undeniable" BOTOX™ look. You know...-can't smile naturally, your eyebrows are paralyzed; you can't even wink anymore at anyone. Of course all of this for only $400 dollars thank you!

Well, we actually have a natural option for you. No more shots, no "dead mask" look, no more paralyzed face.

It is called SkinTox, a natural serum that penetrates your skin quickly and may painlessly increase the volume of the dermis (skin layer) by 15%, erasing those pesky small wrinkles and minimizing the depth of those nasolabial folds, creating a natural, softer, younger, more relaxed look and facial appearance.

Simply apply SkinTox serum onto the small and large wrinkled areas. SkinTox works by quickly and gently washing away the excess accumulated toxins and carbon dioxide from the skin cells, allowing your skin to breath and refresh. You will absolutely love the results - more youthful, even toned, and healthier glowing skin.

This is truly skin deep because of the special one of a kind technology used in this unique product. The SkinTox serum, when applied to the skin, will relax the glabellar muscles and bring your facial skin to its natural beautiful positions.

Go ahead; let your skin be younger, more naturally relaxed, and beautiful!

Directions: On a clean face, apply 2-3 pumps on the wrinkle areas. Use AM & PM daily.

These statements have not been reviewed by the FDA. This product is not intended to diagnose, treat, cure, or prevent any disease.

The Anti-Wrinkles Test:
14 day panel test
30 women ages 35 to 40
Visible wrinkles around the eye
Application of SkinTox serum – twice daily around the eye area for 7 days

Scientific Results:
Moisture content (thickening of skin)
- Gradually increased during the 7 days
- 52% increase in skin moisture content.
- The number of wrinkles, depth, and length of the wrinkle decreased by as much as 50%

If you ever dreamed of a natural serum that is not oily, not a gimmick or trick of lighting but just plain science for your skin, you have found it in **SkinTox**.

Ingredients:
Water, BTX- Perflourohexane, Perfluoroperhydrophenanthrene, Perfluorodecalin, Sodium Hyaluronate, Caprylic Capric Triglycerides, Phenoxyethanol, Ethylhexylglycerin, Dimethicone, Polyacrylamide, Laureth-7, C13-14 Isoparaffin

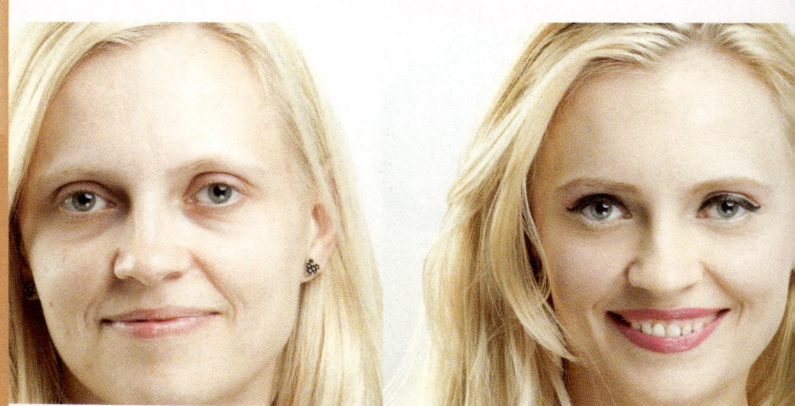

Contraindications:
Do not use product if you are allergic to any of its ingredients.

Side Effects: None

252

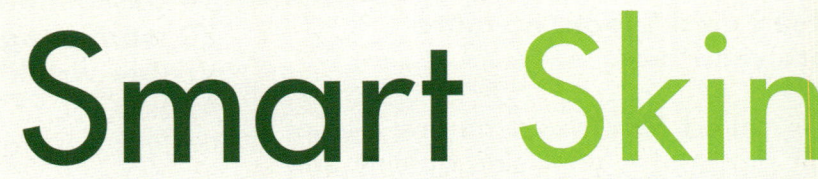

Smart Skin

Most Powerful Skin Rejuvenation Formula

Our U.S. Patent pending skincare product uses natural cucumber extracts to lift the dead skin and remove it without irritation, which may result in stimulating young collagen and elastin. It is smart because it knows just how deep to go as not to cause inflammation to your delicate skin.

Using the age-old wisdom of natural cucumber, coupled with a special extraction technology to empower Smart Skin to lift dead skin and removes without irritation. The result? You may just find yourself gazing at a younger reflection in the mirror! This cream knows just how far to go in stimulating young collagen and elastic, without causing inflammation to delicate skin. Cucumber wisdom has long been used to reduce redness and puffiness by shrinking blood vessels, tightening and lifting the skin.

With daily use you may be able to reveal what has been hidden under up to 250 layers of dead skin all this time: Skin texture soft as a baby's and a brighter skin tone that your face will thank you for!

So we have created Smart Skin! This is **Dr. Tai's** most popular U.S. Patent, which has been in careful development over the last five years. To get under those superficial layers to the real basis of your un-beneficial face-mark, most products use abrasion with small, pointy sediments that do nothing more than irritating your skin by leaving you criss-crossed with microscopic cuts and bruises. The result is not clean smooth skin, but tiny scars making you skin look inflamed and dull. Some even suggest you need amachine with whirring brushes!

The benefits of natural cucumber extract is the within ten seconds of rubbing with your own fingers in a circular motion, it begins to penetrate and lift that crusty grime of dead skin and environmental toxins and dirt. The natural power is so effective that your part in the process will seem effortless, as if you are simply giving yourself a pleasant face massage.

Warning!
The first time you use Smart Skin you may experience shock at the amount of dirt and grime that falls from your face into the sink. Don't be alarmed! This is perfectly normal for most people who have been walking around unaware of the literal mask they wear. Once you get over the shock, let the relief wash over you now that you skin is now, finally, spectacularly cleaned! As you perform this cleaning ritual daily, you will have the most beautiful healthy skin.

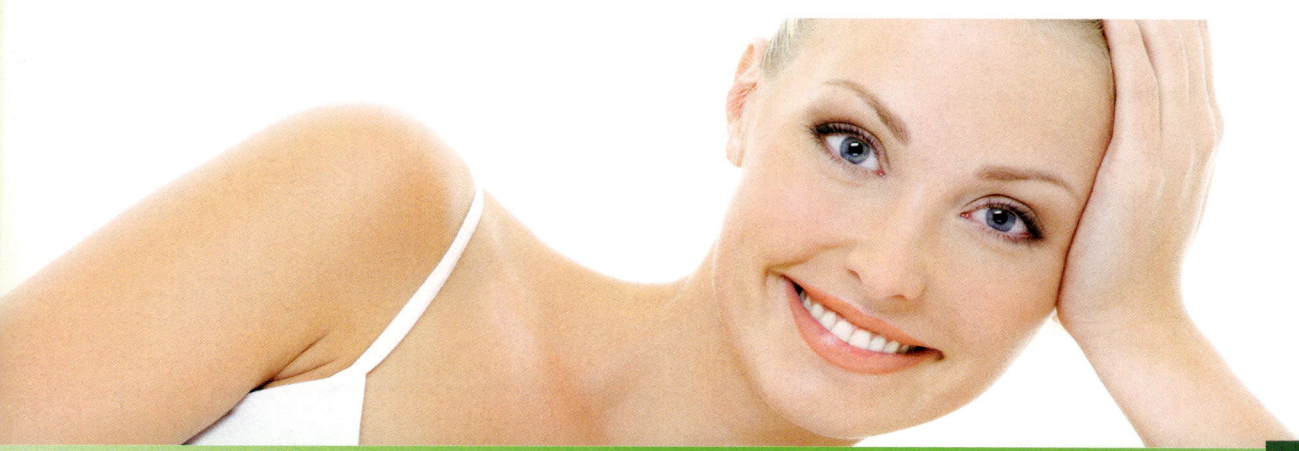

Most Powerful Skin Rejuvenation Formula

Cucumber is a healthy addition to your diet for the wonderful benefits it affords your body in the form of vitamins and minerals, not to enzymes essential for cell growth and antioxidants for cell growth and repair. All of this culminates in the appearance of calm, cool, radiant younger skin.

Q: If I use Smart Skin every day, the mask of dirt of my face will be, well, just about gone. Doesn't that mean I don't have to use every day? I'm afraid of the powerful cleansing action damaging my skin, especially the delicate neck area and décolletage.

- Jennifer, 34

A: The best thing about Mother Nature is that she knows how to be strong and gentle at the same time. Natural cucumber peel extract, while hard on grime, is gentle on skin. To avoid the grimy dirt mask from gathering again, it is recommended to use Smart Skin daily. Cucumber has many benefits for your skin, so the more you use it, the more you can enjoy the cucumber benefits as it doesn't have to work so hard getting through a layer of built-up toxins.

Pamper Procedure:
Smart Skin is the first step in your holistic skincare routine. Apply a small amount from the 50 ml bottle onto dry face and rub briskly until dead skin deposits have formed or the skin surface. Wash with Nattoyan Cleansing Gel and Diamond microdermabrasion, rinse well with water. Use daily for that polished radiant look!

Ingredients:
Deion Water, Carbomer, Glycerin, Glycol Vitamin E, Cucumber peel Extract.

These statements have not been reviewed by the FDA. This product is not intended to diagnose, treat, cure, or prevent any disease..

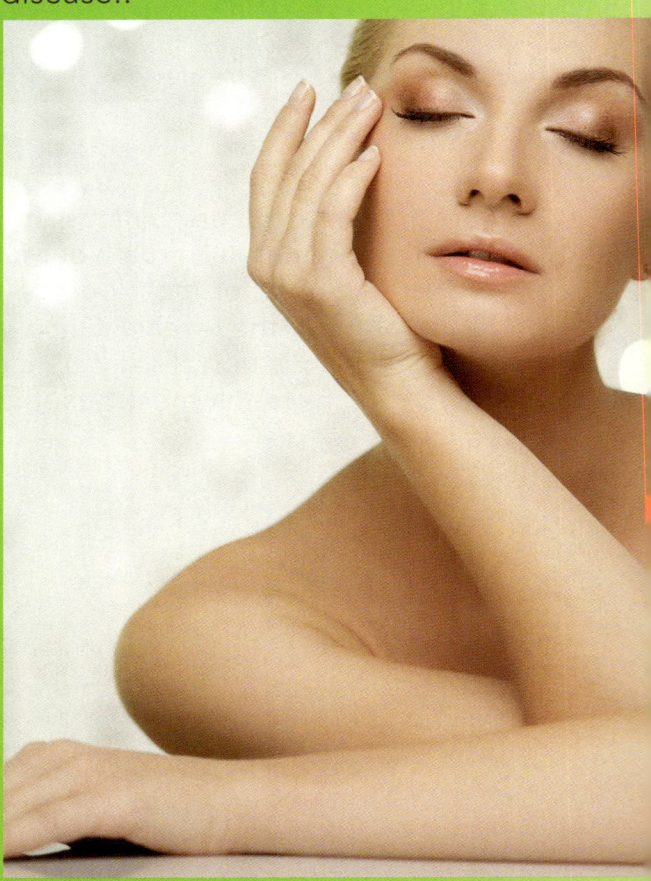

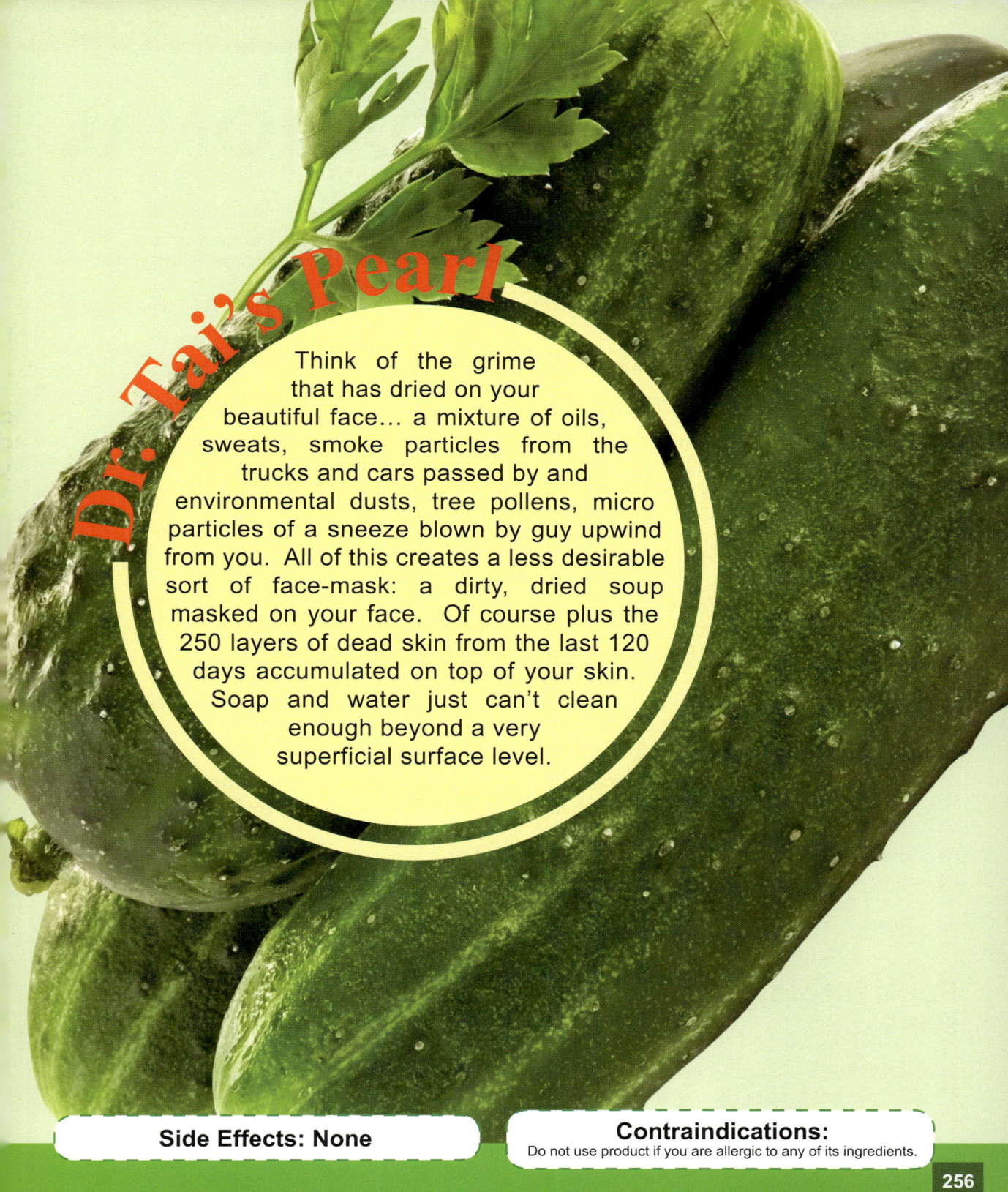

Dr. Tai's Pearl

Think of the grime that has dried on your beautiful face… a mixture of oils, sweats, smoke particles from the trucks and cars passed by and environmental dusts, tree pollens, micro particles of a sneeze blown by guy upwind from you. All of this creates a less desirable sort of face-mask: a dirty, dried soup masked on your face. Of course plus the 250 layers of dead skin from the last 120 days accumulated on top of your skin. Soap and water just can't clean enough beyond a very superficial surface level.

Side Effects: None

Contraindications:
Do not use product if you are allergic to any of its ingredients.

Testing

FOUNDATIONAL

Saliva Hormone Testing

Saliva is used as biological fluid for the detection of different hormone biomarkers. The salivary gland is a natural filter, allowing only unbound and free, useful hormones to come through and provide the most accurate hormone tests.

- Uses 5 samples of saliva
- Explanation of results & support
- Comes with natural treatment recommendations

Full Male Panel - 7 Hormones
Progesterone, Estrone, Estradiol, Testosterone, DHEA, Cortisol AM, Cortisol PM

Full Female Panel - 8 Hormones
Progesterone, Estrone, Estradiol, Estriol, Testosterone, DHEA, Cortisol AM, Cortisol PM

Cancer Discovery & Monitoring Test

Don't wait for Major symptoms to discover Cancer has already spread!!
Catch Cancer at even the earliest stages and metastasis!!
MONITOR YOUR CANCER SPREAD & METASTASIS

Do not risk your health or your life when you can be well informed with this reliable & non-invasive testing. A Great way to **monitor Cancer In Real Time** while you are doing treatment.
(Recommended every 6 months)

It gives great information on undetected spread of Cancer.
Make sure you know your Cancer is under control!

Used to monitor cancer patients on their treatment progress and detect re-occurrence. It checks for circulating Cancer cells present & alive in the patient's blood stream.

This test effectively monitors Cancer progress & prognosis of future Cancer Development.

Food Intolerance
Self-Test Kit

Easy & Immediate Sensitivity Testing!
This simple self-test kit allows you to check for 46 different Food Intolerances.
No shipping samples or waiting days to weeks.

Results within 1 hour!

TESTING

Dried Blood Spot
Testing (DBS) Kits
Convenient & easy to do yourself with a simple prick of the finger!

Vitamin D3 Testing
This deficiency can result in many health-related diseases. Vitamin D3 deficiency is an epidemic even in the 20th century with all our medical advances and is the cause of low immunity and many Cancers

Thyroid Testing
Thyroid disease is linked to over 59 major diseases including Hashimoto's Disease, Graves Disease, Heart Disease, Obesity, Cancer, Hypertension and many more. This simple test detects the TSH, T3, T4 and TPO levels, & the health of your Thyroid Gland unlike other incomplete tests.

ThyroFlex Thyroid Test

The Patented, innovative ThyroFlex Thyroid testing device offers a non-invasive state of the art system for testing for thyroid disease, and the balancing of the core hormones that support and interact with the thyroid.
The ThyroFlex test measures the neurotransmitter speed (brain function), the reflex speed, and the resting metabolic rate (RMR).

As seen on the Dr. Phil Show, Better Arizona, The Today Show, the Global Health Show (New Zealand), Happy Hormone Cottage on Channel 12 News Ohio, and the Holtorf Medical Group by Dr. Petersen on Channel 4 Utah.

BARM is the ONLY authorized, exclusive agent for ThyroFlex.
Get Tested TODAY!

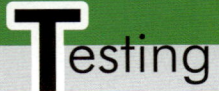

OTHER PANEL

BioFilm Testing - Test for discovering chronic hidden infections & inflammation and evaluating severity of biofilms from Cancer, fungal, candida, bacterial, or viral infections, which is normally not available through mainstream blood testing.

Biofilm is a protective chemical wall that Cancer & Chronic Infections build to protect themselves & Survive the attacks of our body's Immune System.

Used frequently for detection, evaluation, monitoring of Cancer, Lyme Disease, HIV, Infection in Bowels, Epstein Barr and Mononucleosis.

BioFilm Testing is an inexpensive way of monitoring efficacy of therapy.

Elements in Blood III - Panel elements in blood II + mercury, cadmium, arsenic and aluminum in whole blood. Cobalt, molybdenum, lead and gold in serum. Cadmium and lead intracellular.

Elements in Urine II - Calcium, magnesium, copper, zinc, selenium, chromium, manganese, cadmium, lead, mercury, sodium, potassium, iron, nickel, aluminum, vanadium, silver, sulphur, phosphorus, molybdenum, cobalt, arsenic, lithium, iodine, antimony, beryllium, bismuth, bromine, platinum, tin.

Total Vitamin Panel - A, B1, B6, E, B3, Folic Acid, B12, C, Carotene, B2, B5, Biotin, Carnitine, D3, K, CoQ10

Neurotransmitters Panel in Platelets - Dopamine, Epinephrine, Norepinephrine, Metanephrine, Normetanephrine, Serotonin (PRP), MAO (RBC)

COMPONENTS TESTING

Essential Fatty Acids - Omega 3 Series - Alfa-linolenic acid (ALA), Eicosatrienoic acid, Eicosapent acid (EPA), Docosahexaenoic acid, Omega 6 Series – Linoleic acid, Gamma linolenic acid, Eicosadienoic acid, Dihomogammalinolenic acid, Arachidonic acid (AA), Docosatetranoic acid, Ratio AA/EPA, Omega 9 Series – Trans elaidic acid (TEA), Cis oleic acid, Eicosenoic acid, Erucic acid, Nervonic acid, Saturated fatty acids – Palmitic acid, Stearic acid

Amino Acids in Urine - Essential Amino Acids – Threonine, Valine, Methionine, Isoleucine, Leucine, Phenylalanine, Lysine, Histidine, Tryptophaan, Protein Amino Acids – Asparaginezuur, Serine, Asparagine, Glutaminezuur, Glutamine, Proline, Glycine, Alanine, Cystine, Tyrosine, Arginine, Metabolic Amino Acids – Fosfoserine, Taurine, Fosfoethanol-amine, Hydroxyproline, Sarcosine, a-Aminoadipinezuur, Citrulline, a-Aminoboterzuur, Cystathion, B-Alanine, B-Aminoisoboterzuur, Homocystine, Gamma-Aminoboterzuur, Ethanolamine, Hydroxylysine, Ornithine, 1-Methylhistidine, 3-Methylhistidine, Anserine, Carnosine

RESOURCES

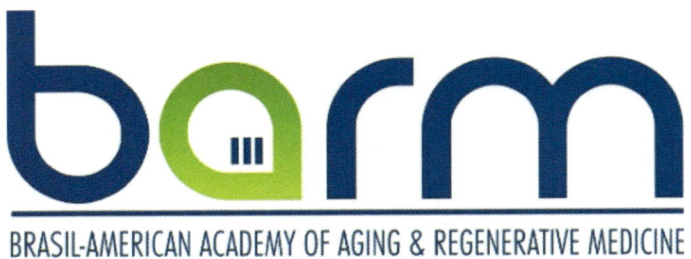

BARM
A Private Membership Society
Brasil-American
Academy of Aging
&
Regenerative Medicine
Sao Paulo, Brasil
www.barm.com.br
www.barmshop.com
webmaster@barm.us

RESOURCES

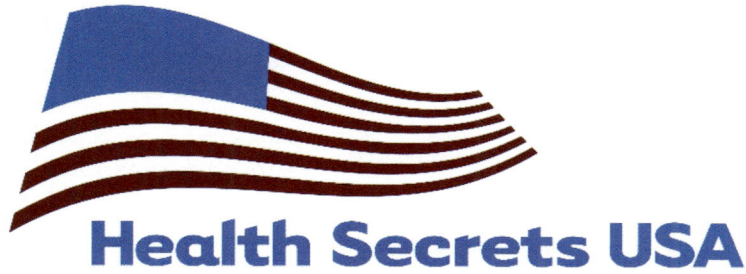

Health Secrets USA
24141 Ann Arbor Trail
Dearborn Heights, MI 48127
www.healthsecretsusa.com
Tel: 313.561.6800
Fax: 313.561.6830
office@healthsecretsusa.com
contact@healthsecretsusa.com

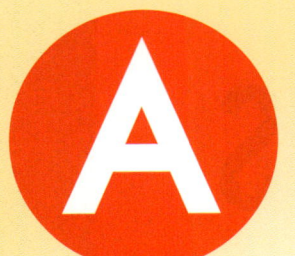
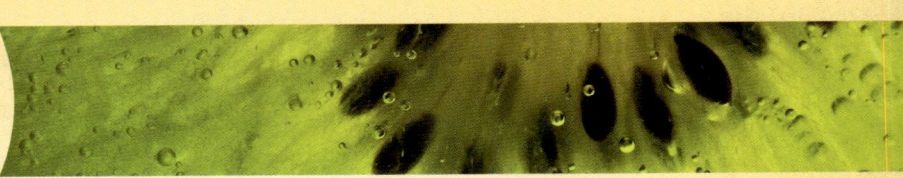

A

Acidity	3, 150, 199
Acne	97, 204, 221, 222, 232, 244, 245
ADHD	15, 42, 45, 46
Adrenal Fatigue	32, 35, 42, 67, 103, 193
AIDS	41, 42
Alzheimer's	134, 136, 155, 161, 164, 165, 209, 210, 212, 214
Amino Acids	8, 24, 35, 41, 99, 104, 180, 183
Angina	15, 98
Anti-Aging	2, 24, 27, 33, 35, 75, 76, 89, 111, 114, 134, 155, 158, 167, 172, 173, 174, 204,
Anti-Bacterial	224
Antibiotics	5, 43, 164
Antifungal	211
Anti-inflammatory	5, 187
	12, 16, 29, 32, 52, 54, 58, 69, 108, 109, 163, 172, 173, 175, 210, 217
Antioxidants	24, 27, 29, 37, 41, 42, 72, 76, 102, 106, 143, 167, 168, 171, 172, 216, 224, 243
Anti-Viral	5, 43, 71, 163, 198
Anxiety	9, 45, 46, 52, 54, 66, 76, 94, 95, 156, 157, 158, 159, 160, 161, 180, 181, 182, 207, 208
Apoptosis	39, 40, 78, 120, 124
Aromatization	115, 117, 118, 123, 124, 128, 186
Arthritis	3, 8, 10, 28, 29, 35, 50, 54, 61, 69, 70, 103, 107, 108, 110, 164, 165, 217
Asthma	164, 170
Astringent	233
Atherosclerosis	12, 15, 42, 103
Autism	15, 42, 45
Autoimmune Diseases	49, 209

B

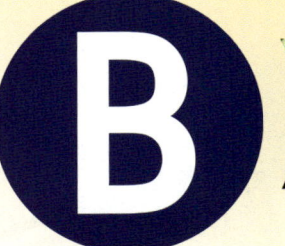
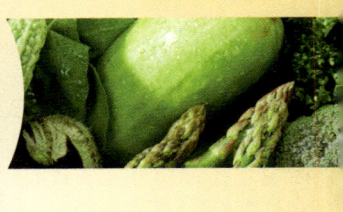

Beauty	70, 88, 171, 174, 223
Bio-Hormones	87
Blood Clots	15, 164
Blood Pressure	15, 27, 35, 66, 68, 70, 80, 141, 145, 161, 162, 190, 195, 202, 209, 215, 218
Bone Health	187, 215, 227, 250
Bone Loss	99, 108, 210
Bronchial Asthma	52
Bruising	8, 60

C

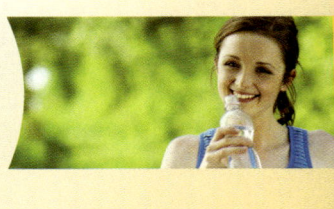

Calcium	3, 19, 20, 22, 23, 74, 80, 82, 83, 84, 99, 126, 127, 186, 203, 209, 210, 211, 214
Cancer	15, 42, 72, 77, 78, 83, 90, 99, 109, 115, 116, 117, 120, 123, 125, 127, 134, 159, 164, 165, 171, 209, 216, 257, 258, 259
Candida	5, 35, 71, 165, 187
Cannabidiol	50, 51, 52, 54

C CONTINUED

Cardiovascular Disease..31, 69, 161, 216
Cataract............................ 37
CBD................................50, 51, 52, 53
Cholesterol.....................11, 12, 13, 14, 24, 75, 99, 102, 127, 155, 156, 164, 165, 187, 209
Chronic Fatigue...............15, 31, 32, 42, 155, 180, 209
Circulation......................12, 15, 24, 27, 28, 37, 56, 69, 70, 80, 151, 154, 166, 173, 174, 186, 189, 190, 202, 212, 224, 239, 240, 247
Cirrhosis..........................111, 210
Clots................................13, 15
Collagen......................... 58, 74, 171, 172, 223, 224, 235, 236, 249, 253
Constipation...................21, 81, 82, 84, 86, 93, 94, 95, 96, 193, 199
CoQ10............................14, 29, 102, 103, 259
Coronary Artery Disease 13
Cortisol...........................10, 31, 65, 67, 68, 136, 155, 192, 198, 214
Cravings......................... 19, 66, 84, 187
Crohn's Disease..............15
Cystic Fibrosis................42

D

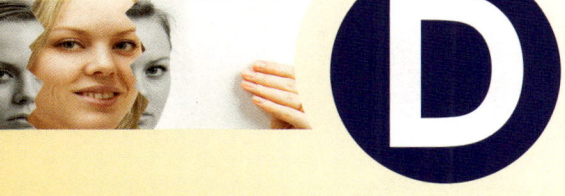

Dead Skin........................ 194, 231, 232, 247, 253, 254, 255, 256
Deep Vein Thrombosis....15
Depression......................8, 9, 31, 50, 52, 66, 79, 94, 98, 103 111, 134, 146, 155, 156, 157, 158, 160, 181, 207, 208, 209
Dermatitis.......................175, 205
Diabetes..........................3, 15, 31, 36, 42, 98, 102, 153, 154, 155, 164, 165, 170, 171, 173, 186, 187, 189, 190, 204, 209, 212, 217, 219

E

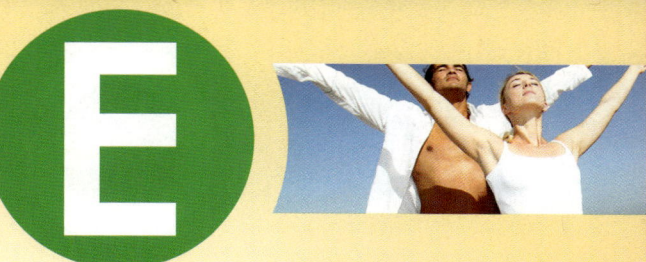

Eczema............................ 86, 175, 205
Elasticity..........................16, 35, 57, 58, 174, 189, 213, 223, 224, 239, 240, 249
Elastin.............................58, 171, 235, 236, 249, 253
Endometriosis.................125, 157, 158
Environmental Toxins..... 170, 172, 254
Erectile Dysfunction....... 117, 185, 203, 204
Estradiol..........................74, 87, 88, 118, 123, 128, 186, 257
Estrogen..........................32, 57, 58, 650 87, 88, 90, 91, 92, 99, 100, 115, 117, 118, 123, 124, 125, 126, 128, 155, 157, 158, 160, 186, 214
Exfoliate.......................... 231

F

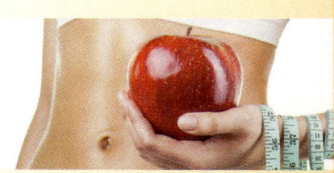

Fat....................................12, 19, 20, 24, 27, 29, 32, 34, 36, 48, 86, 97, 102, 115, 124, 128, 158, 178, 187, 204, 210, 211, 219, 220, 237
Fatigue.............................2, 9, 10, 31, 32, 59, 68, 76, 79, 100, 104, 112, 155, 164, 170, 186, 217, 220
Fibrocystic Breast...........15
Fibromyalgia................... 15, 32, 42, 103, 108, 152, 209
Flu....................................9, 104, 150
Food Cravings.................19
Free Radicals...................24, 27, 37, 41, 42, 143, 164, 167, 168, 220, 223, 224, 243

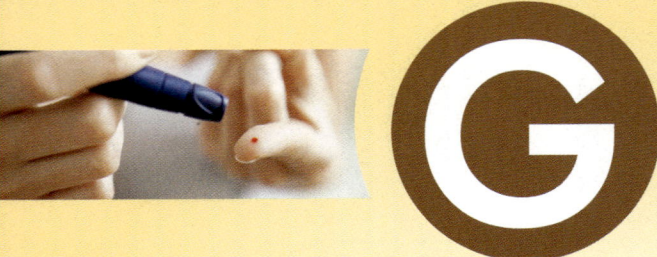
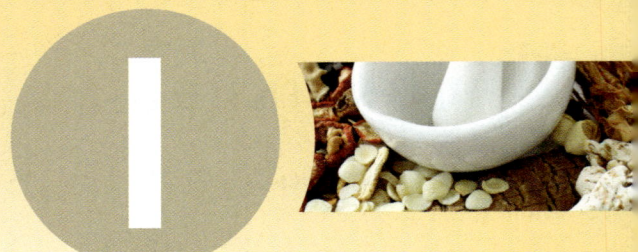

G

Gall Bladder	79, 80, 126
Gastrointestinal	60, 69, 124, 180, 183, 184, 199
Gingivitis	5, 44
Glaucoma	23, 37, 190
Glucose	4, 10, 24, 28, 36, 68, 75, 102, 104, 204
Glutathione	27, 29, 37, 40, 41, 42, 105, 134, 167, 174, 216

I

Immune Disease	189
	3, 8, 27, 31, 48, 49, 83, 100, 104, 155, 216, 217, 258
Immunity	58
Incontinence	5, 8, 15, 18, 48, 52, 54, 58, 60, 85, 86, 90, 113, 131, 132, 165, 170, 173, 259
Inflammation	3, 12, 15, 16, 18, 21, 49, 51, 52, 58, 59, 61, 67, 70, 80, 82, 85, 86, 103, 108, 109, 110, 122, 131, 132, 140, 142, 144, 165, 171, 172, 176, 187, 188, 193, 194, 199, 200, 218, 222, 253, 259
Insomnia	67, 90, 94, 134, 217
Insulin	31, 61, 155, 187, 219
Iodine	8, 25, 129, 130, 147, 148, 173, 194, 195, 259

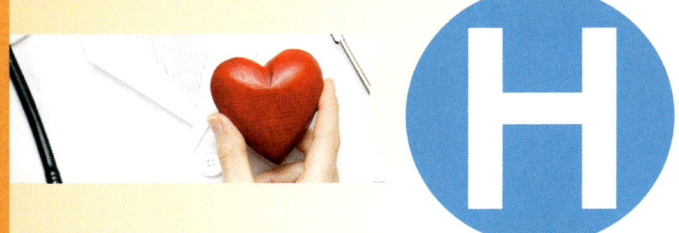

H

Hair	8, 10, 24, 34, 97, 107, 165, 168, 171, 172, 173, 174, 193, 194, 196, 198
Hashimoto's	196, 258
Heart Attack	12, 15, 23, 166
Heart Disease	12, 13, 23, 28, 32, 88, 90, 98, 99, 103, 125, 165, 170, 189, 191, 212, 217, 258
Heavy Metal Toxification	15
Hepatitis	111, 113, 164
Herpes	71, 150
Herpes Zoster	150
Homocysteine	12, 13, 183, 184
Hot Flash	89, 92
Hydration	194, 227
Hyperpigmentation	212
Hypertension	15, 68, 75, 161, 162, 170, 191, 202, 204, 258
Hypothalamus	65, 187, 188, 220
Hypothyroidism	7, 8, 10, 165, 191, 193, 194, 198

J

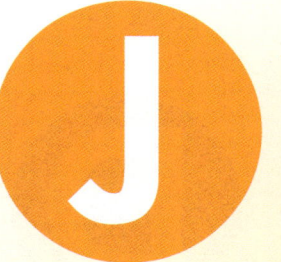

No Entries for Letter J

K

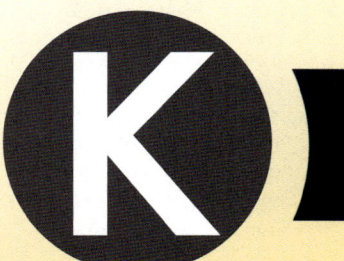

Kidney Failure	60, 218
Kidney Stones	22, 80, 84, 209

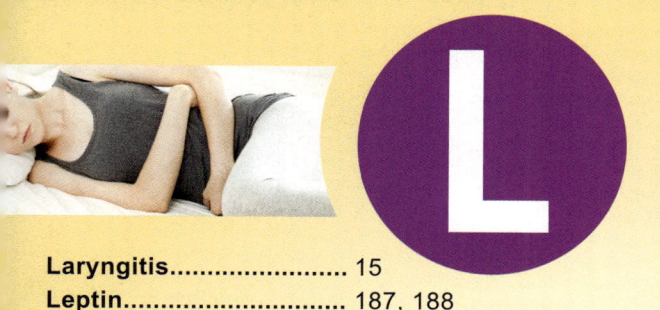

L

Laryngitis..................... 15
Leptin............................ 187, 188
Libido........................... 66, 79, 98, 100, 104, 111, 112, 125, 126, 185, 186, 189, 190, 201, 203, 204
Liver............................. 11, 12, 28, 33, 35, 36, 41, 42, 59, 60, 61, 62, 64, 79, 80, 81, 99, 113, 123, 125, 126, 133, 151, 155, 164, 173, 187, 191, 209, 210, 211, 212, 216, 217

M

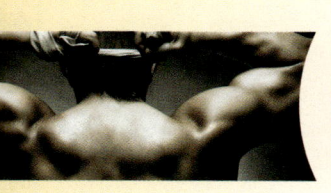
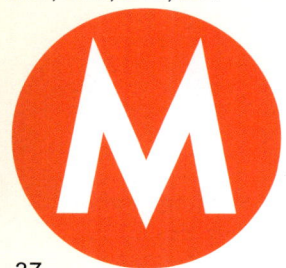

Macular Degeneration..... 37
Male Infertility................. 42
Melatonin....................... 42, 130, 133, 134, 135, 136, 174
Memory......................... 8, 9, 28, 31, 32, 42, 54, 75, 76, 88, 97, 98, 102, 103, 106, 133, 136, 137, 138, 139, 140, 141, 142, 143, 144, 145, 146, 155, 156, 184, 186, 191, 193, 204
Menopause..................... 31, 58, 65, 87, 88, 90, 91, 92, 99, 100, 115, 125, 145, 155, 186, 210
Mental Confusion............ 60, 79
Mercury.......................... 8, 61, 102, 259
Metabolic Acidity............. 4
Metabolism..................... 3, 10, 19, 24, 28, 36, 83, 84, 99, 124, 125, 127, 130, 133, 143, 153, 165, 168, 177, 183, 185, 187, 188, 203, 211, 212, 214, 220

M CONTINUED

Micro-Minerals................. 43, 55, 216
Migraine.......................... 22
Minerals.......................... 147, 148, 213, 227, 243, 249
Mood.............................. 8, 46, 133, 134, 135, 156, 182, 185, 203, 208, 209, 220
Muscle Mass.................... 31, 36, 155, 185, 186, 203, 204
Muscle Pain..................... 151, 152
Muscle Spasm.................. 108, 150, 166

N

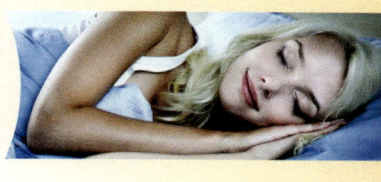

Nails............................... 8, 107, 171, 172, 174, 175, 193, 194
Nerve Growth Factor........ 35, 102
Night Sweats................... 80, 87, 90, 91, 100, 160
Nitric Oxide...................... 76, 154, 189, 190, 201, 202, 204

O

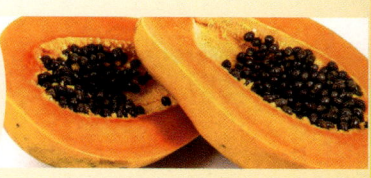

Ocular Diseases............... 37
Omega 3......................... 24, 25, 260
Omega 6......................... 24, 260
Orgasm........................... 57, 58, 65, 189
Osteoarthritis................... 69, 70, 108
Osteoporosis................... 31, 32, 67, 73, 74, 90, 115, 155, 157, 158
Ovarian Cysts.................. 15, 125, 126, 157

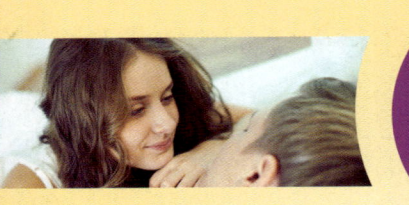  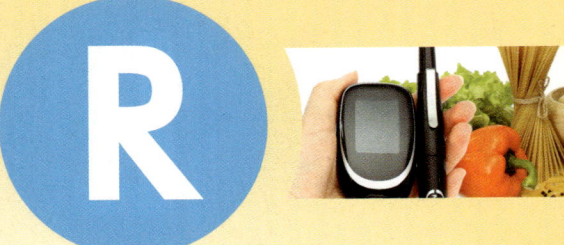

Pain...............................	2, 8, 10, 16, 22, 36, 43, 44, 51, 52, 54, 56, 57, 59, 61, 62, 63, 69, 70, 80, 99, 100, 107, 108, 109, 110, 118, 125, 126, 128, 130, 131, 132, 150, 151, 152, 153, 154, 166, 180, 190, 194, 197, 200, 206, 209
Painful Urination.............	128
Pancreas.........................	81, 134, 210, 219
Parkinson's.....................	42, 98, 161
Penis/Penile Issues	
See Erectile Dysfunction	
pH...................................	3, 4, 57, 82, 85, 86, 150, 199
Phospholipids.................	41, 158, 175
Plaque.............................	12, 13
PMS.................................	79, 99, 100, 125, 157, 158, 160
Pollution.........................	41, 131, 170
Poor Diet.........................	8, 41, 215, 218
Pregnenolone..................	32, 76, 141, 154, 155, 156, 158
Progesterone...................	32, 58, 90, 92, 98, 99, 130, 155, 157, 158, 159, 160, 215, 218, 257
Prostate...........................	23, 72, 90, 98, 115, 116, 117, 118, 119, 120, 122, 123, 124, 125, 126, 158, 160, 209, 212
Prostate Cancer...............	90, 98, 115, 117, 118, 119, 120, 123, 124, 125, 126
Psoriasis..........................	3, 209, 232, 241

Radiation.........................	41, 190
Rejuvenating...................	117, 170, 232
Respiratory.....................	8, 112, 132
Rheumatoid Arthritis.......	108
Rosacea...........................	175, 212

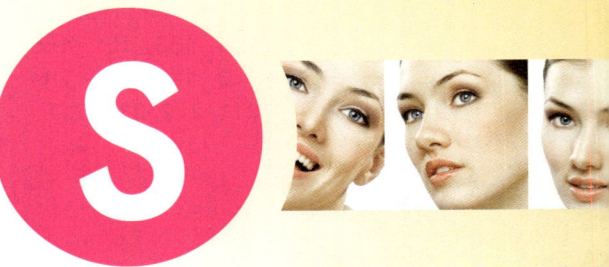

Sagging Skin...................	223, 225
Seizures..........................	50
Self Confidence...............	46, 182, 208
Serotonin.........................	45, 46, 133, 181, 182, 207, 208
Sexual Performance........	97, 116
Sexuality..........................	34, 57, 88, 97
Sinusitis..........................	15, 131, 132
Sleep................................	45, 54, 56, 63, 65, 67, 68, 133, 134, 135, 136, 154, 157, 158, 161, 180, 181, 206, 207, 239, 241
Sleeping Patterns............	46, 182, 208
Spasm..............................	15
Stress...............................	9, 27, 30, 31, 37, 41, 42, 45, 52, 61, 65, 66, 68, 76, 79, 95, 103, 106, 107, 111, 133, 145, 155, 156, 161, 179, 180, 181, 182, 187, 207, 208, 212, 214, 216, 221, 235
Stroke..............................	12, 15, 161, 166, 189, 210, 214, 216
Super Oxide Dismutase..	42, 167, 168
Swelling...........................	16, 58, 61, 108, 109, 110, 142, 190, 200, 216

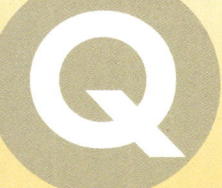

No Entries for Letter Q

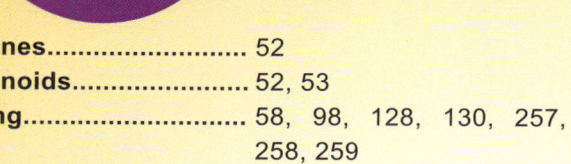
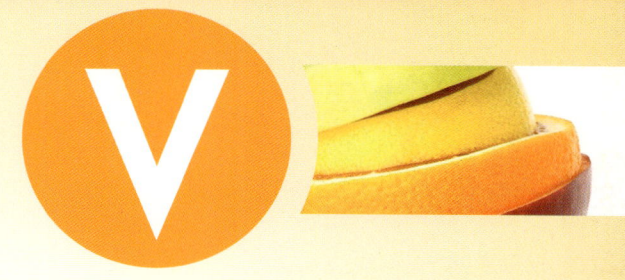

Terpenes...........................	52
Terpenoids......................	52, 53
Testing.............................	58, 98, 128, 130, 257, 258, 259
Testosterone...................	32, 65, 97, 99, 118, 123, 124, 125, 155, 158, 185, 186, 203, 204
Thyroid............................	7, 8, 9, 10, 31, 55, 104, 129, 130, 155, 187, 191, 192, 194, 195, 196, 258
Toothache.......................	44
Topical............................	5, 34, 37, 100, 168, 176, 177, 190, 221
Toxic Metals....................	61, 102
Toxins..............................	23, 28, 51, 59, 61, 82, 102, 168, 170, 172, 173, 216, 218, 224, 233, 235, 247, 252, 255
Transdermal Lyposome...	33, 34, 74, 76, 130, 155, 175, 177, 204

Vaginal Dryness...............	57, 90
Viral Infection..................	5, 131, 189, 259
Vitamin A.........................	23, 38, 98, 159, 173, 178, 223, 224, 238, 241
Vitamin B3.......................	11
Vitamin C.........................	20, 21, 23, 82, 83, 86, 168, 173, 241
Vitamin D........................	23, 84, 209, 212, 215
Vitamin D3......................	21, 96, 104, 174, 209, 213, 214, 215, 258
Vitamin E.........................	23, 29, 98, 134, 159, 178, 224, 232, 241, 245, 255
Vitamin K........................	210, 211, 212, 213, 214

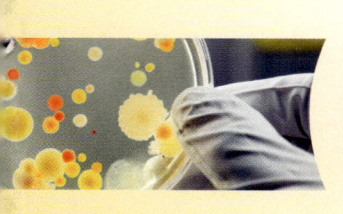

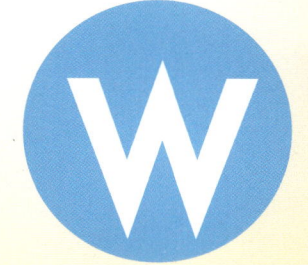
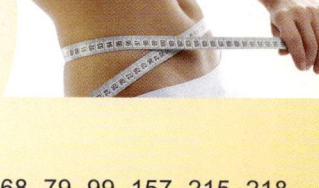

Ulcerative Colitis.............	15, 108
Unwanted Hair Growth....	97
Upset Stomachs..............	187
Uterine Cysts...................	125
Uterine Fibroids...............	15
UVB Rays.........................	209

Water Retention..............	68, 79, 99, 157, 215, 218
Weight Loss....................	9, 20, 83, 102, 104, 128, 177, 187, 220
Wrinkles..........................	89, 90, 171, 173, 174, 223, 224, 239, 240, 249, 251, 252

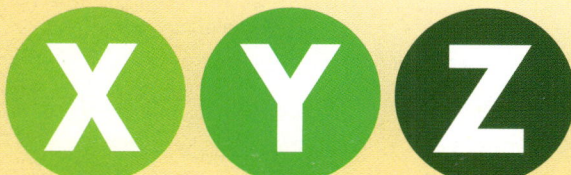

No Entries for Letter X, Y, Z